DEDICATION

This textbook is dedicated to

The pharmacy/medical students of today and tomorrow, whose passion for learning and commitment to patient care will shape the future of our profession. The educators who inspire and mentor the next generation of pharmacists/doctors, imparting not only knowledge but also the values and critical thinking skills essential to pharmaceutical care.

The practicing pharmacists/doctors who daily represent the vital role in healthcare through their clinical expertise, compassionate patient interactions, and tireless advocacy for optimal medication therapy.

The patients whose needs remain at the center of our professional purpose, reminding us that behind every prescription is a person deserving of our best care.

And to all who strive to advance the science and practice of pharmacy in service of human health and wellbeing.

"May this book serve as a trusted companion in your professional journey"

CONTENTS

ACKNOWLEDGMENTS

The creation of this textbook has been a collaborative journey that would not have been possible without the contributions, expertise, and support of the authors. The editors wish to express their sincere gratitude to all the authors who have played a role in bringing this textbook to fruition.

We are grateful to the students who participated in focus groups and pilot testing of educational materials contained within these pages. Their perspective has been crucial in creating a student-centered resource that addresses learning needs at various stages of pharmacy/medical education.

Special recognition is due to the pharmacy/medical organizations and institutions that provided access to resources, clinical practice guidelines, and case studies that enrich this work. Their commitment to advancing pharmacy education aligns with our vision for this textbook.

We acknowledge the editorial and production staff whose attention to detail, design expertise, and tireless efforts have transformed manuscript pages into a polished, accessible educational tool.

Finally, we express our gratitude to our families, colleagues, and mentors who supported us throughout this project with their patience, encouragement, and understanding. Their unwavering support made this collaborative endeavor possible.

While we have strived hard for accuracy and comprehensiveness, we welcome feedback from readers as we continuously seek to improve future editions of this work.

CHAPTER 1

TREATMENT ALGORITHMS FOR CARDIOVASCULAR DISORDERS

Author

Dr. Deepak Shrivastava, Professor and Principal,
IMI Pharmaceutical Studies, Indore, Madhya Pradesh, India

Abstract

Treatment algorithms for cardiovascular disorders rely on evidence-based, stepwise clinical pathways. The management of hypertension begins with accurate diagnosis and ASCVD risk stratification, followed by foundational lifestyle modifications. Pharmacological therapy is then initiated, guided by blood pressure targets and compelling indications, often requiring stepwise addition of first-line agents like diuretics, CCBs, or RAS-blockers. Coronary artery disease management is bifurcated: stable ischemic heart disease is managed with guideline-directed medical therapy (GDMT) for event prevention and symptom control, whereas acute coronary syndromes (ACS) demand time-sensitive reperfusion for STEMI or risk-based invasive strategies for NSTEMI. Heart failure algorithms are stratified by ejection fraction. HFrEF management is built on four concurrent pillar therapies—ARNI/ACEi/ARB, beta-blockers, MRAs, and SGLT2 inhibitors. HFpEF management centers on SGLT2 inhibitors and rigorous comorbidity control. The approach to atrial fibrillation rests on three pillars: anticoagulation based on stroke risk, rate control, and rhythm control strategies. Algorithms for ventricular arrhythmias are dictated by hemodynamic stability, prioritizing defibrillation for unstable patients and ICDs for long-term prevention. Valvular heart disease interventions, whether surgical or transcatheter, are primarily triggered by the onset of symptoms or objective evidence of ventricular dysfunction.

Keywords: *Cardiovascular Algorithms, Guideline-Directed Medical Therapy (GDMT), Hypertension, Acute Coronary Syndrome, Heart Failure*

Learning Objectives

After completion of the chapter, the learners should be able to:

- Identify first-line pharmacological classes for Stage 1 hypertension based on current ACC/AHA guidelines.
- Explain the pathophysiologic differences in the treatment algorithms for Heart Failure with Reduced Ejection Fraction (HFrEF) versus Preserved Ejection Fraction (HFpEF).
- Select the appropriate anticoagulation and rate/rhythm control algorithm for a new patient presenting with atrial fibrillation.
- Differentiate the immediate treatment algorithms for a patient with ST-Elevation Myocardial Infarction (STEMI) versus Non-ST-Elevation Myocardial Infarction (NSTEMI).
- Justify the choice of therapy (e.g., medical management vs. revascularization) for a patient with stable coronary artery disease based on symptoms and risk.

HYPERTENSION

Hypertension, or high blood pressure, is a critical modifiable risk factor for cardiovascular disease, stroke, and chronic kidney disease. Its management algorithm is foundational to preventive cardiology and requires meticulous assessment and long-term stewardship.

Pathophysiology

Essential hypertension is a complex polygenic disorder resulting from a persistent elevation of systemic blood pressure. Its pathophysiology is multifactorial, involving a dysregulation of cardiovascular control systems. Two primary mechanisms are the Sympathetic Nervous System (SNS) and the Renin-Angiotensin-Aldosterone System (RAAS). Overactivity of the SNS leads to increased heart rate, cardiac contractility, and peripheral vasoconstriction. It also stimulates renin release from the kidneys, activating the RAAS. The cascade culminates in Angiotensin II, a potent vasoconstrictor that also stimulates the adrenal cortex to release aldosterone. Aldosterone, in turn, promotes sodium and water reabsorption in the distal nephron, expanding plasma volume. Over time, this sustained pressure load causes endothelial dysfunction and vascular remodeling, leading to arterial stiffness and a "reset" of baroreceptors, which perpetuates the hypertensive state

Diagnosis and Initial Assessment

The therapeutic algorithm begins with accurate diagnosis. This is established from an average of two or more readings taken on two or more separate occasions, ideally using automated oscillometric devices or out-of-office measurements (ambulatory or home blood pressure monitoring) to confirm the diagnosis and rule out white-coat hypertension. Initial assessment involves quantifying the blood pressure stage (e.g., ACC/AHA Stage 1, Stage 2) and performing a comprehensive 10-year atherosclerotic cardiovascular disease (ASCVD) risk calculation. Concurrently, the clinician must evaluate for target-organ damage (e.g., left ventricular hypertrophy, retinopathy, albuminuria) and screen for potential secondary causes, especially in cases of new-onset, resistant, or very high blood pressure.

Differential Diagnosis

While over 90% of hypertension is primary (essential), a crucial early step is to consider secondary causes, particularly in atypical presentations. The differential includes renal parenchymal disease, renovascular disease (renal artery stenosis), primary aldosteronism (which is increasingly recognized as common), obstructive sleep apnea, and substance-induced hypertension (e.g., NSAIDs, decongestants, illicit substances). Less common causes include pheochromocytoma, Cushing's syndrome, and thyroid or parathyroid abnormalities.

Non-pharmacological Interventions

Lifestyle modification is a universal component of all hypertension treatment algorithms and is the primary intervention for elevated blood pressure or Stage 1 hypertension with low ASCVD risk. This includes adherence to a reduced-sodium diet (<1500 mg/day ideally) such as the DASH (Dietary Approaches to Stop Hypertension) eating plan, a diet rich in fruits, vegetables, and low-fat dairy. Regular aerobic exercise (e.g., 90-150 minutes/week), moderation of alcohol consumption, and smoking cessation are equally critical. Weight loss in overweight or obese individuals can have a profound impact.

Treatment Algorithm

The management of hypertension (HTN) is a stepwise process based on accurate blood pressure (BP) measurement, cardiovascular risk stratification, and selection of patient-specific pharmacotherapy.

Step 1: Diagnosis and Risk Stratification

The therapeutic pathway begins with accurate diagnosis, which is confirmed with an average of two or more readings on two or more separate occasions. A reading of BP ≥130/80 mmHg is classified as ACC/AHA Stage 1, while ≥140/90 mmHg is Stage 2. Ambulatory BP monitoring (ABPM) is considered the gold standard to exclude white-coat hypertension.

Following diagnosis, risk stratification is critical. The decision-making process diverges based on the 10-year atherosclerotic cardiovascular disease (ASCVD) risk, often calculated using the Pooled Cohort Equations. For Elevated BP (120-129/<80), the recommendation is non-pharmacological therapy only. For Stage 1 HTN (130-139/80-89), the approach depends on risk: if ASCVD risk is below 10% and the patient has no clinical ASCVD, diabetes (DM), or chronic kidney disease (CKD), non-pharmacological therapy is the sole initial intervention, with reassessment in 3-6 months. However, if the risk is 10% or higher, or these comorbidities are present, both non-pharmacological therapy and a first-line pharmacological agent are initiated. For Stage 2 HTN (≥140/90), the standard of care is to initiate non-pharmacological therapy along with two first-line pharmacological agents from different classes.

Step 2: Non-Pharmacological Interventions (Universal)

Lifestyle modification is a foundational, non-negotiable step in all hypertension management plans. This includes weight loss to aim for a BMI between 18.5-24.9 kg/m^2, adherence to the DASH (Dietary Approaches to Stop Hypertension) diet, and significant sodium restriction to less than 1500 mg/day. Regular aerobic exercise for 90-150 minutes per week, moderation of alcohol (to ≤2 drinks/day for men or ≤1 for women), and smoking cessation are also critical components.

Table 1.1: First-Line Antihypertensive Therapy

Compelling Indication	Preferred First-Line Agent(s)
Heart Failure (HFrEF)	ARNI/ACEi/ARB, Beta-Blocker, MRA, SGLT2i
Post-Myocardial Infarction	Beta-Blocker, ACEi/ARB
Stable Ischemic Heart Disease	Beta-Blocker, ACEi/ARB
Chronic Kidney Disease (CKD)	ACEi or ARB (esp. with albuminuria)
Diabetes Mellitus	ACEi or ARB (esp. with albuminuria)
Stroke (Secondary Prevention)	Thiazide Diuretic, ACEi/ARB
African Ancestry (no CKD/HF)	Thiazide Diuretic or CCB

Step 3: Initial Pharmacological Selection

The first-line classes of medications include thiazide diuretics, Calcium Channel Blockers (CCBs), ACE Inhibitors (ACEi), or Angiotensin II Receptor Blockers (ARBs). The selection process is heavily influenced by patient comorbidities, or "compelling indications."

In patients with no comorbidities, any first-line agent is acceptable, though thiazides or CCBs may demonstrate more effectiveness as initial monotherapy in Black adults. For patients with Chronic Kidney Disease (Stage 3+ or with albuminuria), the therapeutic pathway strongly prefers an ACEi or ARB to slow CKD progression. Similarly, individuals with Diabetes Mellitus and albuminuria should be preferentially started on an ACEi or ARB. In cases of Heart Failure with Reduced Ejection Fraction (HFrEF), the medication choices are dictated by HFrEF's own guidelines, which include ACEi/ARB/ARNI and beta-blockers, but not CCBs as a first-line option. For Stable Ischemic Heart Disease, beta-blockers and an ACEi or ARB are preferred. When initiating therapy for Stage 2 HTN, a two-drug regimen is standard, often using a fixed-dose combination (e.g., ARB + HCTZ) to improve adherence.

Step 4: Follow-up and Titration

After initiation, patients should be reassessed monthly. If the BP goal is not met with one agent, the preferred strategy is to add a second agent from a different class before maximizing the dose of the first. This approach often adds more efficacy with fewer side effects.

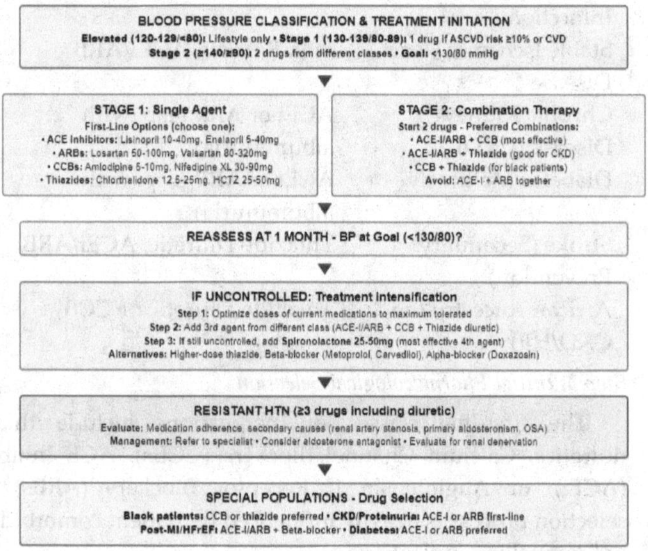

Figure 1.1: Hypertension - Pharmacological Management

When BP remains uncontrolled on three or more agents (including a diuretic), the condition is defined as Resistant Hypertension. The management pathway for this condition involves several checks. First is to confirm adherence and rule out white-coat HTN using ABPM. Second is to identify and screen for secondary causes, such as primary aldosteronism or renal artery stenosis. Third is to optimize the current regimen, for example, by maximizing the diuretic dose or switching from HCTZ to the more potent chlorthalidone. Finally, if BP is still uncontrolled, a fourth-line agent is added. The agent of choice in this situation is typically a mineralocorticoid receptor antagonist (MRA), spironolactone, provided renal function and potassium levels are normal.

Monitoring

Initial monitoring after pharmacological initiation or titration is crucial. Patients should follow up in 2-4 weeks to assess blood pressure response, adherence, and potential adverse effects. Laboratory monitoring is guided by the chosen agent; for example, a basic metabolic panel (BUN, creatinine, potassium) is warranted 1-2 weeks after initiating an ACE inhibitor, ARB, or diuretic. Once the patient is stable and at their goal blood pressure, follow-up visits can be extended to every 3-6 months. At these visits, adherence should be reassessed, and home blood pressure logs should be reviewed. Annual screening for target-organ damage (e.g., EKG, urine albumin-to-creatinine ratio, fundoscopic exam) is a key component of long-term monitoring.

Long-Term Management / Secondary Prevention

The cornerstone of long-term management is lifelong adherence to both non-pharmacological and pharmacological therapies. Hypertension is a chronic condition, not an acute illness, and this "secondary prevention" phase is aimed at preventing the primary complications: stroke, myocardial infarction, heart failure, and chronic kidney disease. This involves consistent home blood pressure monitoring to identify and manage any loss of control. It also requires annual screening for new or worsening target-organ damage and vigilant management of all other co-morbid cardiovascular risk factors, particularly hyperlipidemia and diabetes mellitus.

Patient Counseling Points

Counseling must begin by dispelling the myth that hypertension is curable or can be ignored "if you feel fine." The main points include: 1) Emphasize that hypertension is a "silent killer" and that medication adherence is lifelong and not based on symptoms. 2) Teach proper home blood pressure monitoring, including using a validated, upper-arm cuff of the correct size, resting for 5 minutes before measurement, and keeping a log. 3) Review lifestyle modifications, focusing on sodium restriction as a critical adjuvant to medication. 4) Discuss common medication side effects (e.g., the benign dry cough of an ACE inhibitor, peripheral edema with CCBs) and instruct the patient to report them, not to stop the medication abruptly.

Common Pitfalls in Management

A frequent pitfall is clinical inertia, the failure to initiate or intensify therapy when treatment targets are not met. Another common error is therapeutic fragmentation, where multiple providers prescribe agents without a cohesive plan. Inaccurate BP measurement (e.g., improper cuff size, lack of a rest period) is a foundational error that derails the entire algorithm. Finally, under-dosing diuretics or failing to recognize diuretic resistance in the setting of renal impairment or high sodium intake can lead to perceived treatment failure.

Case Study

A 58-year-old male (Mr. Patel) presents for an annual physical. He has a history of dyslipidemia (on atorvastatin 20mg) and a family history of coronary artery disease. He feels well. You take his blood pressure in the office, and after a 5-minute rest, the average of two readings is **152/94 mmHg.**

Discussion

Mr. Patel's blood pressure places him in **Stage 2 Hypertension** (≥140/90 mmHg). The algorithm for Stage 2 is straightforward: do not just start one medication; you must initiate both non-pharmacological therapy and two first-line pharmacological agents from different classes.

Treatment Algorithm

Diagnosis: Stage 2 Hypertension.
Risk Calculation: You calculate his 10-year ASCVD risk, and it comes back at 16% (High Risk). This reinforces the need for aggressive treatment.
Non-pharmacological: You counsel him on the DASH diet, sodium restriction (<1500 mg/day), and increasing his physical activity.

Pharmacological (Stage 2): You initiate two first-line agents.

Agent 1 (CCB): Amlodipine 5 mg daily.

Agent 2 (ACEi): Lisinopril 10 mg daily. (An ARB like Losartan would also be appropriate).

Follow-up: You schedule a follow-up visit in one month to check his BP response and monitor for side effects (e.g., cough, edema) and labs (potassium, creatinine).

Outcome

You start Mr. Patel on amlodipine and lisinopril and schedule a 1-month follow-up, with a BP goal of <130/80 mmHg .

CORONARY ARTERY DISEASE

Coronary Artery Disease (CAD) manifests as a spectrum from asymptomatic atherosclerosis to stable angina and life-threatening acute coronary syndromes (ACS). The treatment algorithms diverge significantly based on this clinical presentation.

Pathophysiology

Coronary Artery Disease (CAD) is the result of atherosclerosis, an inflammatory process within the coronary artery walls. The process begins with endothelial dysfunction, often caused by risk factors (HTN, smoking, hyperlipidemia). This allows low-density lipoproteins (LDL-C) to enter the sub-endothelial space, where they become oxidized. The oxidized LDL triggers an inflammatory response, attracting monocytes that differentiate into macrophages. These macrophages engulf the LDL, becoming "foam cells." Over decades, these foam cells accumulate, forming a "fatty streak" which progresses into a complex fibro-inflammatory plaque with a lipid core and a fibrous cap. Stable angina occurs when a fixed plaque narrows the lumen by ≥70%, causing a supply-demand mismatch during exertion. An Acute Coronary Syndrome (ACS) occurs when the plaque's fibrous cap ruptures or erodes, exposing the thrombogenic core, which leads to acute thrombus formation and vessel occlusion.

Stable Ischemic Heart Disease

Stable Ischemic Heart Disease (SIHD), or stable angina, is characterized by predictable, exertional chest discomfort relieved by rest or nitrates. The treatment algorithm focuses on two primary goals: mitigating ischemic symptoms and preventing adverse cardiovascular events (MI, death).

Diagnosis and Differential

Diagnosis is based on clinical history and confirmed with non-invasive testing (e.g., stress testing with imaging) or anatomic assessment (coronary computed tomography angiography, CCTA). The differential diagnosis for anginal-type chest pain is broad and includes gastroesophageal reflux disease (GERD), musculoskeletal pain (e.g., costochondritis), pulmonary embolism, and pericarditis.

Treatment Algorithm

Stable Ischemic Heart Disease (SIHD)

The management plan for SIHD has two primary goals: mitigating ischemic symptoms and preventing adverse cardiovascular events like MI and death. Guideline-Directed Medical Therapy (GDMT) is the cornerstone for prevention. This includes antiplatelet therapy, typically low-dose aspirin, and high-intensity statin therapy to lower lipid levels and stabilize plaque. Aggressive risk factor control, including blood pressure management and smoking cessation, is also essential.

For the control of anginal symptoms, beta-blockers are the first-line agents. The dose should be titrated to a resting heart rate of 55-60 bpm. If symptoms persist, a long-acting nitrate or a calcium channel blocker is added. Dihydropyridine CCBs, like amlodipine, are preferred if adding to a beta-blocker. If symptoms still remain, ranolazine can be added as a third-line agent. All patients should also have sublingual nitroglycerin for acute anginal episodes.

Revascularization, either with PCI or CABG, is reserved for patients with refractory symptoms despite maximal medical therapy or those with high-risk anatomic findings, such as left main disease or multi-vessel disease in a patient with diabetes.

Acute Coronary Syndromes (ACS)

The emergent ACS pathway is dictated by 12-lead EKG findings within 10 minutes of presentation.

If the EKG shows ST-Segment Elevation Myocardial Infarction (STEMI), the goal is immediate reperfusion, as "time is muscle." Initial measures include "MONA-B" (Morphine, Oxygen if sat < 90%, Nitrates, Aspirin 324 mg chewed) and a P2Y12 inhibitor. The subsequent reperfusion decision depends on logistics. If at a PCI-capable center, primary PCI is the strategy of choice, with a door-to-balloon time goal of less than 90 minutes. If not at a PCI-capable center, the decision hinges on transfer time. If transfer to a PCI center can be accomplished within 120 minutes, transfer is initiated. If the transfer will exceed 120 minutes, fibrinolytics (e.g., tenecteplase) are administered, with a door-to-needle time goal of less than 30 minutes.

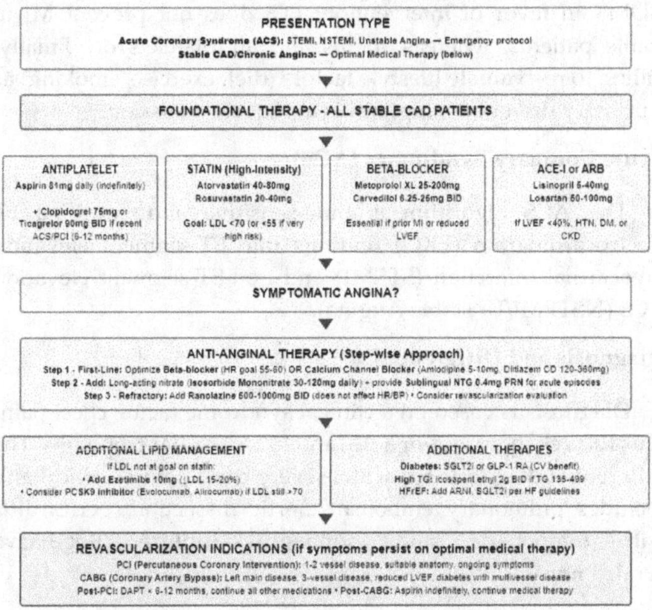

Figure 1.2 Coronary Artery Disease - Pharmacological Management

If the EKG shows Non-ST-Segment Elevation ACS (NSTEMI/Unstable Angina), the initial steps are "MONA-B" plus a P2Y12 inhibitor and systemic anticoagulation (e.g., IV heparin). The next step is risk stratification using a validated score, such as TIMI or GRACE. High-risk patients (e.g., with hemodynamic instability or refractory angina) should proceed to an "early invasive strategy," which involves angiography and potential PCI within 24 hours. Low-risk patients may be managed with an "ischemia-guided strategy," where medical management is continued and a stress test is performed to provoke ischemia before deciding on angiography.

Common Pitfalls

A common pitfall is the "oculo-stenotic reflex," or proceeding to revascularization for an anatomic stenosis without objective evidence of it causing ischemia. Another error is neglecting GDMT in favor of intervention; PCI does not prevent MI in stable patients, whereas statins and antiplatelets do. Finally, failing to re-evaluate lifestyle factors (diet, exercise, smoking) as a primary driver of symptoms is a frequent omission.

Acute Coronary Syndromes (ACS)

The ACS algorithm is time-sensitive and stratified by electrocardiogram (EKG) findings into ST-segment elevation myocardial infarction (STEMI) and non-ST-segment elevation ACS (NSTEMI/Unstable Angina).

Diagnosis and Differential

Diagnosis is based on a clinical syndrome (acute chest pain) plus EKG changes and/or a rise and fall in cardiac troponins. The differential diagnosis for acute, severe chest pain is critical and includes pulmonary embolism, aortic dissection, pericarditis with tamponade, and esophageal rupture (Boerhaave syndrome).

STEMI

Patients with STEMI require an emergent reperfusion strategy. The algorithm is linear: immediate primary PCI is the preferred strategy if it can be performed within guideline-recommended timeframes (e.g., first medical contact-to-device time < 90-120 minutes). If PCI is not available in a timely manner, the algorithm diverts to immediate fibrinolytic therapy (e.g., tenecteplase), followed by transfer to a PCI-capable center. Adjunctive therapy includes immediate dual antiplatelet therapy (DAPT) with aspirin and a P2Y12 inhibitor (e.g., ticagrelor or prasugrel) and anticoagulation (e.g., heparin).

Table 1.2: Acute Coronary Syndrome (ACS) Management Algorithm

Feature	STEMI	NSTEMI / Unstable Angina
EKG Finding	ST-Segment Elevation	ST-Depression, T-Wave Inversion, or Normal
Initial Algorithm	Emergent Reperfusion	Risk Stratification
Primary Goal	Open Artery (PCI < 90 min or Fibrinolysis)	Stabilize, Anti-ischemia, Assess Risk (TIMI/GRACE)
Primary Meds	Aspirin, P2Y12-I (Prasugrel/Ticagrelor), Heparin	Aspirin, P2Y12-I, Anticoagulant, Beta-Blocker, Nitrate
Angio Timing	Immediate	24-48 hrs (if high-risk) or deferred

NSTEMI/Unstable Angina Algorithm

The NSTEMI algorithm begins with immediate anti-ischemic and antithrombotic therapy. This includes DAPT (aspirin and a P2Y12 inhibitor), anticoagulation, nitrates, and beta-blockers (if hemodynamically stable). Subsequent management is guided by risk stratification (e.g., TIMI or GRACE score). High-risk patients (e.g., hemodynamic instability, refractory angina, dynamic EKG changes, high GRACE score) should proceed to an early invasive strategy (angiography and potential PCI within 24-48 hours). Low-risk patients may be managed with a conservative, medical-management-first approach.

Monitoring and Follow-Up

Following an ACS, in-hospital monitoring involves serial EKGs and troponins to ensure resolution of ischemia. After discharge, a follow-up visit should occur within 1-2 weeks to assess for any recurrent angina, dyspnea, medication tolerance, and wound healing (if PCI or CABG was performed). Long-term monitoring for stable CAD involves an annual review of symptoms, risk factor control (BP, lipids, HbA1c), and medication adherence. An annual EKG is reasonable. Stress testing is not routinely needed for asymptomatic, stable patients but is indicated if new or worsening symptoms arise.

Long-Term Management / Secondary Prevention

This is the most critical phase of CAD management. Guideline-Directed Medical Therapy (GDMT) is mandatory to prevent recurrent events. This includes: 1) **Dual Antiplatelet Therapy (DAPT):** Aspirin plus a P2Y12 inhibitor (e.g., clopidogrel, ticagrelor) for 6-12 months post-ACS or post-stenting to prevent stent thrombosis, followed by lifelong single antiplatelet therapy. 2) **High-Intensity Statin:** Atorvastatin 40-80 mg or Rosuvastatin 20-40 mg, regardless of baseline LDL, to stabilize plaque and lower lipids. 3) **Beta-Blocker:** Should be continued for at least 3 years post-MI and lifelong if the patient has concomitant HFrEF or HTN. 4) **ACE Inhibitor/ARB:** Indicated for patients with LVEF ≤ 40%, HTN, DM, or CKD. 5) **Cardiac Rehabilitation:** A structured, monitored exercise and education program is a Class 1 recommendation.

Patient Counseling Points

- DAPT Adherence: The most critical counseling point post-stenting is the absolute necessity of not missing *any* doses of DAPT, as non-adherence can lead to acute, life-threatening stent thrombosis.
- Statin Adherence: Explain that the statin is not just for "cholesterol" but is a vital "plaque-stabilizing" medicine.

- Lifestyle: Aggressive smoking cessation, adherence to a Mediterranean-style diet, and regular exercise.
- Nitroglycerin Use: Teach the patient to use sublingual nitroglycerin for angina: take one, wait 5 minutes; if still chest pain, call emergency services, then take a second.

Common Pitfalls

In STEMI, the most critical pitfall is system-based delay in activating the catheterization lab and achieving reperfusion. In NSTEMI, a common error is inappropriately delaying antiplatelet or anticoagulant therapy. Another pitfall across the ACS spectrum is failing to administer high-intensity statin therapy upon admission or discharge. Finally, neglecting to assess for mechanical complications post-MI (e.g., new murmur indicating papillary muscle rupture) can be a fatal oversight.

Case Study

A 62-year-old female (Mrs. Chen) with a history of hypertension and Type 2 Diabetes calls emergency services for 1 hour of severe, crushing, 10/10 substernal chest pain radiating to her jaw. An EKG is obtained by paramedics 10 minutes from her door. It shows **ST-segment elevations in leads V2-V5**.

Discussion

This is a classic presentation for an **ST-Elevation Myocardial Infarction (STEMI)**. This is the most time-sensitive algorithm in the CAD chapter. The goal is immediate reperfusion, as "time is muscle."

Treatment Algorithm

1. **ACS Classification (EKG):** The EKG shows ST-elevations, confirming **STEMI**.
2. **Immediate Meds:** Paramedics administer Aspirin (324 mg, chewed), Nitroglycerin (sublingual), and establish IV access.
3. **Reperfusion Pathway:** The algorithm mandates immediate reperfusion.
    - The patient is taken to a **PCI-capable hospital**.

   - The cardiac catheterization lab is activated "pre-hospital" based on the paramedic's EKG.
   - **Fibrinolysis is bypassed** because the hospital is PCI-capable and the "first medical contact-to-device" time is expected to be well under 90 minutes.
4. **In-Hospital:** In the ED, she is given a high-dose statin (Atorvastatin 80 mg) and a P2Y12 inhibitor (e.g., Ticagrelor) loading dose. She is taken directly to the cath lab.

Outcome

Mrs. Chen undergoes primary PCI with a drug-eluting stent to her left anterior descending (LAD) artery. Her door-to-balloon time was 52 minutes.

HEART FAILURE

Heart failure (HF) is a clinical syndrome resulting from structural or functional impairment of ventricular filling or ejection of blood. Treatment algorithms are fundamentally stratified by left ventricular ejection fraction (LVEF).

Pathophysiology

Heart failure is a clinical syndrome, not a single disease. It is the final common pathway for many cardiac insults. The pathophysiology is divided by LVEF.

HFrEF (LVEF ≤ 40%)

This is a *systolic* dysfunction. Following an index event (e.g., large MI), the heart's contractility is impaired, leading to a drop in cardiac output. This triggers a *compensatory* but ultimately *maladaptive* neurohormonal response. The SNS and RAAS are activated to maintain blood pressure and perfusion. This leads to vasoconstriction (increased afterload), sodium/water retention (increased preload), and direct cardiotoxic effects (cardiac remodeling, hypertrophy, and fibrosis). This "vicious cycle" causes the heart failure to progress.

HFpEF (LVEF ≥ 50%)

This is a *diastolic* dysfunction. The ventricle becomes stiff, non-compliant, and unable to relax properly. This is often driven by long-standing hypertension, diabetes, and obesity. Because the ventricle cannot relax, filling pressures become very high, which back up into the lungs, causing dyspnea and pulmonary congestion, especially with exertion.

Diagnosis and Classification

Diagnosis is clinical, based on symptoms (e.g., dyspnea, fatigue, edema) and signs (e.g., elevated jugular venous pressure, pulmonary rales). The initial diagnostic algorithm relies on natriuretic peptide levels (BNP or NT-proBNP) to confirm the diagnosis, followed by a transthoracic echocardiogram. The echocardiogram is the main branch point, classifying the patient into HFrEF (LVEF ≤ 40%), HF with mildly reduced EF (HFmrEF, LVEF 41-49%), or HFpEF (LVEF ≥ 50%).

Differential Diagnosis

The differential for a patient presenting with dyspnea and edema is broad. It includes pulmonary disease (COPD, interstitial lung disease), chronic kidney disease (volume overload), cirrhosis (ascites, peripheral edema), and severe anemia. It is crucial to differentiate cardiac causes from non-cardiac causes, as the treatment algorithms are entirely different.

Heart Failure with Reduced Ejection Fraction (HFrEF)

The HFrEF (LVEF ≤ 40%) algorithm is built upon foundational "pillar" therapies that improve survival. The standard-of-care algorithm involves the concurrent initiation and rapid titration of four major drug classes: first, an angiotensin receptor-neprilysin inhibitor (ARNI) is preferred, with an ACE inhibitor or ARB used if ARNI is not tolerated; second, a guideline-directed beta-blocker (carvedilol, metoprolol succinate, or bisoprolol); third, a mineralocorticoid receptor antagonist (MRA) (spironolactone or eplerenone); and fourth, an SGLT2 inhibitor (dapagliflozin or empagliflozin). This approach has superseded the traditional, slow, stepwise sequence. Loop diuretics are used as needed for volume management but do not provide a mortality benefit. The algorithm includes subsequent steps for specific patient populations, such as the addition of hydralazine/isosorbide dinitrate for African American patients with persistent symptoms, or ivabradine for those in sinus rhythm with a persistently elevated heart rate.

Heart Failure with Preserved Ejection Fraction (HFpEF)

The HFpEF (LVEF ≥ 50%) treatment algorithm has historically been less defined, focusing on comorbidity management. The primary approach involves aggressive management of hypertension and atrial fibrillation, and careful use of diuretics for volume control. Recent landmark trials now support the use of SGLT2 inhibitors as a core, first-line therapy to reduce HF hospitalizations in this population. Management of obesity and other metabolic drivers is also a main component.

Table 1.3: Treatment for HFrEF (LVEF ≤ 40%)

Drug Class	Example(s) & Goal
1. RAS Inhibition	Sacubitril/Valsartan (ARNI). *Alt: Lisinopril (ACEi)*. (Neurohormonal blockade)
2. Beta-Blockade	Carvedilol or Metoprolol Succinate. (Block sympathetic overdrive)
3. MRA	Spironolactone or Eplerenone. (Block aldosterone effects)
4. SGLT2 Inhibition	Dapagliflozin or Empagliflozin. (Metabolic/hemodynamic benefits)

Acute Decompensated Heart Failure (ADHF)

The ADHF algorithm is guided by the patient's hemodynamic profile (wet/dry, warm/cold). The initial step is to identify and address precipitants (e.g., ischemia, arrhythmia, non-adherence). Patients presenting as "warm and wet" (euvolemic but congested) are managed primarily with aggressive intravenous loop diuretics. Patients presenting as "cold and wet" (hypoperfused and congested) are in cardiogenic shock and require a more complex algorithm involving inotropes (e.g., dobutamine) or mechanical circulatory support, often necessitating intensive care.

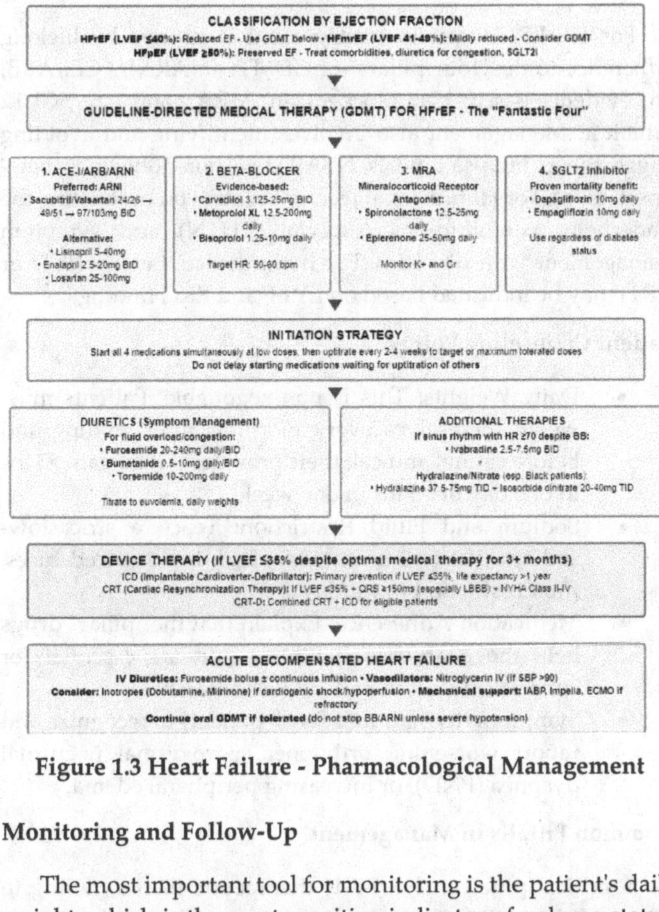

Figure 1.3 Heart Failure - Pharmacological Management

Monitoring and Follow-Up

The most important tool for monitoring is the patient's daily weight, which is the most sensitive indicator of volume status. Clinicians must monitor for signs of congestion (JVP, rales, edema) and hypoperfusion (cool extremities, narrow pulse pressure). After initiating or titrating GDMT, labs (K+ and creatinine) are essential, as the core HFrEF "pillar" drugs (RAASi, MRAs, SGLT2i) and diuretics all affect renal function and electrolytes. GDMT for HFrEF should be titrated every 2-4 weeks as tolerated, with the goal of reaching the target doses used in clinical trials.

Long-Term Management / Secondary Prevention

For HFrEF, long-term management is defined by lifelong adherence to the "four pillars" of GDMT: an ARNI/ACEi/ARB, an evidence-based beta-blocker, an MRA, and an SGLT2 inhibitor. Management also involves identifying and avoiding triggers (e.g., high-salt meals, NSAID use, non-adherence, new-onset AFib). For HFpEF, management centers on controlling the underlying comorbidities (especially HTN) and symptom management with diuretics. For both, device therapy (ICD or CRT) may be indicated based on LVEF and EKG findings.

Patient Counseling Points

- Daily Weights: This is non-negotiable. Patients must weigh themselves every morning, after voiding and before eating, and call their provider if they gain >3 lbs in one day or >5 lbs in one week.
- Sodium and Fluid Restriction: Teach a strict low-sodium diet (< 2 grams/day) and, in advanced cases, fluid restriction (< 2 L/day).
- Medication Adherence: Explain that the "pillar" drugs help the heart remodel *better* and are essential for survival, even if they don't feel different.
- Symptom Recognition: Teach patients to recognize and report worsening orthopnea, paroxysmal nocturnal dyspnea (PND), or increasing peripheral edema.

Common Pitfalls in Management

A critical pitfall in HFrEF is therapeutic inertia; failing to initiate all four pillar therapies, often due to unfounded concerns about transient hypotension or small rises in creatinine. In ADHF, a common error is under-dosing diuretics, leading to incomplete decongestion and early rehospitalization. Another pitfall is the premature discontinuation of GDMT during a hospitalization; beta-blockers, in particular, should be continued unless there is clear evidence of cardiogenic shock.

Case Study

A 68-year-old male (Mr. Johnson) presents to his primary care physician with a 3-month history of progressive shortness of breath on exertion and new 2+ pitting edema in his lower extremities. He has a history of an MI 5 years ago. His BNP is 1200 pg/mL. A transthoracic echocardiogram (TTE) is ordered and shows a **Left Ventricular Ejection Fraction (LVEF) of 30%.**

Discussion

Mr. Johnson's presentation (dyspnea, edema, high BNP) and echo results confirm a new diagnosis of **Heart Failure with Reduced Ejection Fraction (HFrEF)**. The algorithm for HFrEF is built on concurrently initiating the "Four Pillars" of guideline-directed medical therapy (GDMT).

Treatment Algorithm

1. **Classification (Echo):** LVEF is 30% (≤40%), confirming **HFrEF**.
2. **Symptom Management:** To manage his volume overload (edema), you start a loop diuretic:
   - o **Furosemide** 40 mg daily.
3. **GDMT (The "Four Pillars"):** You initiate all four classes, starting at low doses.
   - o **Pillar 1 (ARNI):** Start **Sacubitril/Valsartan** 24/26 mg BID (preferred over an ACEi/ARB).
   - o **Pillar 2 (Beta-Blocker):** Start **Carvedilol** 3.125 mg BID.
   - o **Pillar 3 (MRA):** Start **Spironolactone** 12.5 mg daily.
   - o **Pillar 4 (SGLT2i):** Start **Dapagliflozin** 10 mg daily (regardless of diabetes status).
4. **Follow-up:** You schedule a close follow-up in 1-2 weeks to check his volume status, electrolytes (especially K+), and renal function, and to begin titrating his GDMT doses upwards.

Outcome

Mr. Johnson is started on all four pillar therapies plus a

diuretic. The goal is to titrate these medications to their target doses over the next several months to improve his survival and reduce hospitalizations

ARRHYTHMIAS

The management of arrhythmias depends on the specific type of rhythm disturbance, its hemodynamic consequences, and the underlying substrate.

Atrial Fibrillation

The treatment algorithm for atrial fibrillation (AF) rests on three pillars: anticoagulation, rate control, and rhythm control.

Pathophysiology

Atrial Fibrillation (AF) is a supraventricular tachyarrhythmia characterized by chaotic, disorganized atrial electrical activity (atrial rates of 300-600 bpm) and an irregular ventricular response. This chaos stems from structural and electrical remodeling of the atria, often caused by underlying stressors like hypertension, heart failure, obesity, and age. This atrial remodeling (fibrosis) creates abnormal electrical circuits. The two primary consequences are:

1) Hemodynamic Compromise: The loss of the "atrial kick" (the atrial contribution to ventricular filling) can reduce cardiac output by 20-30%, causing dyspnea and fatigue.

2) Thromboembolism: The fibrillating, non-contracting left atrial appendage allows blood to stagnate, leading to thrombus formation. This clot can dislodge and embolize, most devastatingly to the brain, causing a cardioembolic stroke.

Diagnosis and Differential

Diagnosis is made by EKG or rhythm strip. The algorithm must first differentiate AF from other supraventricular tachycardias (e.g., atrial flutter, AVNRT). It is also critical to evaluate for reversible causes, such as hyperthyroidism, acute alcohol intoxication, or pulmonary embolism.

Treatment Algorithm

The management plan for Atrial Fibrillation (AF) is a three-pronged, parallel approach: stroke prevention, rate control, and rhythm control.

The first pillar, stroke prevention, is paramount. Risk is assessed using the CHA_2DS_2-VASc score. For men with a score of 0 or women with a score of 1, anticoagulation is not needed. For men with a score of 2 or more, or women with 3 or more, oral anticoagulation is strongly indicated. The selection of an agent is the next step. Direct-acting Oral Anticoagulants (DOACs), such as apixaban or rivaroxaban, are preferred over warfarin for their superior safety and efficacy. Warfarin is reserved for patients with mechanical heart valves or moderate-to-severe mitral stenosis.

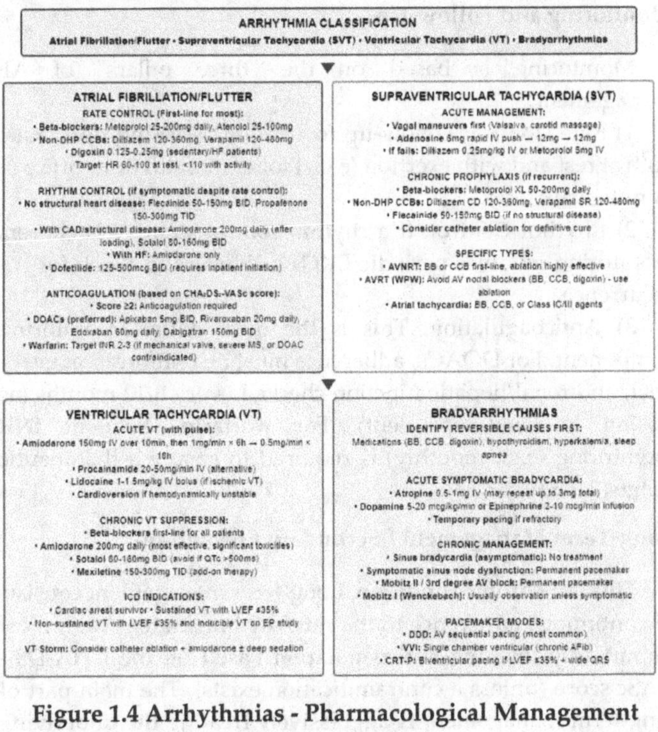
ARRHYTHMIA CLASSIFICATION
Atrial Fibrillation/Flutter • Supraventricular Tachycardia (SVT) • Ventricular Tachycardia (VT) • Bradyarrhythmias
ATRIAL FIBRILLATION/FLUTTER
RATE CONTROL (First-line for most):
• Beta-blockers: Metoprolol 25-200mg daily, Atenolol 25-100mg
• Non-DHP CCBs: Diltiazem 120-360mg, Verapamil 120-480mg
• Digoxin 0.125-0.25mg (sedentary/HF patients)
Target: HR 60-100 at rest, <110 with activity
RHYTHM CONTROL (if symptomatic despite rate control):
• No structural heart disease: Flecainide 50-150mg BID, Propafenone 150-300mg TID
• With CAD/structural disease: Amiodarone 200mg daily (after loading), Sotalol 80-160mg BID
• With HF: Amiodarone only
• Dofetilide: 125-500mcg BID (requires inpatient initiation)
ANTICOAGULATION (based on CHA₂DS₂-VASc score):
• Score ≥2: Anticoagulation required
• DOACs (preferred): Apixaban 5mg BID, Rivaroxaban 20mg daily, Edoxaban 60mg daily, Dabigatran 150mg BID
• Warfarin: Target INR 2-3 (if mechanical valve, severe MS, or DOAC contraindicated)
SUPRAVENTRICULAR TACHYCARDIA (SVT)
ACUTE MANAGEMENT:
• Vagal maneuvers first (Valsalva, carotid massage)
• Adenosine 6mg rapid IV push → 12mg → 12mg
• If fails: Diltiazem 0.25mg/kg IV or Metoprolol 5mg IV
CHRONIC PROPHYLAXIS (if recurrent):
• Beta-blockers: Metoprolol XL 50-200mg daily
• Non-DHP CCBs: Diltiazem CD 120-360mg, Verapamil SR 120-480mg
• Flecainide 50-150mg BID (if no structural disease)
• Consider catheter ablation for definitive cure
SPECIFIC TYPES:
• AVNRT: BB or CCB first-line, ablation highly effective
• AVRT (WPW): Avoid AV nodal blockers (BB, CCB, digoxin) - use ablation
• Atrial tachycardia: BB, CCB, or Class IC/III agents
VENTRICULAR TACHYCARDIA (VT)
ACUTE VT (with pulse):
• Amiodarone 150mg IV over 10min, then 1mg/min × 6h → 0.5mg/min × 18h
• Procainamide 20-50mg/min IV (alternative)
• Lidocaine 1-1.5mg/kg IV bolus (if ischemic VT)
• Cardioversion if hemodynamically unstable
CHRONIC VT SUPPRESSION:
• Beta-blockers first-line for all patients
• Amiodarone 200mg daily (most effective, significant toxicities)
• Sotalol 80-160mg BID (avoid if QTc >500ms)
• Mexiletine 150-300mg TID (add-on therapy)
ICD INDICATIONS:
• Cardiac arrest survivor • Sustained VT with LVEF ≤35%
• Non-sustained VT with LVEF ≤35% and inducible VT on EP study
VT Storm: Consider catheter ablation + amiodarone ± deep sedation
BRADYARRHYTHMIAS
IDENTIFY REVERSIBLE CAUSES FIRST:
Medications (BB, CCB, digoxin), hypothyroidism, hyperkalemia, sleep apnea
ACUTE SYMPTOMATIC BRADYCARDIA:
• Atropine 0.5-1mg IV (may repeat up to 3mg total)
• Dopamine 5-20 mcg/kg/min or Epinephrine 2-10 mcg/min infusion
• Temporary pacing if refractory
CHRONIC MANAGEMENT:
• Sinus bradycardia (asymptomatic): No treatment
• Symptomatic sinus node dysfunction: Permanent pacemaker
• Mobitz II / 3rd degree AV block: Permanent pacemaker
• Mobitz I (Wenckebach): Usually observation unless symptomatic
PACEMAKER MODES:
• DDD: AV sequential pacing (most common)
• VVI: Single chamber ventricular (chronic AFib)
• CRT-P: Biventricular pacing if LVEF ≤35% + wide QRS

Figure 1.4 Arrhythmias - Pharmacological Management

The second pillar is a rate control strategy, which aims for a ventricular rate under 100 bpm (lenient) or under 80 bpm if symptomatic. First-line agents for this are beta-blockers (e.g., metoprolol) or non-dihydropyridine CCBs (e.g., diltiazem). Digoxin can be added as a second-line agent.

The third pillar is a rhythm control strategy, which aims to restore and maintain sinus rhythm. This approach is reserved for patients who remain symptomatic (e.g., with fatigue or dyspnea) despite having an adequately controlled heart rate. Methods for rhythm control include pharmacological cardioversion with antiarrhythmic drugs, electrical cardioversion, or catheter ablation (pulmonary vein isolation), which is the most effective method for maintaining long-term sinus rhythm.

Monitoring and Follow-Up

Monitoring is based on the "three pillars" of AF management.

1) Rate Control: Follow-up focuses on assessing heart rate, both at rest and with exertion (e.g., Holter monitor or in-office 6-minute walk test).

2) Rhythm Control: If a rhythm-control strategy is chosen, monitoring involves periodic EKGs or Holters to check for AF recurrence.

3) Anticoagulation: This is the most critical monitoring component. For DOACs, adherence must be reinforced at every visit, and renal/hepatic function checked every 6-12 months (as dosing is renal-dependent). For warfarin, frequent INR monitoring (e.g., monthly) is required to ensure a therapeutic range (2.0-3.0).

Long-Term Management / Secondary Prevention

This is a chronic condition. Long-term management consists of continuous adherence to the rate/rhythm strategy and, most importantly, lifelong anticoagulation based on the CHA_2DS_2-VASc score (unless a contraindication exists). The main part of long-term management is aggressively treating the underlying conditions that drive atrial remodeling, such as hypertension, heart failure, obesity (weight loss), and obstructive sleep apnea.

Patient Counseling Points

- Stroke Risk: The number one priority is explaining that AF is a major stroke risk and that anticoagulation is not a "blood thinner" but an "anti-clotting" medicine essential for stroke prevention.
- Adherence: Emphasize that DOACs have a short half-life, and missing even one or two doses can leave them unprotected from stroke.
- Bleeding Risk: Counsel on signs of bleeding (e.g., severe bruising, black/tarry stools, hematuria) and the importance of fall prevention. Symptom Reporting: Instruct patients to report dizziness, lightheadedness, or syncope (potential bradycardia from rate-control meds) or new-onset, rapid, irregular palpitations (potential AF recurrence).

Common Pitfalls

The most dangerous pitfall is the failure to anticoagulate an eligible patient, often based on a subjective assessment of "low" fall risk. Another common error is choosing a rhythm-control strategy (e.g., amiodarone) without first ensuring the patient is on therapeutic anticoagulation. Finally, attributing all patient symptoms to AF without ruling out underlying structural heart disease or ischemia is a frequent oversight.

Table 1.4: Management of Atrial Fibrillation

Pillar	Clinical Goal & Agents / Tools
1. Anticoagulation	Prevent Stroke. Use CHA_2DS_2-VASc score. Agents: DOACs (e.g., Apixaban) or Warfarin.
2. Rate Control	Control Symptoms. Set target heart rate. Agents: Beta-Blockers (e.g., Metoprolol) or CCBs (e.g., Diltiazem).
3. Rhythm Control	Restore/Maintain Sinus. For persistent symptoms. Methods: Antiarrhythmic drugs or Catheter Ablation.

Ventricular Arrhythmias

Ventricular arrhythmias range from benign premature ventricular complexes (PVCs) to life-threatening ventricular tachycardia (VT) and ventricular fibrillation (VF).

Diagnosis and Differential

Diagnosis is by EKG. The most critical differential is distinguishing VT from supraventricular tachycardia (SVT) with aberrancy, as the treatment algorithms differ dramatically. Brugada and long-QT syndromes are the main differentials in cases of syncope or sudden death.

Treatment Algorithm

The algorithm is dictated by hemodynamic stability. Unstable VT or any VF is a medical emergency requiring immediate defibrillation according to Advanced Cardiovascular Life Support (ACLS) protocols. Stable, monomorphic VT can be managed pharmacologically with agents like amiodarone or procainamide, often followed by cardioversion. Long-term management for secondary prevention of sudden cardiac death almost universally involves an implantable cardioverter-defibrillator (ICD) and adjunctive antiarrhythmic drug therapy.

Common Pitfalls

The most critical pitfall is misdiagnosing VT as SVT with aberrancy and administering AV nodal blocking agents (e.g., adenosine, verapamil), which can precipitate hemodynamic collapse. Another error is failing to aggressively replete electrolytes (potassium and magnesium), which is a simple and effective measure to reduce ventricular ectopy. Finally, discharging a patient post-VF arrest without a definitive plan for an ICD is a major deviation from the standard of care.

Case Study

A 74-year-old female (Ms. Davis) presents to the ED for palpitations and lightheadedness. Her history is significant for hypertension and Type 2 Diabetes. Her EKG shows an **irregularly irregular rhythm with no P-waves**, at a ventricular rate of 135 bpm, consistent with **Atrial Fibrillation (AFib)**.

Discussion

The algorithm for Atrial Fibrillation is built on three parallel pillars: Anticoagulation (stroke prevention), Rate control (symptom control), and Rhythm control. The most urgent task is stroke risk assessment and rate control.

Treatment Algorithm

1. **Pillar 1 (Anticoagulation):** First, assess stroke risk using the **CHA_2DS_2-VASc** score:
   - **C** (CHF): 0
   - **H** (Hypertension): 1
   - **A_2** (Age ≥75): 0
   - **D** (Diabetes): 1
   - **S_2** (Stroke/TIA): 0
   - **V** (Vascular Disease): 0
   - **A** (Age 65-74): 1
   - **Sc** (Sex, Female): 1

   Total Score = 4. This high score mandates anticoagulation. You start a **DOAC (e.g., Apixaban 5 mg BID)**.
2. **Pillar 2 (Rate Control):** The patient is symptomatic from the rapid rate. You start an IV **beta-blocker (e.g., Metoprolol)** in the ED to lower her heart rate, and then transition to an oral agent.
3. **Pillar 3 (Rhythm Control):** Given her new diagnosis, a "rate control" strategy is chosen first. Rhythm control (e.g., cardioversion) is not needed emergently and can be considered later if she remains symptomatic despite a controlled heart rate.

Outcome

Ms. Davis is started on Apixaban for stroke prevention and Metoprolol for rate control. She is admitted for monitoring and to ensure her heart rate is stable.

VALVULAR HEART DISEASE

Valvular heart disease (VHD) treatment algorithms are determined by the specific valve affected, the severity of the lesion (stenosis or regurgitation), the presence of symptoms, and the impact on ventricular function.

Pathophysiology

The most common cause of Aortic Stenosis (AS) in older adults is degenerative calcification. This is an active inflammatory and fibrotic process, similar to atherosclerosis, that causes valve leaflets to become stiff and thickened. This progressively narrows the aortic valve orifice. To eject blood through this narrowed opening, the left ventricle (LV) must generate extremely high pressures, leading to a state of chronic pressure overload. The LV adapts by developing concentric hypertrophy (thickened walls). While initially compensatory, this hypertrophy makes the ventricle stiff and non-compliant, leading to diastolic dysfunction (HFpEF) and high filling pressures. The hypertrophied muscle also demands more oxygen, leading to angina. Syncope occurs when the fixed cardiac output cannot increase during exertion. If left untreated, the LV eventually fails, leading to systolic dysfunction (HFrEF) and rapid decline.

Diagnosis

Diagnosis and quantification of VHD rely heavily on echocardiography. The algorithm for all VHD involves periodic surveillance. The development of symptoms (angina, syncope, or heart failure) is a primary trigger for intervention. The secondary trigger, in asymptomatic patients, is objective evidence of ventricular decompensation (e.g., reduced LVEF or significant ventricular dilation).

Aortic Stenosis

Treatment Algorithm

The algorithm for asymptomatic severe aortic stenosis (AS) involves vigilant echocardiographic monitoring. Once symptoms develop, prognosis is poor, and intervention is urgently indicated. Intervention is also indicated for asymptomatic patients with severe AS and LVEF < 50%. The choice of intervention is based on a complex algorithm considering patient age, surgical risk, and anatomy, boiling down to surgical aortic valve replacement (SAVR) versus transcatheter aortic valve implantation (TAVI).

Differential and Pitfalls

The main differential is "pseudo-severe" AS, where the valve area is small due to low cardiac output, not true stenosis. This is identified with dobutamine stress echo. A common pitfall is attributing elderly patient symptoms (e.g., dyspnea) to "old age" when they are, in fact, the first sign of severe AS, thereby delaying life-saving intervention.

Mitral Regurgitation

Treatment Algorithm

The algorithm diverges based on etiology. For severe primary (degenerative) mitral regurgitation (MR), the algorithm dictates surgical intervention (preferably repair) for symptomatic patients. Surgery is also indicated for asymptomatic patients if there is evidence of left ventricular systolic dysfunction (LVEF ≤ 60%) or significant left ventricular dilation. For severe secondary (functional) MR, the primary algorithm is optimization of GDMT for the underlying heart failure. Percutaneous transcatheter edge-to-edge repair (TEER) is an evolving option for high-risk surgical patients with persistent symptoms despite maximal GDMT.

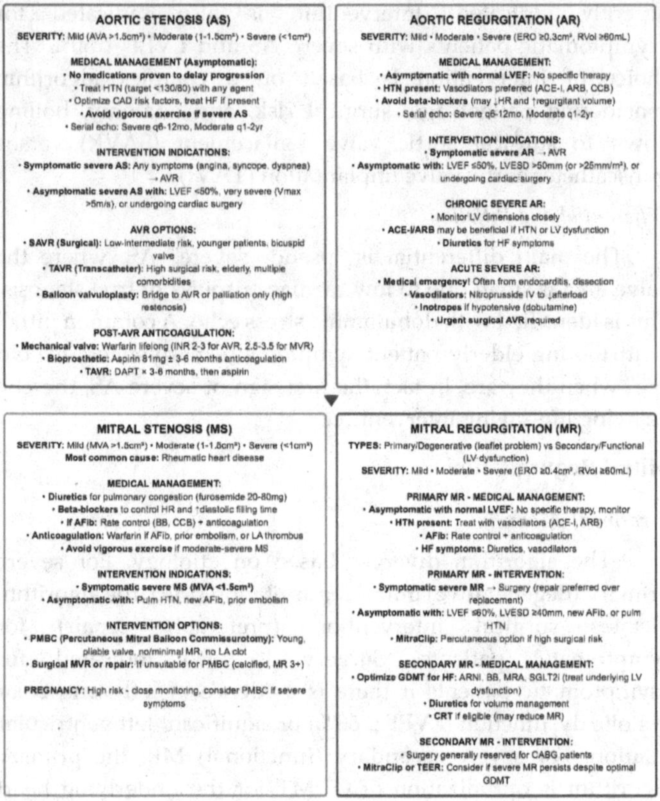
AORTIC STENOSIS (AS)
SEVERITY: Mild (AVA >1.5cm²) • Moderate (1-1.5cm²) • Severe (<1cm²)
MEDICAL MANAGEMENT (Asymptomatic):
• No medications proven to delay progression
• Treat HTN (target <130/80) with any agent
• Optimize CAD risk factors, treat HF if present
• Avoid vigorous exercise if severe AS
• Serial echo: Severe q6-12mo, Moderate q1-2yr
INTERVENTION INDICATIONS:
• Symptomatic severe AS: Any symptoms (angina, syncope, dyspnea) → AVR
• Asymptomatic severe AS with: LVEF <50%, very severe (Vmax >5m/s), or undergoing cardiac surgery
AVR OPTIONS:
• SAVR (Surgical): Low-intermediate risk, younger patients, bicuspid valve
• TAVR (Transcatheter): High surgical risk, elderly, multiple comorbidities
• Balloon valvuloplasty: Bridge to AVR or palliation only (high restenosis)
POST-AVR ANTICOAGULATION:
• Mechanical valve: Warfarin lifelong (INR 2-3 for AVR, 2.5-3.5 for MVR)
• Bioprosthetic: Aspirin 81mg ± 3-6 months anticoagulation
• TAVR: DAPT × 3-6 months, then aspirin
AORTIC REGURGITATION (AR)
SEVERITY: Mild • Moderate • Severe (ERO ≥0.3cm², RVol ≥60mL)
MEDICAL MANAGEMENT:
• Asymptomatic with normal LVEF: No specific therapy
• HTN present: Vasodilators preferred (ACE-I, ARB, CCB)
• Avoid beta-blockers (may ↓HR and ↑regurgitant volume)
• Serial echo: Severe q6-12mo, Moderate q1-2yr
INTERVENTION INDICATIONS:
• Symptomatic severe AR → AVR
• Asymptomatic with: LVEF ≤50%, LVESD >50mm (or >25mm/m²), or undergoing cardiac surgery
CHRONIC SEVERE AR:
• Monitor LV dimensions closely
• ACE-I/ARB may be beneficial if HTN or LV dysfunction
• Diuretics for HF symptoms
ACUTE SEVERE AR:
• Medical emergency! Often from endocarditis, dissection
• Vasodilators: Nitroprusside IV to ↓afterload
• Inotropes if hypotensive (dobutamine)
• Urgent surgical AVR required
MITRAL STENOSIS (MS)
SEVERITY: Mild (MVA >1.5cm²) • Moderate (1-1.5cm²) • Severe (<1cm²)
Most common cause: Rheumatic heart disease
MEDICAL MANAGEMENT:
• Diuretics for pulmonary congestion (furosemide 20-80mg)
• Beta-blockers to control HR and ↑diastolic filling time
• If AFib: Rate control (BB, CCB) + anticoagulation
• Anticoagulation: Warfarin if AFib, prior embolism, or LA thrombus
• Avoid vigorous exercise if moderate-severe MS
INTERVENTION INDICATIONS:
• Symptomatic severe MS (MVA <1.5cm²)
• Asymptomatic with: Pulm HTN, new AFib, prior embolism
INTERVENTION OPTIONS:
• PMBC (Percutaneous Mitral Balloon Commissurotomy): Young, pliable valve, no/minimal MR, no LA clot
• Surgical MVR or repair: If unsuitable for PMBC (calcified, MR 3+)
PREGNANCY: High risk - close monitoring, consider PMBC if severe symptoms
MITRAL REGURGITATION (MR)
TYPES: Primary/Degenerative (leaflet problem) vs Secondary/Functional (LV dysfunction)
SEVERITY: Mild • Moderate • Severe (ERO ≥0.4cm², RVol ≥60mL)
PRIMARY MR - MEDICAL MANAGEMENT:
• Asymptomatic with normal LVEF: No specific therapy, monitor
• HTN present: Treat with vasodilators (ACE-I, ARB)
• AFib: Rate control + anticoagulation
• HF symptoms: Diuretics, vasodilators
PRIMARY MR - INTERVENTION:
• Symptomatic severe MR → Surgery (repair preferred over replacement)
• Asymptomatic with: LVEF ≤60%, LVESD ≥40mm, new AFib, or pulm HTN
• MitraClip: Percutaneous option if high surgical risk
SECONDARY MR - MEDICAL MANAGEMENT:
• Optimize GDMT for HF: ARNI, BB, MRA, SGLT2i (treat underlying LV dysfunction)
• Diuretics for volume management
• CRT if eligible (may reduce MR)
SECONDARY MR - INTERVENTION:
• Surgery generally reserved for CABG patients
• MitraClip or TEER: Consider if severe MR persists despite optimal GDMT

Figure 1.5 Valvular Heart Disease - Management Algorithms

Differential and Pitfalls

The main diagnostic step is differentiating primary from secondary MR, as their treatment paths are opposite (surgery-first vs. medical-first). A common pitfall in secondary MR is intervening on the valve before aggressively titrating HFrEF medical therapy, as the regurgitation may improve significantly with medical optimization alone.

Monitoring and Follow-Up

The management of *asymptomatic* severe AS is "watchful waiting," which requires rigorous monitoring. This involves a clinical visit and a serial echocardiogram every 6-12 months. The echocardiogram is monitored for worsening hemodynamics (valve area, gradient) and, most importantly, for any decline in LVEF (an LVEF < 50% is an indication for intervention, even if asymptomatic). At every visit, the clinician must actively and repeatedly probe for the "cardinal symptoms" of AS.

Long-Term Management / Secondary Prevention

Once symptoms develop or the LVEF drops, medical therapy is ineffective, and the only long-term management is valve replacement (Surgical Aortic Valve Replacement - SAVR, or Transcatheter Aortic Valve Implantation - TAVI). Post-intervention, management depends on the valve type. A bioprosthetic valve (TAVI or SAVR) requires short-term antiplatelet therapy. A mechanical valve (SAVR only) requires lifelong anticoagulation with warfarin. All patients with a prosthetic valve require lifelong prophylaxis against bacterial endocarditis before certain dental or surgical procedures.

Patient Counseling Points

The Cardinal Symptoms: This is the most important counseling point for a patient with asymptomatic severe AS. They *must* be taught to immediately report the onset of the "SAD" symptoms: Syncope (fainting), Angina (chest pain), or Dyspnea (shortness of breath). Explain that the onset of these symptoms is a "game-changer" and an urgent indication for valve replacement.

Activity: Counsel to avoid strenuous, competitive exercise, as it can provoke syncope.

Endocarditis Prophylaxis: After valve replacement, they must inform all doctors and dentists about their prosthetic valve and take antibiotics before all dental procedures.

Warfarin (if mechanical): Explain the necessity of lifelong adherence and regular INR monitoring.

Case Study

An 80-year-old male (Mr. Brown) with a known history of a "heart murmur" presents to his cardiologist for follow-up. He has been "watchfully waiting" for his asymptomatic severe **Aortic Stenosis (AS)**. At his visit, he mentions he has had two episodes in the last month where he felt "woozy" and lightheaded while walking his dog, which he had to stop and rest.

Discussion

This is a critical change in Mr. Brown's status. The algorithm for severe Aortic Stenosis is to monitor closely while asymptomatic, but to intervene immediately upon the onset of **cardinal symptoms (Syncope, Angina, or Dyspnea)**. His "wooziness" is pre-syncope and is a major red flag.

Treatment Algorithm:

- Disease Status: Asymptomatic Severe Aortic Stenosis.
- New Finding: Patient now reports new-onset exertional pre-syncope.
- Algorithm Trigger: The onset of cardinal symptoms (Syncope) is a Class 1 indication for intervention. Medical therapy is ineffective for severe AS.
- Intervention: Given his age (80) and surgical risk, the algorithm points toward a transcatheter (non-surgical) approach. You refer him to the structural heart team for evaluation.

Outcome

Mr. Brown is referred for **Transcatheter Aortic Valve Implantation (TAVI)**. His case has moved from "watchful waiting" to "urgent intervention" because he is no longer asymptomatic.

Summary

Hypertension: The algorithm is stratified by blood pressure stage and ASCVD risk. It prioritizes lifestyle modifications, followed by a stepwise progression of first-line pharmacological agents (diuretics, CCBs, RAS-blockers) based on patient-specific compelling indications.

Coronary Artery Disease: Management is critically bifurcated. Stable disease is managed with GDMT for symptom control and event prevention. Acute coronary syndromes require time-sensitive algorithms: emergent reperfusion (usually PCI) for STEMI, and risk-based invasive strategies for NSTEMI.

Heart Failure: The algorithm is dictated by ejection fraction. HFrEF treatment is built on the concurrent initiation of four pillar therapies (ARNI, beta-blocker, MRA, SGLT2i). HFpEF management focuses on SGLT2i and aggressive comorbidity control.

Arrhythmias: Management for atrial fibrillation follows a three-pillar structure: anticoagulation (based on CHA_2DS_2-VASc score), rate control, and rhythm control. For ventricular arrhythmias, hemodynamic stability dictates the algorithm, prioritizing immediate defibrillation for unstable patients.

Valvular Heart Disease: Treatment algorithms for severe valvular disease (e.g., Aortic Stenosis, Mitral Regurgitation) are primarily driven by the onset of symptoms or the development of objective evidence of ventricular dysfunction (e.g., reduced LVEF), which serve as the main triggers for surgical or transcatheter intervention.

Multiple Choice Questions

1. A 60-year-old male with Type 2 Diabetes and hypertension presents with a blood pressure of 152/94 mmHg. According to standard treatment algorithms, which of the following is the most appropriate initial agent?
   A) Hydrochlorothiazide
   B) Amlodipine
   C) Lisinopril
   D) Carvedilol
2. A 55-year-old female with HFrEF (LVEF 30%) is being seen for follow-up. She is currently on optimal doses of an ARNI, carvedilol, and spironolactone. She has no congestion. Which of the following agents is indicated to be added to her regimen?
   A) Furosemide
   B) Empagliflozin
   C) Digoxin
   D) Hydralazine/Isosorbide Dinitrate
3. A 70-year-old male presents to the emergency department with severe, crushing chest pain. His EKG shows 3mm ST-segment elevations in leads V2-V5. The hospital is PCI-capable. What is the most critical next step in the treatment algorithm?
   A) Administer intravenous fibrinolytics.
   B) Administer sublingual nitroglycerin and wait for troponin results.
   C) Immediate activation of the cardiac catheterization lab for primary PCI.
   D) Start a beta-blocker and heparin infusion.
4. A 68-year-old female with persistent atrial fibrillation and a CHA_2DS_2-VASc score of 4 is intolerant to DOACs. Which of the following is the most appropriate management?
   A) Warfarin with a target INR of 2.0-3.0
   B) Aspirin 325 mg daily
   C) Clopidogrel 75 mg daily

D) No anticoagulation is needed if she is in normal sinus rhythm.

5. A patient presents with acute decompensated heart failure and is found to be hypotensive (BP 80/50 mmHg), with cool extremities and pulmonary rales. How would this patient be classified and what is the indicated treatment?
   A) Warm and Wet; IV Furosemide
   B) Cold and Dry; IV Fluids
   C) Cold and Wet; IV Furosemide and Inotropes (e.g., Dobutamine)
   D) Warm and Dry; Discharge with oral diuretic titration
6. A common and dangerous pitfall in managing a patient with a wide-complex tachycardia (WCT) is misdiagnosing VT as:
   A) Atrial Fibrillation with RVR
   B) SVT with aberrancy, and treating with an AV nodal blocker
   C) Sinus tachycardia, and observing
   D) Atrial flutter, and anticoagulating
7. A 78-year-old asymptomatic patient is found to have severe aortic stenosis on a routine echocardiogram, with a normal LVEF of 60%. What is the next step in the management algorithm?
   A) Immediate surgical aortic valve replacement (SAVR)
   B) Transcatheter aortic valve implantation (TAVI) within 30 days
   C) Initiation of a beta-blocker and ACE inhibitor
   D) Vigilant monitoring with periodic surveillance echocardiography
8. In a patient with stable ischemic heart disease, revascularization with PCI is primarily indicated for which of the following?
   A) Prevention of myocardial infarction

B) Mortality reduction
C) Refractory angina despite maximal guideline-directed medical therapy
D) Treatment of an asymptomatic 80% stenosis

9. Which of the following is considered a "common pitfall" in the management of HFrEF, often leading to poor outcomes?
A) Therapeutic inertia (failure to initiate all four pillar therapies)
B) Aggressively titrating beta-blockers
C) Using an SGLT2i in a patient with diabetes
D) Preferring an ARNI over an ACE inhibitor

10. A patient with severe secondary (functional) mitral regurgitation is symptomatic with dyspnea. The LVEF is 35%. What is the first-line treatment algorithm?
A) Immediate surgical mitral valve repair
B) Optimization of guideline-directed medical therapy for HFrEF
C) Percutaneous transcatheter edge-to-edge repair (TEER)
D) Initiation of rate-control therapy with diltiazem

Self-Assessment Questions

1. What are the main non-pharmacological interventions that form the foundation of the hypertension treatment algorithm?
2. Define "resistant hypertension" and outline the next steps in the treatment algorithm once it is identified.
3. Compare and contrast the primary treatment goals and pharmacological algorithms for Stable Ischemic Heart Disease versus NSTEMI.
4. What are the four "pillar" therapies for Heart Failure with Reduced Ejection Fraction (HFrEF) and why has the algorithm shifted to concurrent initiation?
5. How does the treatment algorithm for Heart Failure with Preserved Ejection Fraction (HFpEF) differ from that of HFrEF?
6. Describe the three-pillar algorithm for managing a patient with new-onset, stable atrial fibrillation.
7. A patient presents with a wide-complex tachycardia. What is the most critical differential diagnosis, and how does hemodynamic stability alter the immediate treatment algorithm?
8. What are the primary triggers for intervention (e.g., SAVR or TAVI) in a patient with asymptomatic severe aortic stenosis?
9. Explain the difference in the management algorithm for primary (degenerative) mitral regurgitation versus secondary (functional) mitral regurgitation.
10. Identify and describe two "common pitfalls" in the management of Acute Decompensated Heart Failure (ADHF)

Bibliography

1. Whelton PK, Carey RM, Aronow WS, Casey DE Jr, Collins KJ, Dennison Himmelfarb C, et al. 2017 ACC/AHA/AAPA/ABC/ACPM/AGS/APhA/ASH/ASPC/NMA/PCN A Guideline for the Prevention, Detection, Evaluation, and Management of High Blood Pressure in Adults: A Report of the American College of Cardiology/American Heart Association Task Force on Clinical Practice Guidelines. J Am Coll Cardiol. 2018 May 15;71(19):e127–248.
2. Fihn SD, Gardin JM, Abrams J, Berra K, Blankenship JC, Dallas AP, et al. 2012 ACCF/AHA/ACP/AATS/PCNA/SCAI/STS Guideline for the Diagnosis and Management of Patients With Stable Ischemic Heart Disease: A Report of the American College of Cardiology Foundation/American Heart Association Task Force on Practice Guidelines. Circulation. 2012 Dec 18;126(25):e354–471.
3. Amsterdam EA, Wenger NK, Brindis RG, Casey DE Jr, Ganiats TG, Holmes DR Jr, et al. 2014 AHA/ACC Guideline for the Management of Patients With Non–ST-Elevation Acute Coronary Syndromes: A Report of the American Heart Association/American College of Cardiology Task Force on Practice Guidelines. J Am Coll Cardiol. 2014 Dec 23;64(24):e139–228.
4. O'Gara PT, Kushner FG, Ascheim DD, Casey DE Jr, Chung MK, de Lemos JA, et al. 2013 ACCF/AHA Guideline for the Management of ST-Elevation Myocardial Infarction: A Report of the American College of Cardiology Foundation/American Heart Association Task Force on Practice Guidelines. J Am Coll Cardiol. 2013 Jan 29;61(4):e78–140.
5. Heidenreich PA, Bozkurt B, Aguilar D, Bress AP, Byun J, Colvin M, et al. 222 AHA/ACC/HFSA Guideline for the Management of Heart Failure: A Report of the American College of Cardiology/American Heart Association Joint Committee on Clinical Practice Guidelines. Circulation. 2022 May 3;145(18):e895–1032.
6. McMurray JJV, Packer M, Desai AS, Gong J, Lefkowitz MP, Rizkala AR, et al. Angiotensin-Neprilysin Inhibition versus Enalapril in Heart Failure. N Engl J Med. 2014 Sep 11;371(11):993–1004.
7. Anker SD, Butler J, Filippatos G, Ferreira JP, Bocchi E, Böhm M, et al. Empagliflozin in Heart Failure with a Preserved Ejection Fraction. N Engl J Med. 2021 Oct 14;385(16):1451–61.
8. January CT, Wann LS, Calkins H, Chen LY, Cigarroa JE, Cleveland JC Jr, et al. 2019 AHA/ACC/HRS Focused Update of the 2014 AHA/ACC/HRS Guideline for the Management of Patients With Atrial Fibrillation: A Report of the American College of Cardiology/American Heart Association Task Force on Clinical Practice Guidelines and the Heart Rhythm Society. J Am Coll Cardiol. 2019 Jul 9;74(1):104–32.
9. Hindricks G, Potpara T, Dagres N, Arbelo E, Bax JJ, Blomström-Lundqvist C, et al. 2020 ESC Guidelines for the diagnosis and management of atrial fibrillation developed in collaboration with the EACTS: The Task Force for the diagnosis and management of atrial fibrillation of the European Society of Cardiology (ESC). Eur Heart J. 2021 Feb 1;42(5):373–498.
10. Al-Khatib SM, Stevenson WG, Ackerman MJ, Bryant WJ, Callans DJ,

Curtis AB, et al. 2017 AHA/ACC/HRS Guideline for Management of Patients With Ventricular Arrhythmias and the Prevention of Sudden Cardiac Death: A Report of the American College of Cardiology/American Heart Association Task Force on Clinical Practice Guidelines and the Heart Rhythm Society. J Am Coll Cardiol. 2018 Oct 2;72(14):e91–220.

11. Otto CM, Nishimura RA, Bonow RO, Carabello BA, Erwin JP 3rd, Gentile F, et al. 2020 ACC/AHA Guideline for the Management of Patients With Valvular Heart Disease: A Report of the American College of Cardiology/American Heart Association Joint Committee on Clinical Practice Guidelines. J Am Coll Cardiol. 2021 Feb 2;77(5):e25–197.
12. James PA, Oparil S, Carter BL, Cushman WC, Dennison-Himmelfarb C, Handler J, et al. 2014 Evidence-Based Guideline for the Management of High Blood Pressure in Adults: Report From the Panel Members Appointed to the Eighth Joint National Committee (JNC 8). JAMA. 2014 Feb 5;311(5):507–20.
13. The SPRINT Research Group. A Randomized Trial of Intensive versus Standard Blood-Pressure Control. N Engl J Med. 2015 Nov 26;373(22):2103–16.
14. Zipes DP, Camm AJ, Borggrefe M, Buxton AE, Chaitman B, Fromer M, et al. ACC/AHA/ESC 2006 Guidelines for Management of Patients With Ventricular Arrhythmias and the Prevention of Sudden Cardiac Death: A Report of the American College of Cardiology/American Heart Association Task Force and the European Society of Cardiology Committee for Practice Guidelines (Writing Committee to Develop Guidelines for Management of Patients With Ventricular Arrhythmias and the Prevention of Sudden Cardiac Death). Circulation. 2006 Sep 5;114(10):e385-484.
15. Packer M, Anker SD, Butler J, Filippatos G, Pocock SJ, Carson P, et al. Cardiovascular and Renal Outcomes with Empagliflozin in Heart Failure. N Engl J Med. 2020 Oct 8;383(15):1413–24.

CHAPTER 2

TREATMENT ALGORITHMS FOR RESPIRATORY DISORDERS

Author

Dr. Basu Venkateswara Reddy,
Professor and Head, Department of Pharmaceutics,
Sri.K.V.College of Pharmacy, Chikkaballapura, Karnataka, India

Abstract

The management of respiratory disorders is structured around algorithms that differentiate disease states and guide stepwise therapeutic intervention. Asthma management follows a control-based approach, stratifying patients into steps that dictate the use of inhaled corticosteroids (ICS) and bronchodilators, with a modern emphasis on ICS-formoterol as both a controller and reliever. The algorithm for Chronic Obstructive Pulmonary Disease (COPD) is based on the GOLD classification, using symptom burden and exacerbation history to guide the use of short- and long-acting bronchodilators (LAMA/LABA), with ICS reserved for patients with eosinophilic phenotypes. Pneumonia treatment algorithms are initiated by assessing severity (e.g., CURB-65) to determine the site of care, followed by empiric antibiotic selection based on likely pathogens and patient risk factors, with a mandate for timely de-escalation. The acute algorithm for pulmonary embolism is driven by hemodynamic stability and right ventricular strain, with risk stratification determining the use of anticoagulation, systemic thrombolysis, or embolectomy. Tuberculosis management is distinctly bifurcated into treatment for latent infection, which is a preventive algorithm, and active disease, which requires a prolonged, multi-drug regimen (RIPE) under directly observed therapy to ensure cure and prevent resistance.

Keywords: *Respiratory Algorithms, Asthma, COPD, Pneumonia, Pulmonary Embolism, Tuberculosis*

Learning Objectives

After completion of the chapter, the learners should be able to:

- List the main components of the stepwise management algorithm for persistent asthma based on GINA guidelines.
- Explain the GOLD classification system and its role in guiding the pharmacological treatment algorithm for COPD.
- Formulate an appropriate empiric antibiotic algorithm for a patient with community-acquired pneumonia (CAP) based on their CURB-65 score and comorbidities.
- Differentiate the management algorithms for latent tuberculosis infection (LTBI) versus active multi-drug-resistant tuberculosis (MDR-TB).
- Prioritize the diagnostic and therapeutic steps in the algorithm for a patient with a suspected massive pulmonary embolism.

ASTHMA

Asthma is a heterogeneous chronic inflammatory disorder of the airways characterized by reversible bronchoconstriction and airway hyperresponsiveness. The treatment algorithm is based on a stepwise, control-based approach to mitigate symptoms and reduce the risk of future exacerbations.

Pathophysiology

The pathophysiology is driven primarily by a T-helper 2 (Th2) cell-mediated immune response. In sensitized individuals, exposure to an allergen triggers IgE production, which coats mast cells. Upon re-exposure, these mast cells degranulate, releasing pre-formed mediators like histamine and leukotrienes. This causes the "early-phase" reaction: acute smooth muscle contraction (bronchoconstriction) and vasodilation. This is followed hours later by a "late-phase" reaction, characterized by a massive influx of eosinophils, which release cytotoxic proteins that damage the airway epithelium and perpetuate inflammation. Over years, this chronic inflammation leads to airway remodeling—a structural change involving bronchial smooth muscle hypertrophy, sub-epithelial fibrosis, and mucus gland hyperplasia—which can make the disease less reversible.

Diagnosis and Classification

Diagnosis is established clinically by a history of variable respiratory symptoms (wheeze, cough, dyspnea) and confirmed by objective measures of variable expiratory airflow limitation, most notably via spirometry. A significant reversible response to a bronchodilator (e.g., FEV1 increase > 12% and 200 mL) is a classic diagnostic finding. Classification has moved from traditional "intermittent" and "persistent" categories to a more practical framework based on the level of therapy required to maintain control, as outlined in the Global Initiative for Asthma (GINA) guidelines.

Differential Diagnosis

The differential for asthma-like symptoms is broad. In adults, it critically includes Chronic Obstructive Pulmonary Disease (COPD), which typically demonstrates non-reversible or poorly reversible airflow obstruction. Other considerations include congestive heart failure ("cardiac asthma"), vocal cord dysfunction, gastroesophageal reflux disease (GERD) with cough, and allergic rhinitis with post-nasal drip. In children, viral bronchiolitis and foreign body aspiration must be considered.

Treatment Algorithm

The modern asthma algorithm is designed to ensure that all patients receive an inhaled corticosteroid (ICS) to manage the underlying inflammation, moving away from short-acting beta-agonist (SABA) monotherapy.

Stepwise Controller Therapy (GINA)

The treatment algorithm is organized into five steps.

Step 1

For patients with infrequent symptoms, the preferred algorithm is as-needed low-dose ICS-formoterol (a long-acting beta-agonist, or LABA, with a fast onset). This single inhaler serves as both the controller and reliever

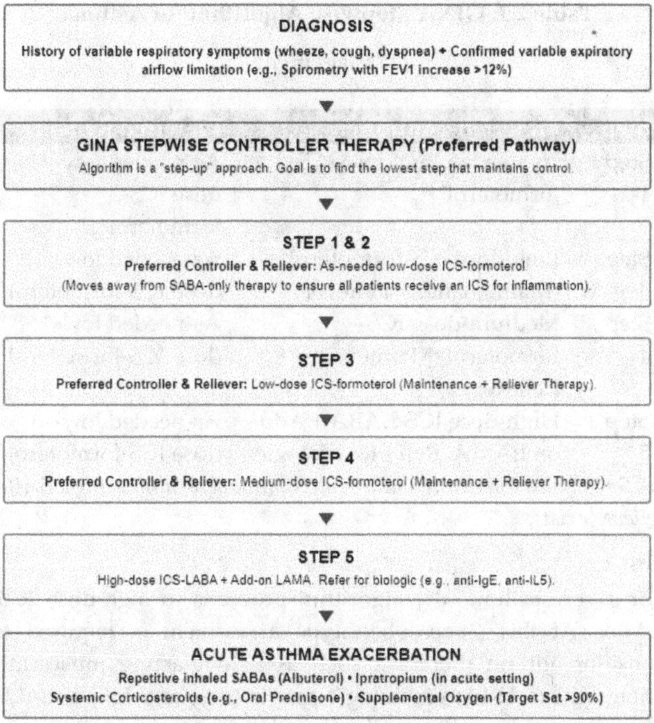

Figure 2.1: Asthma - GINA Stepwise Management

Step 2

For patients with symptoms more frequently, the preferred algorithm is daily low-dose ICS plus as-needed SABA, or the continuation of as-needed low-dose ICS-formoterol.

Step 3

The algorithm advances to a maintenance dose of low-dose ICS-LABA. The ICS-formoterol combination can again be used for both maintenance and relief (known as SMART or MART).

Step 4

This step involves escalating to a medium-dose ICS-LABA combination.

Table 2.1: GINA Stepwise Algorithm for Asthma Management

Step	Preferred Controller	Preferred Reliever
Step 1-2	As-needed low-dose ICS-formoterol*	As-needed low-dose ICS-formoterol*
Step 3	Low-dose ICS-formoterol (Maintenance + Reliever)	As-needed low-dose ICS-formoterol
Step 4	Medium-dose ICS-formoterol (Maintenance + Reliever)	As-needed low-dose ICS-formoterol
Step 5	High-dose ICS-LABA + Add-on LAMA. Refer for biologic.	As-needed low-dose ICS-formoterol

**ICS = Inhaled Corticosteroid. An alternative algorithm using a SABA reliever exists.*

Step 5

For severe asthma, the algorithm proceeds to high-dose ICS-LABA. At this stage, phenotype assessment is required to consider add-on therapies such as a long-acting muscarinic antagonist (LAMA) or biologic agents (e.g., anti-IgE, anti-IL5) for severe eosinophilic or allergic asthma.

Acute Exacerbation Algorithm

The algorithm for an acute asthma exacerbation is time-sensitive. It involves repetitive administration of inhaled SABAs (e.g., albuterol), often with ipratropium bromide in the acute setting, supplemental oxygen to maintain saturation > 90%, and a short course of systemic corticosteroids (e.g., oral prednisone) to control the underlying inflammatory surge.

Monitoring and Follow-Up

The goal of monitoring is to assess asthma control and adjust therapy in a stepwise fashion (e.g., per GINA guidelines). Control is assessed by two domains: symptom control (daytime symptoms, nighttime awakenings, rescue inhaler use, activity limitation) and future risk (exacerbations, lung function decline). Clinically, the "Rule of Twos" is a useful heuristic: if a patient uses their rescue SABA >2 times per week, wakes at night

>2 times per month, or refills their SABA >2 times per year, their asthma is uncontrolled. Objective monitoring involves spirometry (FEV1 and FEV1/FVC ratio) at diagnosis and periodically (e.g., annually) to assess long-term lung function. Peak Expiratory Flow (PEF) monitoring at home can be useful for patients with poor symptom perception or those in the "yellow zone" of their action plan. Follow-up visits should be scheduled every 1-3 months for uncontrolled asthma and every 6-12 months for well-controlled asthma.

Long-Term Management / Secondary Prevention

Long-term management is focused on preventing exacerbations and minimizing symptom burden. The cornerstone of prevention is controlling the underlying inflammation with an inhaled corticosteroid (ICS). The paradigm has shifted away from SABA-only treatment; all patients, even with mild asthma, should receive an ICS, either as a daily controller or as-needed in combination with their rescue bronchodilator. For persistent symptoms, the next step is adding a long-acting beta-agonist (LABA) in a combination inhaler with the ICS. It is critical to note that LABAs should never be used as monotherapy for asthma. Other long-term strategies include trigger avoidance (e.g., dust mite covers, HEPA filters, pet dander control) and the creation of a personalized "Asthma Action Plan." This plan empowers the patient to recognize worsening symptoms (the "yellow zone") and initiate pre-prescribed therapy (e.g., increasing ICS dose or adding oral steroids) to prevent a severe exacerbation.

Patient Counseling Points

- Inhaler Technique: This is the most common cause of treatment failure. The clinician must demonstrate and have the patient demonstrate back the use of their specific device (e.g., MDI with a spacer, or a DPI) and re-check technique at every visit.
- Controller vs. Rescuer: The most important concept to teach is the difference between the "rescuer" (SABA, e.g., albuterol) which opens the tubes immediately, and the "controller" (ICS, e.g., fluticasone) which reduces the

inflammation and prevents attacks. Over-reliance on the rescuer is a red flag for poor control.

- Asthma Action Plan: The patient must understand their "Green," "Yellow," and "Red" zones. They must know what to do when they enter the "Yellow zone" (e.g., "I will add my 'yellow zone' inhaler and call the office") and "Red zone" ("I will use my rescue inhaler, take my oral steroid, and go to the emergency room").
- Trigger Avoidance: Counsel on identifying and mitigating personal triggers, such as dust, pollen, cold air, or exercise-induced bronchospasm.

Common Pitfalls in Management

The most significant pitfall is the historical over-reliance on SABA monotherapy, which manages symptoms but not inflammation, thereby increasing exacerbation risk. Other common errors include poor inhaler technique, failure to identify and mitigate environmental triggers (e.g., allergens, smoke), and misdiagnosing COPD as asthma (or vice-versa), leading to inappropriate therapy.

Case Study

A 22-year-old college student (Ms. Lee) presents with a cough and wheeze. She reports "getting colds" 3-4 times per month that "go to her chest." She has to use her albuterol (SABA) rescue inhaler 4-5 days a week and wakes up with a cough about twice a week. She has no daily controller medication.

Discussion

Ms. Lee's symptoms (rescue inhaler use >2x/week, nighttime awakenings) indicate her asthma is **uncontrolled**. The GINA algorithm has a major paradigm shift: SABA-only therapy is no longer recommended, as it does not treat the underlying inflammation. She is at high risk for an exacerbation. The algorithm dictates she should be on, at minimum, a daily controller or a combination ICS-formoterol reliever.

Treatment Algorithm

- **Classification:** Uncontrolled asthma, consistent with GINA Step 2/3.
- **Algorithm Step-Up:** The patient is currently on SABA-only (an outdated Step 1). She needs to be moved to a therapy that includes an Inhaled Corticosteroid (ICS).
- **Therapeutic Choice:** You select the **GINA "Preferred Pathway"**
- **Option (GINA Step 3):** Low-dose ICS-Formoterol (e.g., budesonide-formoterol) to be used for *both* daily maintenance and as-needed relief (this is the "MART" or "SMART" algorithm).
- **Counseling:** You explain that her new single inhaler is now her "controller" and "reliever" in one. You also provide an "Asthma Action Plan" to help her manage symptoms.
- **Outcome:** Ms. Lee is prescribed a budesonide-formoterol inhaler to use twice daily and as needed for symptoms. You schedule a follow-up in 4 weeks to assess her control, checking her reliever use and nighttime symptoms

CHRONIC OBSTRUCTIVE PULMONARY DISORDER (COPD)

COPD is a common, preventable, and treatable disease characterized by persistent respiratory symptoms and airflow limitation due to airway and/or alveolar abnormalities, usually caused by significant exposure to noxious particles or gases.

Pathophysiology

Chronic Obstructive Pulmonary Disease (COPD is caused by an abnormal inflammatory response to noxious particles, primarily cigarette smoke. The pathophysiology encompasses two overlapping phenotypes:

Emphysema

This is a disease of the acinus (the gas-exchanging units).

Oxidative stress from smoke leads to an imbalance between proteases (like neutrophil elastase) and anti-proteases (like alpha-1-antitrypsin). This protease activity destroys alveolar walls, creating large, non-functional air sacs (bullae). This reduces the surface area for gas exchange and causes loss of elastic recoil, leading to "air trapping" and lung hyperinflation.

Chronic Bronchitis

This is a disease of the conducting airways. It is defined clinically by a productive cough for ≥3 months in ≥2 consecutive years. Pathologically, it involves neutrophilic inflammation (distinct from the eosinophilic inflammation of asthma), smooth muscle hypertrophy, and profound goblet cell and mucus gland hyperplasia, leading to chronic airway obstruction and a productive cough.

Diagnosis and Classification

Diagnosis is confirmed by spirometry in a patient with appropriate symptoms (dyspnea, chronic cough) and risk factors (e.g., tobacco smoke). A post-bronchodilator FEV1/FVC ratio < 0.70 confirms the presence of persistent airflow limitation. The GOLD (Global Initiative for Chronic Obstructive Lung Disease) classification system is the cornerstone of the management algorithm. It classifies patients into groups (A, B, E) based on symptom burden (using mMRC or CAT scores) and exacerbation history, which guides initial therapy.

Differential Diagnosis

The primary differential diagnosis for COPD is asthma. The main distinguishing features include age of onset (COPD typically > 40), smoking history, and the significant reversibility of airflow limitation seen in asthma. Other differentials include heart failure, bronchiectasis, and, in younger patients or non-smokers, alpha-1 antitrypsin deficiency, which must be screened for.

Treatment Algorithm

The COPD algorithm focuses on symptom reduction, risk reduction (exacerbations), and slowing disease progression.

Stable COPD Algorithm

The algorithm begins universally with smoking cessation and pulmonary rehabilitation.

- **Group A:** Patients with low symptoms and low exacerbation risk. The algorithm starts with a short- or long-acting bronchodilator (SABA or LABA/LAMA).
- **Group B:** Patients with high symptoms but low exacerbation risk. The algorithm dictates initial therapy with a long-acting bronchodilator. Dual therapy with a LAMA + LABA is often used if symptoms are severe.
- **Group E:** Patients with high exacerbation risk (e.g., ≥ 2 moderate exacerbations or ≥ 1 hospitalization in the past year). The algorithm mandates initial therapy with a LAMA + LABA combination. If the patient has a high blood eosinophil count (≥ 300 cells/μL), indicating an "asthma-like" inflammatory component, the algorithm supports the addition of an ICS (triple therapy: LAMA+LABA+ICS).

Table 2.2: Pharmacological Algorithm for Stable COPD (GOLD Groups)

Patient Group	Symptoms	Exacerbation Risk	Initial Pharmacotherapy
Group A	Low (mMRC 0-1)	Low (0-1)	A Bronchodilator (SABA or SAMA)
Group B	High (mMRC ≥ 2)	Low (0-1)	A Long-Acting Bronchodilator (LABA or LAMA)
Group C	Low (mMRC 0-1)	High (≥ 2 or ≥ 1 hosp.)	LAMA (Long-Acting Muscarinic Antagonist)
Group D	High (mMRC ≥ 2)	High (≥ 2 or ≥ 1 hosp.)	LAMA or LAMA + LABA (or LABA + ICS if eos ≥ 300)

Acute Exacerbation Algorithm

Management of an acute exacerbation of COPD (AECOPD)

involves an intensified regimen of short-acting bronchodilators (SABA/SAMA), a 5-7-day course of oral corticosteroids (e.g., prednisone 40 mg), and supplemental oxygen. Antibiotics are added to the algorithm if the patient exhibits all three cardinal symptoms (increased dyspnea, sputum volume, and sputum purulence) or two symptoms if one is sputum purulence.

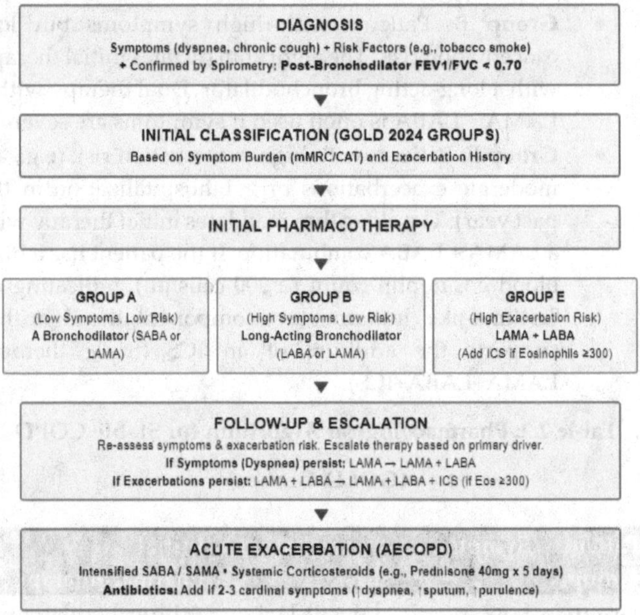

Figure 2.2: COPD - GOLD Pharmacological Management

Monitoring and Follow-Up

COPD management (per GOLD guidelines) is guided by assessing two factors: symptom burden (using the mMRC dyspnea scale or the CAT score) and the history of exacerbations. Annual spirometry (FEV1) is required to make the initial diagnosis and track long-term disease progression, but therapeutic adjustments are based on symptoms and exacerbations, not FEV1. Follow-up visits, typically every 3-6 months, should re-assess mMRC/CAT scores, exacerbation frequency, and oxygen saturation. Inhaler technique must be re-checked at every visit.

Long-Term Management / Secondary Prevention

1. **Smoking Cessation:** This is the single most important intervention. It is the only strategy proven to slow the progressive decline in FEV1.
2. **Pharmacotherapy:** The mainstay is bronchodilation with long-acting agents. This includes Long-Acting Muscarinic Antagonists (LAMAs, e.g., tiotropium) and Long-Acting Beta-Agonists (LABAs, e.g., salmeterol). Dual LAMA/LABA therapy is used for patients with persistent symptoms. Inhaled corticosteroids (ICS) are *not* first-line and are reserved for patients with a high exacerbation risk *and* evidence of eosinophilic inflammation (e.g., blood eosinophils ≥300).
3. **Non-Pharmacological:** Pulmonary rehabilitation is a critical, high-value intervention that improves exercise tolerance and quality of life. Long-term oxygen therapy is indicated for patients with chronic hypoxemia (PaO_2 ≤55 mmHg or SpO_2 ≤88% at rest).
4. **Vaccinations:** Annual influenza and routine pneumococcal vaccination (e.g., PCV20) are essential to prevent exacerbations.

Patient Counseling Points

- Smoking Cessation: This must be the primary counseling point at every single encounter. Use the "5 A's" (Ask, Advise, Assess, Assist, Arrange).
- Exacerbation Recognition: Teach the patient the three cardinal signs of an acute exacerbation: worsening dyspnea, increased sputum volume, and increased sputum purulence. Many patients will have an "at-home" prescription for antibiotics and oral steroids to start immediately upon recognition.
- Inhaler Technique: As with asthma, this is a frequent point of failure. Patients must be taught how to use their specific devices (e.g., HandiHaler, Ellipta).
- Oxygen Safety: For patients on home O_2, it is a life-or-death counseling point: Oxygen is an accelerant. There can be *no smoking* and no open flames in the home.

Common Pitfalls in Management

A common pitfall is the inappropriate use of ICS in patients without a high exacerbation risk and eosinophilia, which unnecessarily increases the risk of pneumonia. Conversely, a frequent error is failing to add an ICS in a patient with frequent exacerbations and eosinophilia. Other pitfalls include under-utilization of pulmonary rehabilitation, failure to screen for alpha-1 antitrypsin deficiency, and therapeutic inertia in escalating bronchodilator therapy.

Case Study

A 68-year-old male (Mr. Evans) with a 40-pack-year smoking history presents with significant, progressive shortness of breath. His main complaint is being "too winded" to walk to his mailbox. He has a chronic cough but has had no "flares" or hospitalizations in the last year. His mMRC dyspnea score is 3. His FEV1/FVC ratio is 0.62.

Discussion

Mr. Evans has a confirmed diagnosis of COPD. The treatment algorithm is guided by the **GOLD classification**, which is based on symptom burden (mMRC or CAT score) and exacerbation history.

- **Symptoms:** His mMRC is 3 (high symptoms, ≥2).
- **Exacerbations:** He has had 0 hospitalizations and no moderate exacerbations (low risk).
- This places him in **GOLD Group B** (High Symptoms, Low Risk).

Treatment Algorithm

1. **Classification:** GOLD Group B.
2. **Initial Therapy:** The algorithm for Group B is to start a long-acting bronchodilator to manage his high symptom burden.
    - o A **LAMA** (Long-Acting Muscarinic Antagonist) or a **LABA** (Long-Acting Beta-Agonist) is appropriate.
    - o Given his significant symptoms, starting with

a **dual-therapy LAMA/LABA combination inhaler** is also a primary option and often more effective.

3. **Non-pharmacological:** You refer him to Pulmonary Rehabilitation and counsel him on smoking cessation.
4. **Note:** An ICS (inhaled corticosteroid) is **not** indicated, as he is not in Group E (high exacerbation risk).

Outcome

You start Mr. Evans on a combination LAMA/LABA inhaler (e.g., tiotropium/olodaterol) to maximize bronchodilation and improve his dyspnea. You also give him a referral for pulmonary rehab.

PNEUMONIA

Pneumonia is an acute infection of the pulmonary parenchyma. Treatment algorithms are stratified by the site of acquisition (community-acquired vs. hospital-acquired) and disease severity, which dictate the site of care and the empiric antibiotic regimen.

Pathophysiology

Pneumonia occurs when a pathogen (e.g., *Streptococcus pneumoniae, Haemophilus influenzae*) bypasses the upper airway defense mechanisms (e.g., cough reflex, mucociliary escalator) and establishes itself in the distal lung. This is often facilitated by aspiration of oropharyngeal contents. The pathogen multiplies rapidly in the alveolar space, triggering an intense host inflammatory response. Neutrophils are recruited, and capillaries leak, flooding the alveoli with fluid, pus, red blood cells, and fibrin. This process, known as consolidation, prevents the affected lung segments from participating in gas exchange, leading to a V/Q (ventilation/perfusion) mismatch and systemic hypoxemia.

Diagnosis and Classification

Diagnosis is based on a clinical syndrome (e.g., fever, cough, pleuritic chest pain) combined with the presence of a new infiltrate on chest radiography. Community-Acquired Pneumonia (CAP) is distinguished from Hospital-Acquired Pneumonia (HAP) and Ventilator-Associated Pneumonia (VAP), as the latter are associated with more resistant pathogens. A critical first step in the CAP algorithm is assessing severity using a validated score, such as the CURB-65 (Confusion, Urea, Respiratory rate, Blood pressure, age ≥ 65) or the Pneumonia Severity Index (PSI), to determine the appropriate site of care (outpatient, inpatient ward, or ICU).

Differential Diagnosis

The differential for a patient presenting with fever and a new pulmonary infiltrate is broad. It includes acute bronchitis (which typically lacks an infiltrate), acute exacerbation of COPD, heart failure (which can mimic pneumonia with pulmonary edema), pulmonary embolism (which can cause infiltrates and fever), and non-infectious causes like drug toxicity or diffuse alveolar hemorrhage.

Treatment Algorithm

The algorithm is time-sensitive, with a "door-to-dose" goal for antibiotic administration.

Community-Acquired Pneumonia (CAP)

- Outpatient (no comorbidities): The algorithm targets the most common typical and atypical pathogens. First-line therapy is amoxicillin or doxycycline.
- Outpatient (with comorbidities): For patients with conditions like heart, lung, liver, or renal disease, the algorithm broadens coverage. A combination of a beta-lactam (e.g., amoxicillin-clavulanate or a cephalosporin) plus a macrolide (e.g., azithromycin) or doxycycline is recommended. Respiratory fluoroquinolone (e.g., levofloxacin) monotherapy is an alternative.
- Inpatient (Non-ICU): The standard algorithm is a beta-lactam (e.g., ceftriaxone) plus a macrolide, or respiratory fluoroquinolone monotherapy.
- Inpatient (ICU): A beta-lactam plus either a macrolide

or a respiratory fluoroquinolone is required. If risk factors for *Pseudomonas* or MRSA are present (e.g., prior isolation, recent hospitalization), the algorithm expands to include agents like piperacillin-tazobactam and vancomycin, respectively.

Table 2.3: Pneumonia Site-of-Care Algorithm (CURB-65 Score)

CURB-65 Criteria (1 point each)	Score	Site-of-Care
Confusion (New)	0-1	Outpatient
Urea (BUN > 20 mg/dL)	2	Inpatient (General Ward)
Respiratory Rate (≥ 30/min)	3-5	Inpatient (ICU) (Consider)
Blood Pressure (SBP < 90 or DBP ≤ 60)		
Age ≥ 65 years		

HAP/VAP

The algorithm for HAP/VAP is more complex and must be guided by local antibiograms and patient-specific risk factors for multi-drug resistant (MDR) organisms. Empiric therapy typically requires broad-spectrum coverage for *Pseudomonas* and other Gram-negatives, plus MRSA coverage.

Monitoring and Follow-Up

For outpatients, telephone or in-person follow-up should occur within 48-72 hours to ensure clinical improvement (e.g., fever reduction, symptom improvement). For inpatients, monitoring involves daily assessment of vital signs (Temp, HR, RR, BP, SpO2), oxygen requirement, and WBC count. Clinical improvement is expected within 48-72 hours. Failure to improve in this timeframe (non-responding pneumonia) should trigger a search for complications (e.g., empyema, abscess) or consideration of a non-responsive pathogen (e.g., MRSA, *Pseudomonas*) or a non-infectious diagnosis. A follow-up chest X-ray in 6-8 weeks is essential for all patients (especially smokers) to ensure complete radiographic resolution and to rule out an underlying malignancy that may have caused a post-obstructive pneumonia.

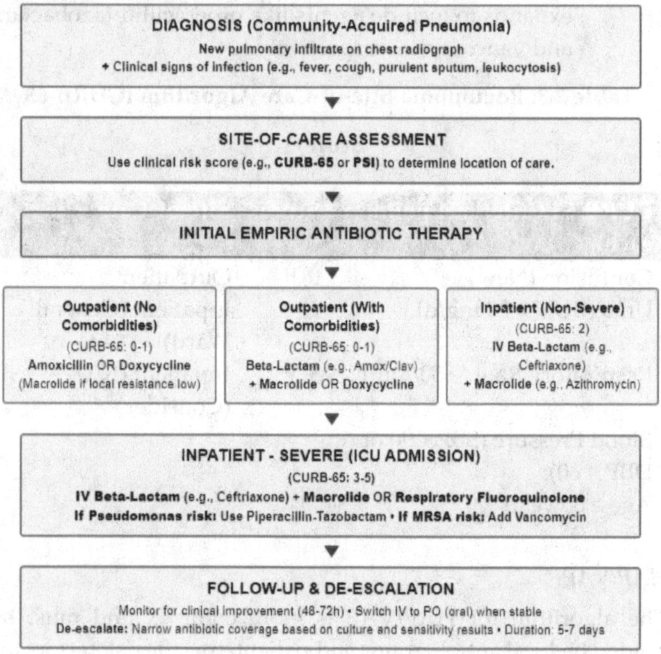

Figure 2.3: Pneumonia - Treatment Algorithm (CAP)

Long-Term Management / Secondary Prevention

For most healthy individuals, pneumonia is an acute, resolved event. Secondary prevention is focused on risk reduction.

1. **Vaccination:** This is the most effective preventive strategy. All adults ≥65 (or younger with comorbidities) should receive pneumococcal vaccination (PCV20 or PCV15+PPSV23), and all individuals should receive an annual influenza vaccine.
2. **Smoking Cessation:** Tobacco smoke paralyzes the cilia in the airways, crippling the mucociliary escalator and dramatically increasing the risk of pneumonia.

3. **Aspiration Precautions:** For high-risk patients (e.g., post-stroke, dementia, severe GERD), this may involve a swallow evaluation, speech therapy, and modifying diet consistency.

Patient Counseling Points

- **Complete the Full Course:** The most important point is to take the *entire* course of antibiotics as prescribed, even if they start to feel better after a few days. Stopping early can lead to treatment failure or antibiotic resistance.
- **Symptom Timeline:** Counsel the patient that while the fever and "sick" feeling should resolve in a few days, the cough and fatigue may linger for several weeks. This is a normal part of recovery.
- **When to Return:** Teach "red flag" symptoms that warrant an immediate return to care: worsening shortness of breath, new or worsening chest pain, a high fever that returns, or confusion.
- **Vaccination:** Use the acute illness as a "teachable moment" to strongly recommend future influenza and pneumococcal vaccination.

Common Pitfalls in Management

A critical pitfall is a delay in antibiotic administration in severe pneumonia or septic shock. Another is the failure to correctly apply severity scores, leading to high-risk patients being undertreated as outpatients. Failing to obtain appropriate cultures before initiating antibiotics in severe CAP, and conversely, over-testing in low-risk outpatient CAP, are common errors. Finally, a significant pitfall is the failure to de-escalate or narrow antibiotic therapy once culture and sensitivity data are available.

Case Study

A 72-year-old female (Mrs. Rodriguez) with diabetes and mild CKD is brought to the ED from home with a 2-day history of fever, productive cough (yellow sputum), and new confusion. Her vitals are: T 101.8°F, HR 112, BP 105/60, **RR 32**, O2 Sat 91%

on room air. Her BUN is 25 mg/dL.

Discussion

This is a classic presentation for **Community-Acquired Pneumonia (CAP)**. The first step in the algorithm is to determine the site of care (outpatient vs. inpatient) using a severity score like **CURB-65.**

Treatment Algorithm

1. **Severity Score (CURB-65):**
    - **C** (Confusion): 1
    - **U** (Urea > 20): 1
    - **R** (Resp. Rate ≥ 30): 1
    - **B** (BP < 90/60): 0
    - **Age** (≥ 65): 1
    - **Total Score = 4.** (A score of 3-5 indicates severe pneumonia and warrants ICU consideration).
2. **Site of Care:** Her score of 4 means she requires **Inpatient (ICU) admission.**
3. **Diagnostic Workup:** You order blood cultures (x2), a sputum culture, a urine legionella/strep antigen, and a chest X-ray (which confirms a RLL infiltrate).
4. **Empiric Antibiotics (Inpatient, Severe):** The algorithm for severe CAP is a beta-lactam *plus* a macrolide OR a beta-lactam *plus* a respiratory fluoroquinolone.
    - **Regimen:** You start **Ceftriaxone 1g IV** and **Azithromycin 500mg IV.**
5. **De-escalation:** 48 hours later, her cultures are negative, but she is improving. You de-escalate her to oral antibiotics to complete a 5-day course.

Outcome

Mrs. Rodriguez is admitted to the ICU, started on IV ceftriaxone and azithromycin, and recovers. She is discharged on day 4 to complete her antibiotic course.

PULMONARY EMBOLISM

Pulmonary Embolism (PE) is the obstruction of the pulmonary arteries by a thrombus, typically originating from the deep veins of the legs. The management algorithm is entirely dependent on initial risk stratification and hemodynamic stability.

Pathophysiology

The pathophysiology has two major components:

Respiratory

The obstruction blocks blood flow to a segment of the lung. This lung tissue is still *ventilated* but is not *perfused,* creating "alveolar dead space." This is a profound V/Q mismatch that impairs gas exchange and leads to hypoxemia.

Hemodynamic

The clot acutely increases pulmonary vascular resistance (PVR). The right ventricle (RV), which is a thin-walled, volume-compliant chamber, is not designed to pump against this high pressure. This causes acute RV strain, dilation, and failure. In a "massive" PE, the RV fails, leading to obstructive shock (hypotension) as it cannot pump blood forward to the left side of the heart.

Diagnosis and Risk Stratification

The diagnostic algorithm begins with clinical suspicion. Pre-test probability is assessed using a validated score (e.g., Wells' score).

- **Low Probability:** The PERC (Pulmonary Embolism Rule-out Criteria) score can be used. If all are negative, PE is reasonably excluded. If PERC is positive, the algorithm proceeds to a D-dimer test. A negative D-dimer rules out PE.
- **Intermediate/High Probability:** The algorithm proceeds directly to definitive imaging. A CT Pulmonary Angiography (CTPA) is the diagnostic test of choice. A V/Q (ventilation/perfusion) scan is an alternative, particularly in patients with

contraindications to CT contrast.

Differential Diagnosis

The differential for acute pleuritic chest pain and dyspnea is extensive. It includes acute coronary syndrome, pericarditis, pneumonia, pneumothorax, musculoskeletal pain, and aortic dissection. Differentiating these is a critical emergent task.

Treatment Algorithm

Once PE is diagnosed, the algorithm is stratified by hemodynamic stability.

- **Massive PE (Hemodynamically Unstable):** This is defined by persistent hypotension (SBP < 90 mmHg). This is a life-threatening emergency. The algorithm mandates immediate reperfusion, most commonly with systemic thrombolysis (e.g., alteplase). Catheter-directed thrombolysis or surgical embolectomy are alternatives.
- **Submassive PE (Hemodynamically Stable, RV Strain):** These patients are stable but have evidence of right ventricular dysfunction on echocardiogram or elevated biomarkers (troponin, BNP). The algorithm for this group is anticoagulation. Systemic thrombolysis is considered on a case-by-case basis if the patient shows signs of hemodynamic deterioration.
- **Low-Risk PE (Stable, No RV Strain):** The standard of care is anticoagulation alone. Direct-acting oral anticoagulants (DOACs) like apixaban or rivaroxaban are preferred over warfarin due to their rapid onset and ease of use.

The duration of anticoagulation is the final step, typically 3-6 months for a provoked PE (e.g., post-surgery) and extended or indefinite for an unprovoked PE.

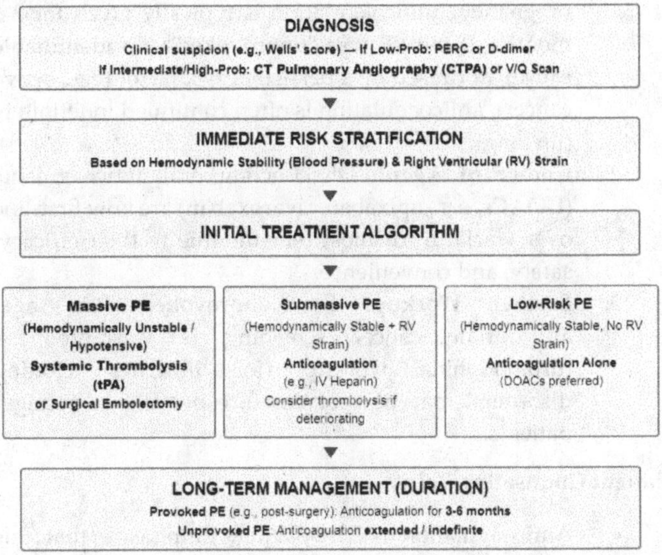

Figure 2.4: Pulmonary Embolism - Treatment Algorithm

Monitoring and Follow-Up

In the acute phase (in-hospital), monitoring is focused on hemodynamics (BP, HR), oxygenation, and signs of RV strain (e.g., serial troponins, EKG, or formal echocardiogram). The patient must also be monitored for bleeding complications from high-dose anticoagulation (e.g., drop in hemoglobin, new-onset headache). For "submassive" PEs, monitoring for any clinical deterioration is key, as this may trigger a move to thrombolysis. Outpatient follow-up should occur within 1-2 weeks to ensure adherence to the anticoagulant, check for any bleeding complications, and assess for resolution of dyspnea and hypoxemia.

Long-Term Management / Secondary Prevention

The primary goal is to prevent a recurrent DVT/PE. The main decision is the duration of anticoagulation.

1. **Duration of Therapy:** If the PE was "provoked" by a major, transient risk factor (e.g., recent major surgery,

pregnancy), anticoagulation is typically given for 3-6 months. If the PE was "unprovoked" (no identifiable cause), or caused by a persistent risk factor (e.g., active cancer), anticoagulation is often continued indefinitely (lifelong).

2. **Choice of Agent:** Direct-acting oral anticoagulants (DOACs, e.g., apixaban, rivaroxaban) are now first-line over warfarin for most patients due to their efficacy, safety, and convenience.
3. **Further Workup:** For unprovoked PEs, age-appropriate cancer screening is warranted. A thrombophilia workup (for inherited clotting disorders) may be considered, especially in younger patients.

Patient Counseling Points

- Anticoagulation is Life-Saving: Emphasize that this medication is not just for symptoms; it is to prevent a new clot, which can be fatal. Adherence is non-negotiable.
- Bleeding Risk: This is the primary side effect. Teach the patient to report any serious falls (especially head injuries), black or tarry stools, red urine, or severe, unstoppable bleeding. They must inform all providers, including dentists, that they are on an anticoagulant.
- DOACs vs. Warfarin: If on a DOAC, counsel that there is no routine blood monitoring, which makes adherence even more critical. If on warfarin, explain the need for frequent INR checks and the importance of a consistent diet (especially Vitamin K).
- Prevention: Counsel on risk-reduction for long-haul travel, such as frequent ambulation, calf exercises, and compression stockings.

Common Pitfalls in Management

A common diagnostic pitfall is ordering a D-dimer in a high-probability patient; the test has a high false-negative rate in this setting, and a positive result is non-diagnostic, so imaging should be the first step. A major therapeutic pitfall is the inappropriate use of thrombolysis in low-risk PE, which carries a significant risk of intracranial hemorrhage with no mortality benefit. Conversely, failing to recognize subtle signs of RV strain and impending decompensation in a submassive PE can be a fatal error.

Case Study

A 45-year-old male (Mr. Singh) presents to the ED with a 1-day history of acute-onset dyspnea and sharp, right-sided chest pain that is worse when he takes a deep breath. He returned from an 8-hour flight from India 3 days ago. His HR is 105, O2 Sat 94%.

Discussion

This presentation (acute pleuritic chest pain, dyspnea, tachycardia, recent long-haul flight) is highly suspicious for a **Pulmonary Embolism (PE)**. The algorithm is to first assess pre-test probability.

Treatment Algorithm

1. **Pre-test Probability (Wells' Score):**
   - Tachycardia (>100): 1.5
   - Immobilization (flight): 1.5
   - PE as #1 diagnosis: 3.0
   - **Total Score = 6.0 (High Probability)**.
2. **Diagnostic Test:** Because his Wells' score is high, the algorithm dictates **skipping the D-dimer** (which is only for *ruling out* PE in low-risk patients) and proceeding directly to definitive imaging.
   - **Test:** A **CT Pulmonary Angiography (CTPA)** is ordered.
3. **Diagnosis:** The CTPA confirms a **subsegmental PE** in the right lower lobe. His vitals are stable (SBP > 90) and his troponin/BNP are normal (no RV strain).
4. **Treatment (Low-Risk PE):** The algorithm for a hemodynamically stable, low-risk PE is **anticoagulation alone.**
   - **Therapy:** You start a **DOAC (e.g., Rivaroxaban 15mg BID)**, which is preferred

over warfarin for its rapid onset and ease of use. Thrombolysis is contraindicated.

Outcome

Mr. Singh is diagnosed with a low-risk, provoked PE. He is started on Rivaroxaban and discharged from the ED (or after a 23-hour observation) with a plan to continue anticoagulation for 3-6 months.

TUBERCULOSIS

Tuberculosis (TB) is a chronic granulomatous infection caused by *Mycobacterium tuberculosis*. The treatment algorithm is highly structured, lengthy, and fundamentally different for latent versus active disease.

Pathophysiology

Tuberculosis is transmitted via aerosolized droplets from an individual with active pulmonary TB.

1. **Primary TB:** When inhaled, the bacilli reach the alveoli and are ingested by alveolar macrophages. The bacillus's unique cell wall allows it to survive and multiply *inside* the macrophage. This triggers a cell-mediated immune response, where T-cells and macrophages form a granuloma (a "wall" of immune cells) to contain the infection. This walled-off lesion, often with central caseous (cheesy) necrosis, is called a "Ghon complex."
2. **Latent TB (LTBI):** In >90% of individuals, the immune system successfully contains the bacilli within these granulomas, and the person remains asymptomatic and non-infectious.
3. **Active TB:** If the immune system weakens (e.g., HIV, malnutrition, immunosuppressive drugs like TNF-alpha inhibitors), the granuloma can break down. The bacilli are released, multiply rapidly, and cause necrotizing, cavitary lesions (classically in the oxygen-rich upper lobes), leading to the symptoms of active disease (cough, fever, night sweats, weight loss) and

infectiousness

Diagnosis

- **Latent TB Infection (LTBI):** Diagnosis is based on evidence of an immune response to *M. tuberculosis* in an asymptomatic patient. This is established via a tuberculin skin test (TST) or an interferon-gamma release assay (IGRA). A positive test does not distinguish latent from active disease.
- **Active TB Disease:** Diagnosis in a symptomatic patient (e.g., chronic cough, fever, night sweats, weight loss) requires identifying the organism. This algorithm involves chest radiography (showing typical findings like apical cavitations) and obtaining sputum for AFB (acid-fast bacilli) smear, mycobacterial culture, and nucleic acid amplification testing (NAAT), which provides rapid confirmation.

Differential Diagnosis

The differential for active pulmonary TB includes other causes of chronic cough and constitutional symptoms. The main considerations are lung cancer (which can also be apical), fungal pneumonias (e.g., histoplasmosis, blastomycosis), bacterial lung abscess, and non-tuberculous mycobacterial infections.

Treatment Algorithm

Latent TB Infection (LTBI)

The algorithm provides several preferred regimens for preventing progression to active disease:

- Isoniazid (INH) and Rifapentine weekly for 3 months (12 doses).
- Rifampin (RIF) daily for 4 months.
- Isoniazid (INH) and Rifampin (RIF) daily for 3 months.
- Isoniazid (INH) daily for 6 or 9 months (an older, less-preferred regimen).

Table 2.4: Core Treatment Algorithms for PE and TB

Condition	Primary Goal	Initial Treatment Algorithm
Pulmonary Embolism (PE)	Anticoagulation & Hemodynamic Support	Low-Risk: DOAC or LMWH. Submassive: Anticoagulation ± advanced therapy. Massive (Shock): Systemic Thrombolysis (tPA) or Embolectomy.
Tuberculosis (TB)	Bacterial Eradication & Prevent Resistance	Intensive Phase (2 mo): RIPE (Rifampin, Isoniazid, Pyrazinamide, Ethambutol). Continuation Phase (4 mo): RI (Rifampin, Isoniazid).

Active TB Disease (Drug-Susceptible)

The standard algorithm is a 6-month, two-phase regimen.

- Intensive Phase (2 months): Consists of four drugs: Rifampin (RIF), Isoniazid (INH), Pyrazinamide (PZA), and Ethambutol (EMB). This is known as the "RIPE" regimen.
- Continuation Phase (4 months): Consists of two drugs: Rifampin (RIF) and Isoniazid (INH). This entire algorithm is ideally administered via Directly Observed Therapy (DOT) to ensure adherence. Ethambutol can be discontinued once susceptibility to INH and RIF is confirmed.

Drug-Resistant TB

If resistance to INH (INH-monoresistance) or both INH and RIF (Multi-Drug Resistant TB, or MDR-TB) is identified, the algorithm shifts to specialized, longer regimens (often 18-24 months) involving second-line agents (e.g., fluoroquinolones, bedaquiline) managed by TB specialists.

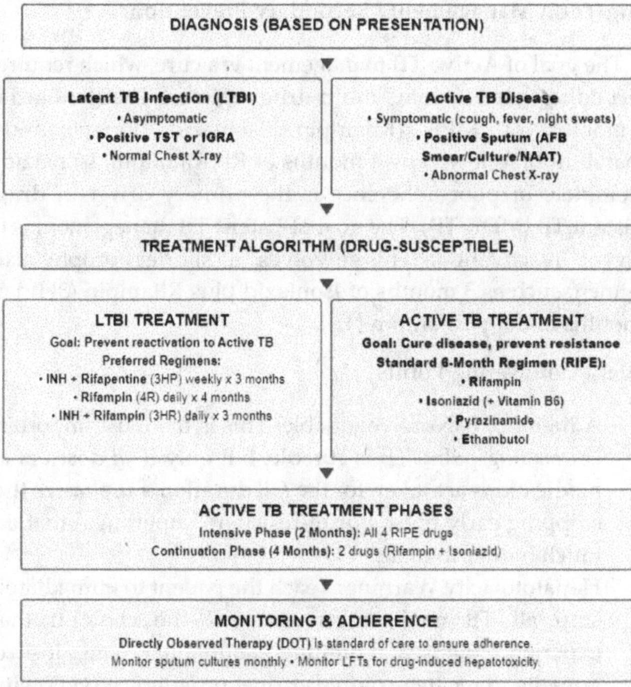

Figure 2.5: Tuberculosis - Treatment Algorithm

Monitoring and Follow-Up

Monitoring for **Active TB** is intensive and often involves Directly Observed Therapy (DOT). Sputum smears and cultures are collected monthly to confirm conversion to negative, which indicates treatment response. The most critical monitoring is for drug toxicity, especially hepatotoxicity from Isoniazid, Rifampin, and Pyrazinamide. Baseline LFTs are mandatory, with regular (e.g., monthly) follow-up labs, especially for high-risk patients. Monitoring for **Latent TB** is simpler, involving a baseline LFT check and monthly clinical follow-up to assess for side effects (hepatotoxicity, neuropathy) and ensure treatment adherence.

Long-Term Management / Secondary Prevention

The goal of **Active TB** management is a cure, which requires strict adherence to a long, multi-drug regimen. The standard is 2 months of RIPE (Rifampin, Isoniazid, Pyrazinamide, Ethambutol), followed by 4 months of RI (Rifampin, Isoniazid). Incomplete or poor adherence is the primary driver of drug-resistant TB (MDR-TB). The goal of **Latent TB** management is to prevent reactivation. This involves a shorter prophylactic regimen, such as 3 months of Isoniazid plus Rifampin (3HP) or 4 months of daily Rifampin (4R).

Patient Counseling Points

- Adherence is Non-Negotiable: This is the most important counseling point. TB is curable, but only if *all* doses of *all* medications are taken for the *full* duration. Emphasize that stopping early breeds drug-resistant "superbugs" that are much harder to treat.
- Hepatotoxicity Warning: Teach the patient to immediately stop all TB medications and call the clinic if they experience nausea, vomiting, abdominal pain, loss of appetite, dark (tea-colored) urine, or jaundice (yellowing of the skin or eyes).
- Rifampin Side Effects: Warn the patient that Rifampin will turn all body fluids (urine, sweat, tears) a harmless orange-red color. This is expected and not dangerous, but it will permanently stain soft contact lenses.
- Isoniazid Side Effects: Explain that Isoniazid (INH) can cause nerve damage (peripheral neuropathy). They must take their prescribed Vitamin B6 (pyridoxine) every day to prevent this.
- Infection Control (Active TB): The patient must understand they are infectious. They need to wear a mask in public, cough into a tissue, and remain in respiratory isolation (e.g., stay home from work/school) until they have provided 3 consecutive negative sputum smears.

Common Pitfalls in Management

The most significant pitfall in TB management is patient non-adherence to the long therapeutic course, which is the primary driver of treatment failure and drug resistance. Another critical error is the failure to monitor for and manage drug toxicities, particularly RIPE-induced hepatotoxicity. In diagnosis, a common pitfall is ruling out active TB based on a negative AFB smear alone, as culture is more sensitive. Finally, failing to perform meticulous contact tracing and evaluation for LTBI in close contacts of an active case perpetuates the spread of the disease.

Case Study

A 34-year-old male (Mr. Tsegaye), who immigrated from Ethiopia 2 years ago, presents with a 3-month history of a persistent, productive cough, 15-lb unintentional weight loss, and drenching night sweats. A chest X-ray shows a **cavitary lesion in the right upper lobe**.

Discussion

This is the classic "B-symptom" presentation of **Active Tuberculosis (TB)** in a patient from an endemic country, with the hallmark radiographic finding of an apical cavity. The algorithm is to confirm the diagnosis and initiate multi-drug therapy immediately.

Treatment Algorithm

- **Diagnosis:** The clinical and radiographic suspicion is extremely high.
- **Isolation:** The patient is placed in **airborne respiratory isolation** immediately.
- **Diagnostic Workup:** You obtain 3 sputum samples (8 hours apart) for **AFB smear, mycobacterial culture, and NAAT (PCR)**. The NAAT comes back positive for *M. tuberculosis* complex.
- **Treatment (Active TB):** The algorithm is the 6-month, two-phase RIPE regimen.
    1. **Intensive Phase (2 months):** You initiate all four drugs: **Rifampin**, **Isoniazid** (with Vitamin B6), **Pyrazinamide**, and **Ethambutol**.
    2. **Continuation Phase (4 months):** Once

susceptibilities return, you will stop PZA and EMB and continue RI for 4 months.

- **Public Health:** The case is reported to the Department of Health for contact tracing.

Outcome

Mr. Tsegaye is started on RIPE therapy under Directly Observed Therapy (DOT) to ensure adherence. He will remain in isolation until he has three consecutive negative sputum smears.

Summary

Asthma: The algorithm is a stepwise approach (GINA) focused on inflammation control. The modern standard is to use an ICS-containing inhaler (e.g., ICS-formoterol) for all patients, either daily or as-needed, to avoid SABA-monotherapy.

COPD: The algorithm (GOLD A, B, E) is guided by symptom burden and exacerbation risk. LAMA/LABA combinations are foundational, with ICS added only for the eosinophilic (Group E) phenotype.

Pneumonia: The algorithm is driven by severity assessment (CURB-65/PSI) to determine site of care (outpatient vs. inpatient). Empiric antibiotics are chosen to cover likely pathogens and narrowed based on culture data.

Pulmonary Embolism: This is a risk-stratified algorithm. Hemodynamic instability (massive PE) mandates thrombolysis. Stable, high-risk (submassive PE) patients require anticoagulation and close monitoring. Low-risk PE is managed with anticoagulation alone (DOACs preferred).

Tuberculosis: Management follows two distinct algorithms. Latent TB involves short-course preventive monotherapy or combination therapy. Active TB requires a prolonged (6-month) four-drug intensive phase (RIPE) followed by a two-drug continuation phase, ideally with DOT

Multiple Choice Questions

1. According to the 2024 GINA guidelines, what is the preferred "reliever" therapy for a patient with mild asthma (Step 1)?
   A) As-needed albuterol (SABA)
   B) As-needed low-dose inhaled corticosteroid (ICS)
   C) As-needed low-dose ICS-formoterol
   D) Daily low-dose ICS
2. A 68-year-old male with COPD (FEV1 45% predicted) reports significant daily dyspnea (CAT score 22) but has had no exacerbations in the past year. According to the GOLD classification, what is his group?
   A) Group A
   B) Group B
   C) Group E
   D) Group D (outdated)
3. What is the first-line treatment algorithm for a patient in GOLD Group B?
   A) SABA as needed
   B) LAMA + LABA
   C) LAMA + LABA + ICS
   D) A long-acting bronchodilator (LAMA or LABA)
4. A 70-year-old patient with CAP has a CURB-65 score of 3. What is the most appropriate site of care according to the treatment algorithm?
   A) Outpatient
   B) Outpatient with home health
   C) Inpatient (general ward) or observation
   D) Inpatient (ICU)
5. A 30-year-old healthy male is diagnosed with outpatient CAP. He has no comorbidities and has not taken antibiotics recently. What is the most appropriate first-line empiric antibiotic algorithm?
   A) Amoxicillin
   B) Azithromycin

C) Levofloxacin

D) Ceftriaxone

6. A 45-year-old female presents with acute pleuritic chest pain. Her Wells' score for PE is 5.0 (intermediate probability). What is the next step in the diagnostic algorithm?

   A) Order a D-dimer.

   B) Order a V/Q scan.

   C) Order a CT pulmonary angiography (CTPA).

   D) Start empiric anticoagulation.

7. A 60-year-old male is diagnosed with a massive pulmonary embolism and is hypotensive (SBP 80/50 mmHg). What is the indicated treatment?

   A) Systemic thrombolysis (e.g., alteplase)

   B) IV heparin infusion only

   C) Surgical embolectomy (as first-line)

   D) Placement of an IVC filter

8. Which of the following is a preferred, short-course treatment algorithm for latent tuberculosis infection (LTBI)?

   A) Rifampin daily for 4 months

   B) Isoniazid daily for 12 months

   C) RIPE therapy for 2 months

   D) Levofloxacin daily for 6 months

9. A common and dangerous pitfall in asthma management is:

   A) Over-reliance on SABA monotherapy

   B) Using an ICS-LABA combination

   C) Stepping down therapy in a well-controlled patient

   D) Prescribing pulmonary rehabilitation

10. A patient is started on RIPE therapy for active pulmonary TB. Which of the following drugs necessitates counseling on potential orange discoloration of bodily fluids?

    A) Isoniazid

B) Rifampin
C) Pyrazinamide
D) Ethambutol

Self-Assessment Questions

1. Explain the GINA Step 1 algorithm for asthma and why it represents a major shift from traditional SABA-only "reliever" therapy.
2. A patient with COPD has an mMRC score of 3 and 1 exacerbation in the past year. How would they be classified according to GOLD, and what is the appropriate initial pharmacological algorithm?
3. A patient has high exacerbation risk (GOLD Group E) and a blood eosinophil count of 350 cells/μL. How does this finding alter the standard COPD treatment algorithm?
4. Describe the CURB-65 criteria and explain how the resulting score dictates the treatment algorithm (site of care) for Community-Acquired Pneumonia.
5. What is the first-line empiric antibiotic algorithm for an outpatient with CAP who has no comorbidities, versus an outpatient who has significant comorbidities (e.g., diabetes, CKD)?
6. A patient presents with acute dyspnea. The Wells' score is low, and the PERC score is negative. What is the next step in the diagnostic algorithm for PE?
7. Compare and contrast the immediate treatment algorithm for a patient with massive PE versus a patient with low-risk PE.
8. What is the main diagnostic difference between latent TB and active TB?
9. Outline the standard 6-month, 4-drug algorithm (RIPE) for drug-susceptible active tuberculosis.
10. Identify two common pitfalls in the management of COPD and two in the management of acute pulmonary embolism.

Bibliography

1. Global Initiative for Asthma. Global Strategy for Asthma Management and Prevention, 2024. [Accessed 2024 Oct 24]. Available from: https://ginasthma.org/gina-reports/
2. Global Initiative for Chronic Obstructive Lung Disease. Global Strategy for the Diagnosis, Management, and Prevention of Chronic Obstructive Pulmonary Disease, 2024 Report. [Accessed 2024 Oct 24]. Available from: https://goldcopd.org/2024-gold-report/
3. Metlay JP, Waterer GW, Long AC, Anzueto A, Brozek J, Crothers K, et al. Diagnosis and Treatment of Adults with Community-acquired Pneumonia. An Official Clinical Practice Guideline of the American Thoracic Society and Infectious Diseases Society of America. Am J Respir Crit Care Med. 2019 Oct 1;200(7):e45–e67.
4. Konstantinides SV, Meyer G, Becattini C, Bueno H, Geersing GJ, Harjola VP, et al. 2019 ESC Guidelines for the diagnosis and management of acute pulmonary embolism developed in collaboration with the European Respiratory Society (ERS). Eur Heart J. 2020 Jan 21;41(4):543–603.
5. Sterling TR, Njie G, Zenner D, Cohn DL, Reves R, Ahmed A, et al. Guidelines for the Treatment of Latent Tuberculosis Infection: Recommendations from the National Tuberculosis Controllers Association and CDC, 2020. MMWR Recomm Rep. 2020 Feb 14;69(1):1–11.
6. Nahid P, Dorman SE, Alipanah N, Barry PM, Brozek JL, Cattamanchi A, et al. Official American Thoracic Society/Centers for Disease Control and Prevention/Infectious Diseases Society of America Clinical Practice Guidelines: Treatment of Drug-Susceptible Tuberculosis. Clin Infect Dis. 2016 Oct 15;63(7):e147–e195.
7. Lipson DA, Barnhart F, Brehm N, Brooks J, Criner GJ, Day NC, et al. Once-Daily Single-Inhaler Triple versus Dual Therapy in Patients with COPD. N Engl J Med. 2018 Jun 14;378(24):2267–80.
8. O'Donoghue M, Boden WE, Braunwald E, Cannon CP, Clayton TC, de Winter RJ, et al. Early invasive vs. conservative strategy in patients with unstable angina or non-ST-elevation myocardial infarction: a meta-analysis. JAMA. 2008 Jul 23;300(4):401–11.
9. Rodrigo GJ, Neffen H, Plaza V. The role of single-inhaler therapy with budesonide/formoterol in the management of asthma. Expert Opin Pharmacother. 2008 Sep;9(13):2287–97.
10. Wells PS, Anderson DR, Rodger M, Ginsberg JS, Kearon C, Gent M, et al. Derivation of a simple clinical model to categorize patients probability of pulmonary embolism: increasing the models utility with the SimpliRED D-dimer. Thromb Haemost. 2000 Mar;83(3):416–20.
11. Rabe KF, Martinez FJ, Ferguson GT, Wang C, Singh D, Wedzicha JA, et al. Triple Inhaled Therapy at Two Glucocorticoid Doses in Moderate-to-Very-Severe COPD. N Engl J Med. 2020 Sep 10;383(11):1040–51.
12. The PERC Rule Writing Group. Clinical criteria to prevent unnecessary diagnostic testing in emergency department patients with suspected pulmonary embolism. J Thromb Haemost. 2004 Aug;2(8):1247–55.

13. Lim WS, van der Eerden MM, Laing R, Boersma WG, Karalus N, Town GI, et al. Defining community acquired pneumonia severity on presentation to hospital: an international derivation and validation study. Thorax. 2003 May;58(5):377–82.
14. Suissa S, Patenaude V, Lapi F, Ernst P. Inhaled corticosteroids in COPD and the risk of serious pneumonia. Thorax. 2013 Nov;68(11):1029–36.
15. Meyer G, Vicaut E, Danays T, Agnelli G, Becattini C, Beyer-Westendorf J, et al. Fibrinolysis for patients with intermediate-risk pulmonary embolism. N Engl J Med. 2014 Apr 10;370(15):1402–11.

CHAPTER 3

TREATMENT ALGORITHMS FOR GASTROINTESTINAL DISORDERS

Author

Mr. Gourab Saha, Associate Professor,
Department of Pharmaceutics, College of Pharmaceutical Sciences, Berhampur, Mohada, Odisha, India

Abstract

Gastrointestinal treatment algorithms focus on resolving symptoms, healing mucosal damage, and managing underlying etiology. The algorithm for gastroesophageal reflux disease (GERD) is a stepwise approach, commencing with lifestyle modifications and proceeding to an 8-week trial of proton pump inhibitors (PPIs). Failure of this trial, or the presence of alarm features, triggers endoscopic evaluation. Peptic ulcer disease (PUD) management is bifurcated by cause: *H. pylori*-positive ulcers are treated with an eradication algorithm (e.g., bismuth quadruple therapy), while NSAID-induced ulcers require PPI therapy and cessation of the offending agent. The algorithm for inflammatory bowel disease (IBD) is stratified by disease type (Crohn's vs. Ulcerative Colitis) and severity, utilizing a "step-up" or "top-down" approach with 5-ASAs, corticosteroids, immunomodulators, and biologics to induce and maintain remission. Celiac disease management is a singular algorithm centered on a strict, lifelong gluten-free diet and nutritional monitoring. Hepatitis algorithms are virus-specific: Hepatitis A is managed supportively; chronic Hepatitis B treatment is guided by viral load and liver inflammation, using nucleos(t)ide analogs for long-term suppression; and Hepatitis C is managed with a curative, pangenotypic direct-acting antiviral (DAA) regimen.

Keywords: *Gastrointestinal Algorithms, GERD, Peptic Ulcer Disease, Inflammatory Bowel Disease, Celiac Disease, Hepatitis*

Learning Objectives

After completion of the chapter, the learners should be able to:

- Identify the first-line triple and quadruple therapy regimens for H. pylori eradication in peptic ulcer disease.
- Explain the "step-up" versus "top-down" therapeutic algorithms for managing Inflammatory Bowel Disease (IBD).
- Select the appropriate treatment algorithm (lifestyle, H2RA, or PPI) for a patient with GERD based on symptom severity and frequency.
- Differentiate the diagnostic and management algorithms for Crohn's disease versus ulcerative colitis.
- Justify the decision to initiate or defer antiviral therapy for a patient with chronic Hepatitis C based on genotype and liver function

GASTROESOPHAGEAL REFLUX DISEASE (GERD)

GERD is a highly prevalent condition characterized by symptoms or mucosal complications resulting from the reflux of gastric contents into the esophagus. The treatment algorithm is stepwise, focusing on symptom control and prevention of complications like esophagitis and Barrett's esophagus.

Pathophysiology

GERD is a condition of chronic mucosal damage produced by the abnormal reflux of gastric contents into the esophagus. This is fundamentally a failure of the anti-reflux barrier. The pathophysiology is centered on the lower esophageal sphincter (LES), a high-pressure zone that should remain closed except during swallowing. In GERD, this barrier fails, often due to transient LES relaxations (T-LES-Rs), where the sphincter relaxes inappropriately, unconnected to swallowing. Other contributing factors include a chronically hypotensive (weak) LES, the presence of a hiatal hernia (which displaces the LES from the supportive diaphragm), delayed gastric emptying, and impaired esophageal acid clearance. This repeated acid and pepsin exposure damages the squamous epithelium of the esophagus, causing inflammation (esophagitis) and leading to the classic symptoms of heartburn and regurgitation.

Diagnosis and Classification

Diagnosis is most often made clinically based on a classic symptom presentation (heartburn, regurgitation). An 8-week empiric trial of a proton pump inhibitor (PPI) is a common diagnostic and therapeutic first step. Endoscopy (EGD) is not required for diagnosis but is a key part of the algorithm if alarm features are present (dysphagia, odynophagia, weight loss, anemia, gastrointestinal bleeding) or if patients fail to respond to PPI therapy. Ambulatory 24-hour pH monitoring is the gold standard for diagnosis in patients with refractory, atypical, or extraesophageal symptoms.

Differential Diagnosis

The differential for GERD symptoms is broad. It is critical to first exclude cardiac chest pain. Other considerations include peptic ulcer disease, non-ulcer dyspepsia, eosinophilic esophagitis (especially in patients with refractory symptoms and dysphagia), motility disorders like achalasia, and pill esophagitis.

Treatment Algorithm

The algorithm for GERD proceeds in a stepwise fashion.

- **Step 1: Lifestyle and Dietary Modification:** All patients are advised to lose weight (if overweight), elevate the head of the bed, and avoid late-night meals. Trigger food avoidance (e.g., caffeine, alcohol, fatty foods) is recommended if a clear association with symptoms exists.
- **Step 2: Empiric PPI Trial:** For patients with typical GERD symptoms, a standard-dose PPI once daily for 8 weeks is the first-line pharmacological algorithm.
- **Step 3: Management of Response:**
    - **Successful Response:** The algorithm dictates stepping down to the lowest effective dose, which may include low-dose PPI, an H2-receptor antagonist (H2RA), or on-demand therapy.

    - **No Response/Partial Response:** The algorithm requires optimization (e.g., ensuring correct timing before a meal) or escalating to twice-daily PPI dosing. Failure of this step defines refractory GERD.
- **Step 4: Refractory GERD:** These patients require referral for upper endoscopy to rule out other etiologies. If endoscopy is unrevealing, ambulatory pH monitoring (on or off therapy) is used to confirm the diagnosis and correlate symptoms with reflux events. Surgical options, such as laparoscopic Nissen fundoplication or magnetic sphincter augmentation (LINX), are considered for confirmed refractory GERD.

Table 3.1: Stepwise Management Algorithm for GERD

Step	Intervention	Rationale / Goal
Step 1	Lifestyle Modifications + PRN Antacids/H2RAs	For intermittent, mild symptoms.
Step 2	Scheduled H2RA or Daily PPI (4-8 wks)	For persistent or frequent symptoms.
Step 3	Optimize PPI (e.g., BID dosing)	For refractory symptoms.
Step 4	Refer for EGD / pH testing	Investigate for complications or alternative diagnoses.

Monitoring and Follow-Up

Initial monitoring is based on symptom response to an empiric 8-week trial of a proton pump inhibitor (PPI). If symptoms resolve, the diagnosis is confirmed. If symptoms are refractory, adherence and PPI timing (30-60 min before the first meal) must be reassessed. The primary diagnostic tool for refractory or "alarm" symptoms (dysphagia, weight loss, bleeding) is an upper endoscopy (EGD) to rule out complications. For patients on long-term PPIs, monitoring involves periodic assessment for the lowest effective dose. While routine monitoring for micronutrient deficiencies (e.g., B12, magnesium) is controversial, it should be considered in high-risk patients. For patients diagnosed with Barrett's esophagus (a precancerous complication), long-term monitoring involves a surveillance EGD with biopsies every 3-5 years.

Long-Term Management / Secondary Prevention

The goal of long-term management is to control symptoms and prevent complications. This begins with foundational lifestyle modifications. For many, this is a chronic, relapsing condition requiring maintenance therapy. The standard of care is the lowest effective dose of a PPI, taken daily or on-demand. For patients who wish to avoid long-term medication or who have refractory symptoms (especially volume regurgitation), anti-reflux surgery (e.g., Nissen fundoplication) or a magnetic sphincter augmentation procedure (LINX) are options. Secondary prevention is focused on the management of Barrett's esophagus, where long-term PPIs are mandatory to reduce the risk of progression to esophageal adenocarcinoma.

Patient Counseling Points

1. **PPI Timing:** This is a critical counseling point. PPIs are proton-pump *inhibitors,* not acid *blockers*. They must be taken 30-60 minutes *before* the first meal of the day to inhibit the actively secreting pumps.
2. **Lifestyle & Diet:** Counsel on weight loss (if overweight), smoking cessation, and avoiding meals 2-3 hours before lying down. Common trigger foods include caffeine, chocolate, alcohol, and spicy/fatty foods.
3. **Alarm Symptoms:** The patient must be taught to report "red flag" symptoms immediately: dysphagia (difficulty swallowing), odynophagia (painful swallowing), unintentional weight loss, or signs of bleeding (anemia, black stools).
4. **Risks vs. Benefits:** Discuss that while long-term PPI use is generally safe, it is associated with a small increased risk of C. difficile colitis and community-acquired pneumonia. The goal is always to use the lowest effective dose.

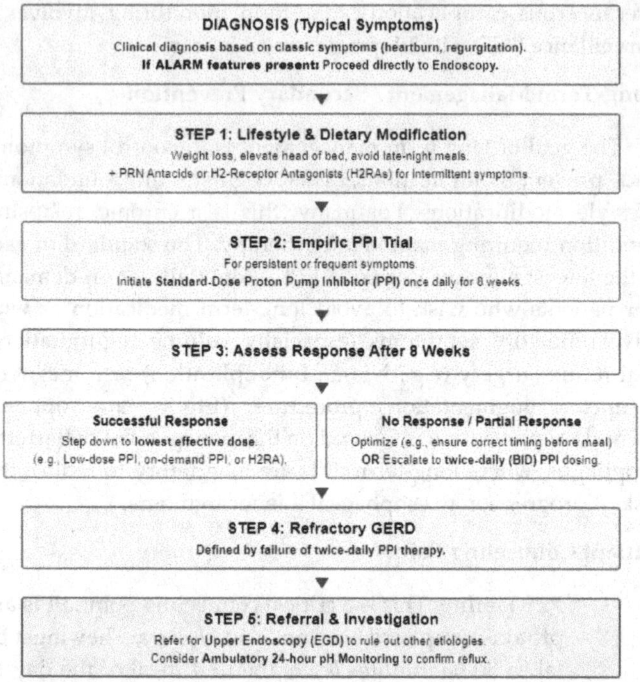

Figure 3.1: Gastroesophageal Reflux Disease (GERD)

3.1.4 Common Pitfalls in Management

A critical pitfall is misattributing cardiac chest pain to GERD, delaying cardiovascular workup. Another is the indefinite continuation of high-dose PPIs without attempting to step down therapy, leading to potential long-term risks (e.g., *C. difficile* infection, micronutrient malabsorption). Failing to investigate "alarm features" with prompt endoscopy is a major error that can delay a cancer diagnosis. Finally, overlooking eosinophilic esophagitis as a cause of refractory symptoms is a common diagnostic omission.

Case Study

A 48-year-old male (Mr. Chen) presents with a 3-month history of burning, substernal chest pain ("heartburn") and a sour taste in his mouth (regurgitation). Symptoms are worse after large meals and when he lies down at night. He has no "alarm features" (no dysphagia, weight loss, or bleeding).

Discussion

This is a classic clinical presentation of **Gastroesophageal Reflux Disease (GERD)**. Because there are no alarm features, the management algorithm does not begin with an EGD (endoscopy). Instead, the standard of care is an empiric trial of the most effective medication.

Treatment Algorithm

1. **Diagnosis:** Clinical diagnosis of GERD.
2. **Algorithm Step 1 (Lifestyle):** You counsel Mr. Chen on lifestyle modifications: avoid late-night meals, elevate the head of his bed, and reduce trigger foods (he identifies coffee and spicy food).
3. **Algorithm Step 2 (Empiric Trial):** You initiate the first-line pharmacological algorithm:
    - **Proton Pump Inhibitor (PPI) Trial:** Start **Omeprazole 20 mg once daily**, taken 30 minutes *before* breakfast.
4. **Follow-up:** The plan is to continue this for a full 8-week course.
5. **Algorithm Step 3 (Management):** You schedule a follow-up call in 4 weeks. If his symptoms are resolved, the diagnosis is confirmed. After 8 weeks, the algorithm dictates "stepping down" to the lowest effective dose (e.g., omeprazole 20 mg as-needed or switching to an H2RA like famotidine).

Outcome

Mr. Chen is started on an 8-week trial of Omeprazole 20 mg daily. He is to report back if symptoms do not improve, which would trigger the next step in the algorithm (e.g., optimizing the dose or referring for EGD).

PEPTIC ULCER DISEASE

PUD refers to defects in the gastric or duodenal mucosa that extend through the muscularis mucosae. The treatment algorithm is critically dependent on identifying and eradicating the underlying cause, most commonly *Helicobacter pylori* infection or NSAID use.

Pathophysiology

The pathophysiology is a fundamental imbalance between aggressive factors (gastric acid, pepsin) and protective factors (mucus layer, bicarbonate, mucosal blood flow, prostaglandins). Over 90% of PUD is caused by one of two etiologies:

Helicobacter pylori Infection

This spiral-shaped bacterium colonizes the gastric mucus. It survives the acidic environment by producing urease, which creates a neutral ammonia cloud. It induces a chronic inflammatory response (gastritis) and releases toxins (e.g., CagA, VacA) that disrupt the mucosal barrier, making it susceptible to acid damage.

NSAID Use

Nonsteroidal anti-inflammatory drugs (e.g., ibuprofen, naproxen, aspirin) inhibit cyclooxygenase (COX-1 and COX-2) enzymes. COX-1 is crucial for gastro-protection, as it synthesizes prostaglandins that maintain the mucosal barrier, stimulate bicarbonate secretion, and preserve mucosal blood flow. Blocking prostaglandins renders the stomach vulnerable to its own acid.

Diagnosis

The gold standard for diagnosis is upper endoscopy (EGD), which allows for direct visualization, localization, and biopsy of the ulcer. Biopsy is mandatory for gastric ulcers to rule out malignancy. Concurrently, all patients should be tested for *H. pylori* infection. This can be done via endoscopic biopsy (rapid urease test, histology) or non-invasively (urea breath test, stool antigen test). Serology is less useful as it cannot distinguish active from past infection.

Differential Diagnosis

The differential for epigastric pain includes GERD, functional dyspepsia, gastritis, pancreatitis, biliary colic, and gastric cancer. A sudden onset of severe, diffuse abdominal pain in a patient with PUD should raise suspicion for perforation, a surgical emergency.

Treatment Algorithm

The PUD algorithm is bifurcated based on etiology.

- **Algorithm 1: *H. pylori*-Positive PUD:** The primary goal is eradication. First-line therapy is guided by local clarithromycin resistance rates and patient allergies.
    - **High Clarithromycin Resistance (>15%):** Bismuth quadruple therapy (Bismuth, PPI, tetracycline, metronidazole) for 14 days is the preferred algorithm.
    - **Low Clarithromycin Resistance (<15%):** Clarithromycin-based triple therapy (PPI, clarithromycin, amoxicillin or metronidazole) for 14 days is an option. Following therapy, a PPI is continued for 4-8 weeks to ensure ulcer healing. Eradication *must* be confirmed ≥ 4 weeks after therapy completion, typically with a urea breath test or stool antigen test.
- **Algorithm 2: NSAID-Induced PUD:** The primary algorithm is cessation of the offending NSAID. If this is not possible, the NSAID should be reduced to the lowest effective dose and co-prescribed with a PPI. In either case, standard-dose PPI therapy is initiated and continued for 4-8 weeks to promote healing.
- **Algorithm 3: Bleeding Ulcer:** This is a medical emergency. The algorithm involves hemodynamic resuscitation, IV PPI infusion, and urgent upper endoscopy for hemostatic therapy (e.g., clipping, thermal coagulation).

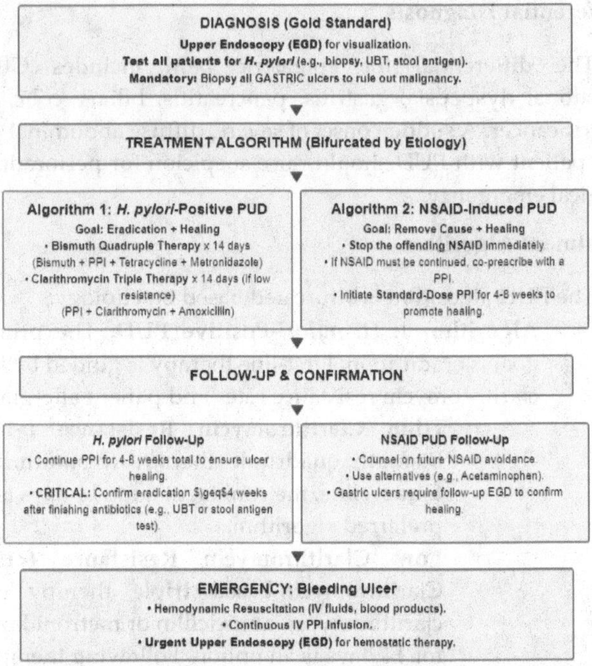

Figure 3.2: Peptic Ulcer Disease (PUD)

Table 3.2: Algorithm for Peptic Ulcer Disease Treatment

Etiology	Diagnostic Test(s)	Treatment Algorithm
H. pylori	Urea Breath Test, Stool Antigen, Biopsy	Triple/Quadruple Therapy (e.g., PPI + Clarithro + Amox) for 14 days + PPI for 4-8 wks.
NSAID-Induced	History of NSAID use; negative *H. pylori* test.	Stop NSAID. Treat with PPI for 8 wks.
Refractory	Ulcer non-healing after 8-12 wks of PPI.	Evaluate for non-adherence, *H. pylori* resistance, or Zollinger-Ellison Syndrome.

Monitoring and Follow-Up

The most important monitoring step after treatment is to confirm *H. pylori* eradication. This must be done ≥4 weeks after completing antibiotic therapy and after holding PPIs for 1-2 weeks. Non-invasive eradication tests include the urea breath test (UBT) or a fecal antigen test. For complicated ulcers (e.g., bleeding) or any *gastric* ulcer (which carries a small risk of malignancy), a follow-up EGD in 8-12 weeks is mandatory to confirm healing and to re-biopsy if necessary. Duodenal ulcers are almost never malignant and do not require routine follow-up EGD.

Long-Term Management / Secondary Prevention

Secondary prevention is entirely dependent on the underlying cause. If the ulcer was from *H. pylori,* successful eradication is curative. If the ulcer was from NSAIDs, the primary strategy is to stop the offending agent immediately. If an NSAID (e.g., aspirin for cardiovascular protection) must be continued, long-term co-therapy with a PPI or misoprostol is required to prevent recurrence. All patients should be advised to quit smoking, as it impairs ulcer healing and increases recurrence.

Patient Counseling Points

1. **Adherence to Eradication Therapy:** For *H. pylori,* the patient must complete the full 14-day, multi-drug (e.g., "quadruple therapy") regimen. Non-adherence is the primary cause of treatment failure.
2. **Stop NSAIDs:** The patient must understand the direct link between their ulcer and NSAID use. They should be counseled to use alternative analgesics, such as acetaminophen, in the future.
3. **Alarm Symptoms:** Teach the patient to seek immediate care for "red flag" signs of a complicated ulcer: sudden, severe abdominal pain (perforation), hematemesis (vomiting blood or "coffee grounds"), or melena (black, tarry stools).
4. **Smoking Cessation:** Emphatically counsel that

smoking directly harms the stomach lining, prevents healing, and makes ulcers more likely to return.

Common Pitfalls in Management

The most critical pitfall is the failure to confirm *H. pylori* eradication after treatment, leading to ulcer recurrence. Another is failing to biopsy gastric ulcers or ensure their healing with a follow-up EGD, which can result in a missed gastric cancer diagnosis. Finally, simply prescribing a PPI for an NSAID-induced ulcer without addressing the causative agent (i.e., stopping or reducing the NSAID) is an incomplete and often ineffective strategy.

Case Study

A 55-year-old female (Ms. Jones) presents with a 2-month history of gnawing epigastric pain. The pain is *better* after she eats. She has no history of NSAID use. You refer her for an EGD, which reveals a 1.5 cm ulcer in the duodenal bulb. A biopsy rapid urease test is **positive.**

Discussion

This patient has a ***H. pylori*-positive duodenal ulcer**. The management algorithm for PUD is bifurcated by cause. Since she is *H. pylori*-positive and does not use NSAIDs, the algorithm is clear: the primary goal is *H. pylori* eradication.

Treatment Algorithm

1. **Diagnosis:** *H. pylori*-positive duodenal ulcer.
2. **Eradication Algorithm:** You select a first-line therapy. Assuming your local clarithromycin resistance is high (>15%), the preferred algorithm is **Bismuth Quadruple Therapy**:
   - **PPI** (e.g., Omeprazole 20 mg) BID
   - **Bismuth** Subcitrate QID
   - **Tetracycline** QID
   - **Metronidazole** QID
   - **Duration:** 14 days.
3. **Healing Algorithm:** After the 14-day eradication, you continue the **Omeprazole 20 mg daily for 4-6 more**

weeks to ensure the ulcer itself heals.

4. **Confirmation (Critical Step):** You instruct her to return 4 weeks *after* completing all antibiotics (and after holding her PPI for 1-2 weeks) for a **Urea Breath Test** to confirm eradication.

Outcome

Ms. Jones is prescribed 14 days of Bismuth Quadruple Therapy, followed by 6 weeks of omeprazole. A urea breath test is scheduled to confirm a cure.

INFLAMMATORY BOWEL DISEASE (IBD)

IBD encompasses two primary chronic inflammatory conditions of the gastrointestinal tract: Ulcerative Colitis (UC) and Crohn's Disease (CD). Treatment algorithms are complex, aiming to induce and maintain long-term, steroid-free remission.

Pathophysiology

The pathophysiology is a complex, dysregulated immune response to intestinal microbes in a genetically susceptible individual.

Ulcerative Colitis

The inflammation is superficial, limited to the mucosa and submucosa. It is *continuous,* starting in the rectum (proctitis) and extending proximally, but is *confined* to the colon. The inflammation is characterized by neutrophilic infiltration, leading to crypt abscesses and friable, bleeding mucosa.

Crohn's Disease

The inflammation is *transmural,* meaning it affects the entire thickness of the bowel wall. This can lead to strictures (narrowing), fistulas (abnormal connections between organs), and abscesses. It is characterized by *skip lesions* (patches of healthy bowel alternating with inflamed segments) and can affect *any* part of the GI tract, from "mouth to anus," though it most commonly involves the terminal ileum.

Diagnosis and Classification

Diagnosis is made through a combination of clinical, endoscopic, histologic, and radiologic findings. UC is characterized by continuous, circumferential inflammation confined to the colonic mucosa, starting from the rectum. CD is characterized by discontinuous, "skip lesions," transmural inflammation, and can affect any part of the GI tract from mouth to anus. IBD is classified by location, severity (mild, moderate, severe), and behavior (e.g., inflammatory vs. fistulizing CD).

Differential Diagnosis

The primary differential is infectious colitis, especially *C. difficile, E. coli* O157:H7, and *Campylobacter,* which must be ruled out at initial presentation. Other considerations include Irritable Bowel Syndrome (IBS) (which lacks inflammation), celiac disease, ischemic colitis, and microscopic colitis.

Treatment Algorithm

The treatment algorithm is stratified by disease type and severity.

Ulcerative Colitis (UC)

- **Mild-Moderate (Proctitis/Proctosigmoiditis):** The algorithm begins with topical 5-aminosalicylic acid (5-ASA) agents (e.g., mesalamine suppositories or enemas).
- **Mild-Moderate (Extensive):** The algorithm combines oral 5-ASA with topical 5-ASA.
- **Moderate-Severe:** Flares are induced into remission with oral corticosteroids (e.g., prednisone). For maintenance of remission, the algorithm advances to immunomodulators (e.g., azathioprine) or biologic agents (e.g., anti-TNF [infliximab], anti-integrin [vedolizumab], or JAK inhibitors [tofacitinib]).

Crohn's Disease (CD)

- **Mild (Ileal/Right-Sided):** The algorithm for inducing remission often uses oral budesonide (a corticosteroid with high first-pass metabolism) for 8-12 weeks.

- **Moderate-Severe:** Flares are induced with systemic corticosteroids (e.g., prednisone). Maintenance is achieved with immunomodulators or biologics. The "top-down" algorithm, initiating biologics early, is favored in patients with high-risk features (e.g., fistulizing disease, deep ulcers, young age at diagnosis).

Table 3.3: Comparison of IBD Management Goals

Feature	Crohn's Disease	Ulcerative Colitis
Location	Mouth to Anus ("Skip lesions")	Colon only (Continuous)
Inflammation	Transmural (full thickness)	Mucosal (superficial)
Mild-Mod Tx	5-ASA (e.g., Mesalamine), Budesonide (ileal)	5-ASA (Rectal or Oral Mesalamine)
Mod-Severe Tx	Systemic Steroids (flare); Biologics (e.g., TNFα-I) or Immunomodulators (maintenance).	Systemic Steroids (flare); Biologics or Immunomodulators (maintenance).

Monitoring and Follow-Up

IBD requires lifelong, active monitoring. Clinical monitoring involves assessing flare-up symptoms (e.g., stool frequency, bleeding, abdominal pain). Objective monitoring is crucial and includes inflammatory markers (CRP) and, most importantly, fecal calprotectin, a stool test that is highly sensitive for intestinal inflammation. Therapeutic drug monitoring (e.g., biologic trough levels) is often used to optimize dosing. Endoscopic monitoring (colonoscopy) is performed to assess disease activity, gauge response to therapy, and, critically, to conduct long-term surveillance for colorectal cancer, which should begin 8-10 years after diagnosis.

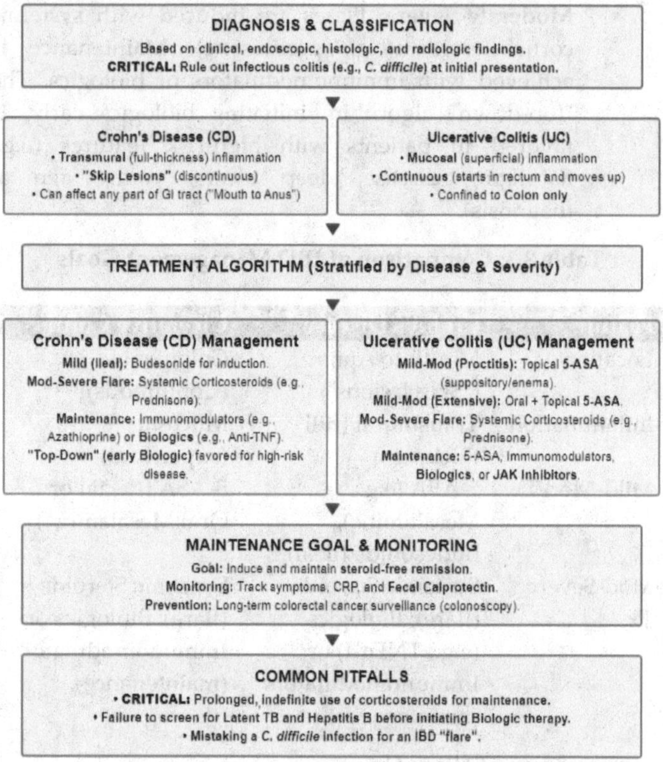

Figure 3.3: Inflammatory Bowel Disease (IBD)

Long-Term Management / Secondary Prevention

The goal is to maintain remission. This is achieved with long-term maintenance therapy. For mild-to-moderate UC, this is often a 5-ASA agent (e.g., mesalamine). For moderate-to-severe UC or any Crohn's disease, maintenance involves immunomodulators (e.g., azathioprine, methotrexate) or, more commonly, biologic agents (e.g., anti-TNF agents like infliximab or anti-integrins like vedolizumab). Secondary prevention is focused on preventing complications. This includes colorectal cancer surveillance, monitoring and treating nutritional deficiencies, and bone density monitoring (DEXA scans) due to high-risk from steroid use and chronic inflammation.

Patient Counseling Points

1. **Adherence to Maintenance:** This is the most important concept. The goal of therapy is not just to treat flares, but to *prevent* them. Stopping maintenance medication, even when feeling well, will lead to a flare-up.
2. **Smoking Cessation (Crohn's):** Smoking is a major risk factor for Crohn's disease. It makes the disease more aggressive, increases flare frequency, and reduces medication efficacy. Smoking cessation is a primary therapeutic goal.
3. **Recognizing a Flare:** Teach the patient the signs of their specific flare (e.g., increased stool frequency, bleeding, pain, fever) and to contact their provider early.
4. **Cancer Risk:** The patient must understand they are at an increased risk for colorectal cancer and must adhere to their long-term surveillance colonoscopy schedule.

Common Pitfalls in Management

A major pitfall is the prolonged, indefinite use of systemic corticosteroids for maintenance, which provides no long-term benefit and carries severe side effects. The goal is always steroid-free remission. Another critical error is the failure to screen for latent tuberculosis and hepatitis B before initiating anti-TNF biologic therapy, which can lead to reactivation of these infections. Finally, failing to rule out C. *difficile* infection as the cause of a "flare" in a patient with established IBD is a common and dangerous oversight.

Case Study

A 24-year-old male (Mr. Al-Jamil) presents with a 6-month history of intermittent, non-bloody diarrhea, crampy right-lower-quadrant abdominal pain, and a 10-lb weight loss. A colonoscopy reveals patchy, deep, linear ulcers (cobblestoning) in the terminal ileum and ascending colon, with a normal rectum. Biopsies confirm **Crohn's Disease.**

Discussion

This patient has moderate-to-severe **Crohn's Disease (CD)**. The algorithm for CD is different from Ulcerative Colitis (UC). It is not just about superficial inflammation (like in UC), but about transmural (full-thickness) disease. Given his weight loss and deep ulcerations, he is at high risk for complications (strictures, fistulas).

Treatment Algorithm

1. **Diagnosis:** Moderate-to-severe, inflammatory ileocolonic Crohn's Disease.
2. **Algorithm Step 1 (Induce Remission):** He is in an active flare. The algorithm to induce remission is:
    - **Oral Corticosteroids:** Start **Prednisone 40 mg daily** with a slow taper over several weeks.
3. **Algorithm Step 2 (Maintain Remission):** Steroids are not for long-term use. The algorithm requires a steroid-sparing maintenance agent. Given his high-risk features, a "Top-Down" approach (starting with a biologic) is favored.
    - **Initiate Biologic:** You start **Adalimumab (a TNF-inhibitor)** via subcutaneous injection (after screening for latent TB and hepatitis).
4. **Safety Screening:** Before starting the biologic, you perform the mandatory safety algorithm: PPD/Quantiferon-Gold and Hepatitis B serologies.

Outcome

Mr. Al-Jamil is started on a prednisone taper to control his flare and given his first loading doses of Adalimumab for long-term, steroid-free maintenance.

CELIAC DISEASE

Celiac disease is a chronic, immune-mediated enteropathy triggered by gluten ingestion in genetically susceptible individuals. It is characterized by small intestinal mucosal inflammation, villous atrophy, and nutrient malabsorption.

Pathophysiology

Celiac disease is a T-cell-mediated autoimmune disorder of the small intestine caused by an intolerance to gluten in genetically predisposed individuals (those carrying HLA-DQ2 or HLA-DQ8 genes). When gluten (a protein in wheat, barley, and rye) is ingested, its gliadin component is deamidated by tissue transglutaminase (tTG). This modified gliadin is then presented to T-cells, triggering an intense inflammatory and autoimmune response. This response attacks the small bowel mucosa, leading to the characteristic finding of villous atrophy—the flattening of the finger-like projections that absorb nutrients. This destruction of the absorptive surface area leads to malabsorption, nutritional deficiencies, and a wide range of gastrointestinal and extra-intestinal symptoms.

Diagnosis

The diagnostic algorithm begins with serologic testing in a patient who is actively consuming a gluten-containing diet. The preferred test is IgA anti-tissue transglutaminase (tTG) antibody, with a total serum IgA level to rule out selective IgA deficiency. If serology is positive, the diagnosis is confirmed by upper endoscopy with multiple duodenal biopsies demonstrating characteristic findings (e.g., villous atrophy, crypt hyperplasia, increased intraepithelial lymphocytes).

Differential Diagnosis

The differential for malabsorptive diarrhea includes Crohn's disease, small intestinal bacterial overgrowth (SIBO), tropical sprue, and autoimmune enteropathy. It is also critical to differentiate celiac disease from non-celiac gluten sensitivity (NCGS), a clinical diagnosis where patients have symptoms in response to gluten but lack the serologic and histologic findings of celiac disease.

Treatment Algorithm

The sole treatment algorithm for celiac disease is the initiation and lifelong adherence to a strict gluten-free diet (GFD). This involves eliminating all foods containing wheat, barley, and rye.

- **Step 1: Dietary Education:** Formal consultation with a dietitian skilled in celiac disease is a mandatory part of the algorithm to ensure correct GFD implementation and avoidance of cross-contamination.
- **Step 2: Nutritional Monitoring:** At diagnosis, patients should be screened for micronutrient deficiencies, particularly iron, vitamin B12, folate, vitamin D, and zinc, with repletion as necessary.
- **Step 3: Disease Monitoring:** The algorithm involves follow-up serologic testing (tTG-IgA) 6-12 months after GFD initiation, which should normalize with dietary adherence.
- **Step 4: Bone Health:** A baseline bone density scan (DEXA) is recommended due to the high risk of osteopenia and osteoporosis from malabsorption.

Monitoring and Follow-Up

After diagnosis, monitoring has two goals: assessing adherence to the diet and screening for complications. Adherence is monitored by assessing symptom resolution and by serologic testing. The main antibody, anti-tTG IgA, should be checked 6-12 months after starting the diet. If the patient is adherent, the antibody titer should decrease significantly or normalize. Persistent or recurrent symptoms, or failure of serology to normalize, warrants referral to a dietician and re-evaluation for unintentional gluten exposure. Patients must also be monitored for nutritional deficiencies (e.g., iron, folate, B12, vitamin D, calcium) and for bone disease (a baseline DEXA scan is recommended).

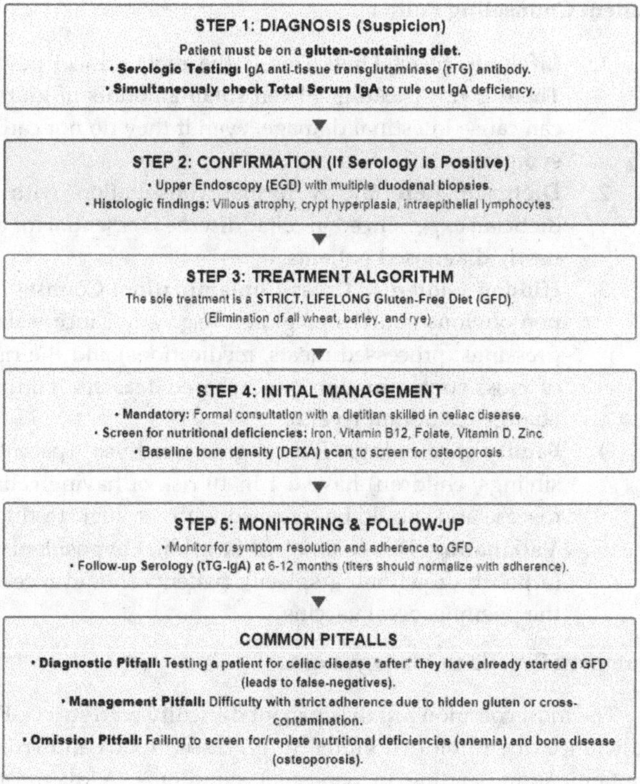

Figure 3.4: Celiac Disease

Long-Term Management / Secondary Prevention

The *only* treatment for celiac disease is a strict, 100% gluten-free diet for life. There are no pharmacological agents to prevent or treat the disease. This diet allows the intestinal villi to heal and prevents the long-term complications of untreated disease, which include osteoporosis, infertility, and, most seriously, an increased risk of small bowel lymphoma (Enteropathy-Associated T-cell Lymphoma).

Patient Counseling Points

1. **Lifelong, Strict Diet:** This is the most critical point. There is no "cheating." Even small amounts of gluten can cause intestinal damage, even if they do not cause symptoms.
2. **Dietician Referral:** A formal consultation with a dietician experienced in celiac disease is essential for all newly diagnosed patients.
3. **Hidden Gluten & Cross-Contamination:** Counsel on non-obvious sources of gluten (e.g., soy sauce, salad dressings, processed meats, medications) and the risk of cross-contamination (e.g., shared toasters, cutting boards, restaurant fryers).
4. **Family Screening:** First-degree relatives (parents, siblings, children) have a 1 in 10 risk of having celiac disease and should be screened with serologic testing.
5. **Vaccination:** Due to a risk of functional hyposplenism (a poorly functioning spleen), patients should receive the pneumococcal vaccine.

Common Pitfalls in Management

The most common pitfall is patient difficulty with strict GFD adherence due to hidden gluten in processed foods and cross-contamination, leading to persistent symptoms. A diagnostic pitfall is testing a patient for celiac disease *after* they have already initiated a GFD, which leads to false-negative serology and histology. Finally, failing to screen for and replete common nutritional deficiencies can lead to long-term complications like anemia and osteoporosis.

Case Study

A 31-year-old female (Ms. O'Brien) presents with a 1-year history of chronic bloating, flatulence, and anemia (Hgb 10.5 g/dL) with a low iron and ferritin. She mentions she also has an itchy, blistering rash on her elbows (dermatitis herpetiformis).

Discussion

This combination of GI symptoms, iron deficiency anemia, and dermatitis herpetiformis is highly specific for **Celiac Disease**. The diagnostic algorithm must be followed *before* the patient stops eating gluten.

Treatment Algorithm

1. **Diagnosis (Algorithm Step 1):**
   - **Serology:** While she is still eating a normal (gluten-containing) diet, you order an **IgA anti-tissue transglutaminase (tTG) antibody** and a total IgA level. Her tTG-IgA comes back very high (>10x upper limit of normal).
   - **Confirmation (Step 2):** Given the high antibody level and classic rash, the diagnosis is confirmed. (An EGD with duodenal biopsies showing villous atrophy is the gold standard but may be omitted in cases like this).
2. **Treatment (Algorithm Step 1):** The *only* treatment is a lifelong, strict gluten-free diet.
   - **Referral:** You place a formal consultation with a **dietitian skilled in celiac disease** to provide education on the gluten-free diet and avoiding cross-contamination.
3. **Monitoring (Algorithm Step 2/3):**
   - **Nutrition:** You screen her for other deficiencies (B12, Folate, Vitamin D) and start her on oral iron.
   - **Bone Health:** You order a baseline DEXA scan.
   - **Follow-up:** You plan to re-check her tTG-IgA serology in 6-12 months, which should normalize with dietary adherence.

Outcome

Ms. O'Brien is diagnosed with Celiac Disease. She is started on an iron supplement and has an urgent referral to a dietitian to begin her lifelong gluten-free diet.

HEPATITIS

Hepatitis, or inflammation of the liver, has a broad etiology, but treatment algorithms are most clearly defined for viral hepatitis (A, B, and C). These algorithms are etiology-specific, with goals ranging from supportive care to long-term suppression or cure.

Pathophysiology

Hepatitis refers to inflammation of the liver, most commonly caused by a group of distinct viruses.

Hepatitis A (HAV)

This is an acute, self-limiting infection caused by an RNA virus. It is transmitted via the fecal-oral route, often through contaminated food or water. It does *not* cause chronic disease.

Hepatitis B (HBV)

This is a DNA virus transmitted via blood and body fluids (e.g., sexual contact, perinatal). The risk of chronic infection is inversely related to the age at acquisition; >90% of infected newborns will develop chronic HBV, whereas <5% of adults will. Chronic HBV infection integrates into the host DNA and can lead directly to cirrhosis and hepatocellular carcinoma (HCC).

Hepatitis C (HCV)

This is an RNA virus transmitted primarily via blood (e.g., IV drug use, pre-1992 blood transfusions). HCV is highly prone to chronicity, with 70-80% of those infected developing chronic hepatitis. This chronic inflammation is the primary driver of progressive liver fibrosis, which leads to cirrhosis and HCC over 20-30 years.

Diagnosis

Diagnosis is made via a hepatitis serology panel, which can identify the causative virus and the phase of infection (acute vs. chronic).

Hepatitis A (HAV)

Diagnosed by positive anti-HAV IgM antibody (acute infection).

Hepatitis B (HBV)

Diagnosed by hepatitis B surface antigen (HBsAg) and anti-HBc IgM (acute) or anti-HBc total (chronic exposure).

Hepatitis C (HCV)

Diagnosed by a positive anti-HCV antibody, followed by a quantitative HCV RNA test to confirm active, chronic infection.

Differential Diagnosis

The differential for acute hepatitis (elevated aminotransferases) is extensive and includes alcoholic hepatitis, drug-induced liver injury (DILI) (e.g., from acetaminophen), autoimmune hepatitis, Wilson's disease, and acute obstruction or ischemia (shock liver).

Treatment Algorithm

The algorithms are virus-specific.

- **Hepatitis A:** The algorithm is entirely supportive. No antiviral therapy is indicated. Management involves rest, hydration, and avoidance of hepatotoxins. Prevention via vaccination is key.
- **Acute Hepatitis B:** The algorithm is also primarily supportive. Antiviral therapy (e.g., tenofovir, entecavir) is reserved for the small subset of patients who develop fulminant hepatic failure.
- **Chronic Hepatitis B:** This algorithm is complex. Treatment is indicated for patients with evidence of active liver inflammation (elevated ALT) and significant viral replication (high HBV DNA). The goal is viral *suppression,* not cure. First-line therapies are nucleos(t)ide analogs with a high barrier to resistance, such as Tenofovir or Entecavir.
- **Chronic Hepatitis C:** The goal is a curative_ sustained virologic response (SVR). The modern algorithm is simple:
    1. Confirm active infection (HCV RNA positive).
    2. Assess for cirrhosis (using non-invasive

fibrosis scores like FIB-4 or elastography).

3. Prescribe an 8-12 week course of a pangenotypic direct-acting antiviral (DAA) regimen (e.g., sofosbuvir/velpatasvir or glecaprevir/pibrentasvir).
4. Confirm SVR (undetectable HCV RNA) 12 weeks after treatment completion.

Table 3.4: Treatment Goals for Chronic Viral Hepatitis

Virus	Primary Goal	Drug Classes
Hepatitis B (HBV)	Suppression. (Sustained undetectable HBV DNA, HBeAg loss/seroconversion).	Nucleos(t)ide Analogs (e.g., Tenofovir, Entecavir)
Hepatitis C (HCV)	Cure. (Sustained Virologic Response, SVR)	Direct-Acting Antivirals (DAAs). (e.g., Sofosbuvir/Velpatasvir)

Monitoring and Follow-Up

Monitoring for **Hepatitis A** is supportive, tracking LFTs until they normalize. Monitoring for **Chronic HBV** is lifelong. It involves periodic (e.g., every 6-12 months) measurement of LFTs, HBeAg/anti-HBe status, and HBV DNA (viral load) to determine if the patient is in an active or inactive carrier state and if treatment is warranted. Monitoring for **Hepatitis C** is focused on achieving a cure. After completing an 8-12 week course of Direct-Acting Antivirals (DAAs), the single most important follow-up test is an HCV RNA (viral load) 12 weeks *after* finishing therapy. If this is undetectable, the patient is considered cured (a "Sustained Virologic Response," or SVR).

Long-Term Management / Secondary Prevention

For **Chronic HBV**, management may involve lifelong antiviral therapy (e.g., tenofovir, entecavir) to suppress the viral load, normalize LFTs, and reduce the risk of HCC. For **Chronic HCV**, management *is* a cure, achieved with 8-12 weeks of DAA therapy. **For both chronic HBV and HCV**, the most critical secondary prevention measure is lifelong surveillance for **Hepatocellular Carcinoma (HCC)**. All patients with cirrhosis, and some chronic HBV patients even without cirrhosis, must receive a screening abdominal ultrasound every 6 months to detect HCC at an early, curable stage. All hepatitis patients should be vaccinated against Hepatitis A and B (if not already immune) and counseled to avoid all hepatotoxins, especially alcohol.

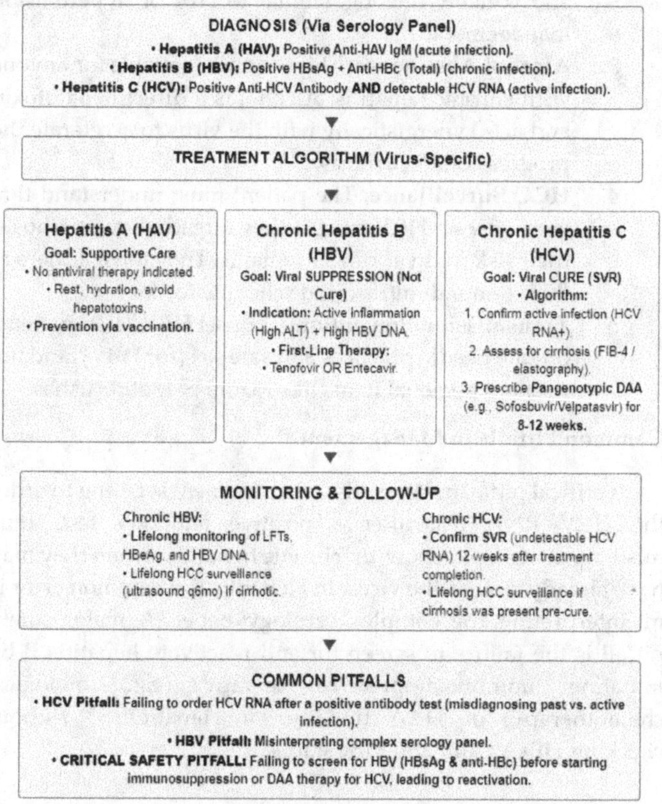
DIAGNOSIS (Via Serology Panel)
• Hepatitis A (HAV): Positive Anti-HAV IgM (acute infection).
• Hepatitis B (HBV): Positive HBsAg + Anti-HBc (Total) (chronic infection).
• Hepatitis C (HCV): Positive Anti-HCV Antibody AND detectable HCV RNA (active infection).
TREATMENT ALGORITHM (Virus-Specific)
Hepatitis A (HAV)
Goal: Supportive Care
• No antiviral therapy indicated.
• Rest, hydration, avoid hepatotoxins.
• Prevention via vaccination.
Chronic Hepatitis B (HBV)
Goal: Viral SUPPRESSION (Not Cure)
• Indication: Active inflammation (High ALT) + High HBV DNA.
• First-Line Therapy:
• Tenofovir OR Entecavir.
Chronic Hepatitis C (HCV)
Goal: Viral CURE (SVR)
• Algorithm:
1. Confirm active infection (HCV RNA+).
2. Assess for cirrhosis (FIB-4 / elastography).
3. Prescribe Pangenotypic DAA (e.g., Sofosbuvir/Velpatasvir) for 8-12 weeks.
MONITORING & FOLLOW-UP
Chronic HBV:
• Lifelong monitoring of LFTs, HBeAg, and HBV DNA.
• Lifelong HCC surveillance (ultrasound q6mo) if cirrhotic.
Chronic HCV:
• Confirm SVR (undetectable HCV RNA) 12 weeks after treatment completion.
• Lifelong HCC surveillance if cirrhosis was present pre-cure.
COMMON PITFALLS
• HCV Pitfall: Failing to order HCV RNA after a positive antibody test (misdiagnosing past vs. active infection).
• HBV Pitfall: Misinterpreting complex serology panel.
• CRITICAL SAFETY PITFALL: Failing to screen for HBV (HBsAg & anti-HBc) before starting immunosuppression or DAA therapy for HCV, leading to reactivation.

Figure 3.5: Pharmacological Management of Viral Hepatitis

Patient Counseling Points

1. **HCV is Curable:** This is a profoundly important message. Unlike HBV, modern DAA therapy is a *cure* for over 95% of patients, with a simple, well-tolerated 8-12 week oral regimen.
2. **HBV is Controllable:** For chronic HBV, patients must understand that therapy is *suppressive,* not curative, and is likely lifelong, similar to HIV or hypertension management.
3. **Alcohol Abstinence:** This is non-negotiable for anyone with chronic hepatitis. Alcohol is a direct hepatotoxin and acts synergistically with the virus to accelerate the progression to cirrhosis.
4. **HCC Surveillance:** The patient must understand that even *after* an HCV cure, if they already have cirrhosis, their risk for liver cancer remains. They must adhere to their 6-month ultrasound schedule for life.
5. **Transmission Prevention:** Counsel HBV/HCV patients on safe needle practices and safe sex (for HBV), and not to share personal items like razors or toothbrushes.

Common Pitfalls in Management

A critical pitfall in Hepatitis C management is failing to order the HCV RNA test after a positive antibody test, thus misdiagnosing a patient with "chronic hepatitis" when they may have already cleared the virus. In Hepatitis B, a common error is misinterpreting the complex serology panel. A major safety pitfall is the failure to screen for and reactivate hepatitis B by initiating immunosuppressive therapy (e.g., biologics, chemotherapy) or DAA therapy for Hepatitis C without checking HBsAg and anti-HBc status.

Case Study

A 45-year-old male (Mr. Evans) has a routine physical. His labs are notable for a mildly elevated ALT (52 U/L). He has no symptoms. As part of a workup, you order a viral hepatitis panel. The results are:

- Anti-HCV: **Positive**
- HBsAg: Negative
- Anti-HBs: Positive (from vaccination)
- Anti-HAV: Positive (from prior exposure)

Discussion

The positive Anti-HCV antibody indicates exposure to **Hepatitis C**. It does not confirm *active* infection. The algorithm requires a second test to see if the virus is still present.

Treatment Algorithm

1. **Diagnosis (Algorithm Step 1):**
    - **Confirm Active Infection:** You order an **HCV RNA (viral load)** test. It comes back **Positive** (detected).
    - **Staging:** You calculate his FIB-4 score (using age, AST, ALT, platelets), which is low, suggesting no cirrhosis.
    - **Diagnosis:** Chronic Hepatitis C, non-cirrhotic.
2. **Treatment (Algorithm Step 2):** The goal is a **cure (SVR)**. The modern algorithm is simple:
    - **Therapy:** You prescribe a pangenotypic Direct-Acting Antiviral (DAA) regimen.
    - **Regimen: Sofosbuvir/Velpatasvir (Epclusa)**, one pill daily.
    - **Duration:** 12 weeks.
3. **Monitoring (Algorithm Step 3):**
    - **Confirm Cure:** You schedule labs for 12 weeks *after* he finishes his medication to check for a **Sustained Virologic Response (SVR)** (an undetectable HCV RNA).
4. **Counseling:** You counsel him to abstain from alcohol

and get vaccinated for Hepatitis A (though he is already immune).

Outcome

Mr. Evans is started on a 12-week curative regimen of Sofosbuvir/Velpatasvir. He is expected to be fully cured (SVR12) of his Hepatitis

Summary

GERD: The algorithm is a stepwise "step-up" and "step-down" approach, starting with lifestyle changes, advancing to an 8-week PPI trial, and reserving endoscopy for alarm features or refractory symptoms.

Peptic Ulcer Disease: Management is a bifurcated algorithm targeting the underlying cause. *H. pylori* requires an eradication regimen (e.g., quadruple therapy) and confirmation of cure. NSAID-induced ulcers require PPI therapy and removal of the offending agent.

Inflammatory Bowel Disease: The algorithm is stratified by disease (UC vs. CD) and severity. It involves inducing remission (often with corticosteroids) and maintaining remission with steroid-sparing agents (5-ASAs, immunomodulators, or biologics).

Celiac Disease: The treatment algorithm is singular: a strict, lifelong gluten-free diet, coupled with nutritional screening and formal dietetic counseling.

Hepatitis: Algorithms are virus-specific. Hepatitis A is supportive. Chronic Hepatitis B is managed with long-term viral suppression (tenofovir/entecavir). Chronic Hepatitis C is managed with a curative, short-course (8-12 weeks) pangenotypic direct-acting antiviral (DAA) regimen.

Multiple Choice Questions

1. A 50-year-old male with heartburn and regurgitation has no alarm features. According to the standard GERD algorithm, what is the most appropriate initial step?
   A) 24-hour ambulatory pH monitoring
   B) Upper endoscopy (EGD)
   C) 8-week trial of a standard-dose PPI
   D) Surgical consultation for fundoplication
2. A 45-year-old female has refractory GERD symptoms despite twice-daily PPI therapy. EGD is normal. What is the gold standard test to confirm the diagnosis?
   A) Barium swallow
   B) Esophageal manometry
   C) Ambulatory pH monitoring
   D) Repeat EGD with biopsy
3. A 60-year-old male is diagnosed with a 1.5 cm gastric ulcer. Biopsies are benign, and the rapid urease test is positive. What is the most appropriate management algorithm?
   A) 14 days of bismuth quadruple therapy, followed by confirmation of eradication.
   B) 8 weeks of PPI therapy, then stop.
   C) 14 days of clarithromycin triple therapy, no follow-up needed.
   D) 8 weeks of H2-receptor antagonist therapy.
4. Which of the following is the most critical pitfall in the management of gastric ulcers?
   A) Failing to check a urea breath test
   B) Failing to biopsy the ulcer to rule out malignancy
   C) Using a PPI for more than 4 weeks
   D) Prescribing quadruple therapy instead of triple therapy

5. What is the first-line treatment algorithm for a patient newly diagnosed with mild-to-moderate ulcerative proctitis?
   A) Oral prednisone
   B) Oral mesalamine (5-ASA)
   C) Topical mesalamine (suppository or enema)
   D) Infliximab (anti-TNF)
6. A 22-year-old is diagnosed with fistulizing Crohn's disease. This is considered high-risk. What treatment algorithm is favored?
   A) A "step-up" approach starting with 5-ASA
   B) A "top-down" approach, initiating a biologic agent early C) Long-term budesonide therapy
   D) On-demand SABA inhaler
7. A patient is starting infliximab for severe Ulcerative Colitis. Which of the following screening tests must be performed as part of the safety algorithm?
   A) Colonoscopy
   B) Latent tuberculosis and Hepatitis B serology
   C) Celiac disease serology
   D) Stool antigen test for H. pylori
8. The only treatment algorithm for confirmed celiac disease is:
   A) A lifelong, strict gluten-free diet
   B) An 8-week trial of oral budesonide
   C) On-demand PPI therapy
   D) A pangenotypic direct-acting antiviral
9. A 30-year-old patient is diagnosed with chronic Hepatitis C (genotype 1, no cirrhosis). What is the standard-of-care treatment algorithm?
   A) Supportive care and observation
   B) Lifelong tenofovir
   C) A 12-week course of pangenotypic direct-acting antivirals (DAAs)
   D) A 48-week course of pegylated-interferon and ribavirin

10. A 40-year-old female is diagnosed with acute Hepatitis A. What is the correct management algorithm?

    A) 12 weeks of sofosbuvir/velpatasvir

    B) A 7-day course of amoxicillin-clavulanate

    C) Supportive care

    D) Immediate hospitalization for IV antiviral therapy

Self-Assessment Questions

1. A patient with typical GERD symptoms fails an 8-week, once-daily PPI trial. What are the next two steps in the management algorithm?
2. What are the "alarm features" that mandate prompt upper endoscopy in a patient with GERD symptoms?
3. A patient is diagnosed with a H. pylori-positive duodenal ulcer. Outline the first-line treatment algorithm in an area with high clarithromycin resistance.
4. Why is it a mandatory part of the PUD algorithm to confirm H. pylori eradication and to biopsy all gastric ulcers?
5. Compare and contrast the typical "step-up" algorithm for mild-to-moderate Ulcerative Colitis with the "top-down" approach for high-risk Crohn's Disease.
6. What is the most significant long-term pitfall in IBD management, and what class of medications is used to avoid it?
7. A patient has positive anti-tTG IgA serology. What is the definitive next step in the diagnostic algorithm for celiac disease?
8. A patient with chronic Hepatitis B has a high HBV DNA level but persistently normal ALT. What is the general approach to this "immune-tolerant" phase?
9. Describe the simple, 3-step modern algorithm for curing a patient with chronic Hepatitis C.
10. What critical safety screening must be performed before initiating DAA therapy for Hepatitis C?

Bibliography

1. Katz PO, Dunbar KB, Schnoll-Sussman FH, Pfeifer K, Kavitt RT, Gerson LB. ACG Clinical Guideline for the Diagnosis and Management of Gastroesophageal Reflux Disease. Am J Gastroenterol. 2022 Jan 1;117(1):27–56.
2. Laine L, Yang H, Chang SC, Datto C. Trends in Endoscopy for Uncomplicated GERD in the Era of PPIs. Am J Med. 2008 Nov;121(11):1010.e1–7.
3. Fallone CA, Chiba N, van Zanten SV, Fischbach L, Gisbert JP, Hunt RH, et al. The Toronto Consensus for the Treatment of Helicobacter pylori Infection in Adults. Gastroenterology. 2016 Jul;151(1):51–69.
4. Laine L, Jensen DM. Management of patients with ulcer bleeding. Am J Gastroenterol. 2012 Mar;107(3):345–60.
5. Rubin DT, Ananthakrishnan AN, Siegel CA, Sauer BG, Long MD. ACG Clinical Guideline: Ulcerative Colitis in Adults. Am J Gastroenterol. 2019 Mar;114(3):384–413.
6. Lichtenstein GR, Loftus EV, Isaacs KL, Regueiro MD, Gerson LB, Sands BE. ACG Clinical Guideline: Management of Crohn's Disease in Adults. Am J Gastroenterol. 2018 Apr;113(4):481–517.
7. Rubio-Tapia A, Hill ID, Kelly CP, Calderwood AH, Murray JA. ACG Clinical Guidelines: Diagnosis and Management of Celiac Disease. Am J Gastroenterol. 2013 May;108(5):656–76.
8. Husain N, Zaka-ur-Rab Z, Khan S. Celiac disease: A diagnostic pitfall. J Pak Med Assoc. 2007 Aug;57(8):403–5.
9. Terrault NA, Lok ASF, McMahon BJ, Chang KM, Hwang JP, Jonas MM, et al. Update on Prevention, Diagnosis, and Treatment of Chronic Hepatitis B: AASLD 2018 Hepatitis B Guidance. Hepatology. 2018 Apr;67(4):1560–99.
10. AASLD-IDSA. HCV Guidance: Recommendations for Testing, Managing, and Treating Hepatitis C. [Accessed 2024 Oct 25]. Available from: https://www.hcvguidelines.org
11. Chey WD, Leontiadis GI, Howden CW, Moss SF. ACG Clinical Guideline: Treatment of Helicobacter pylori Infection. Am J Gastroenterol. 2017 Feb;112(2):212–39.
12. Shah SC, Iyer PG, Moss SF. AGA Clinical Practice Update on the Management of Refractory GERD: Expert Review. Gastroenterology. 2021 Oct;161(4):1365–71.
13. Feuerstein JD, Isaacs KL, Schneider Y, Siddique SM, Falck-Ytter Y, Singh S. AGA Clinical Practice Guidelines on the Management of Moderate to Severe Ulcerative Colitis. Gastroenterology. 2020 Apr;158(5):1450–61.
14. Falck-Ytter Y, Neelam B, Johanna M, Shahnaz S, Tuan T, John JW. ACG Clinical Guideline: Diagnosis and Management of Celiac Disease. Am J Gastroenterol. 2013 May;108(5):656–76.
15. WGO. World Gastroenterology Organisation Global Guidelines: Hepatitis B. [Accessed 2024 Oct 25]. Available from: https://www.worldgastroenterology.org/guidelines/hepatitis-b.

CHAPTER 4

TREATMENT ALGORITHMS FOR ENDOCRINE DISORDERS

Author

Miss Hyndavi Trylockya Nagumantri, Pharm D Scholar, Koringa College of Pharmacy, Korangi, Tallarevu, Andhra Pradesh, India

Abstract

Endocrine disorder management involves correcting hormonal excesses or deficiencies to restore physiologic balance, with algorithms guided by laboratory thresholds and clinical targets. The algorithm for Type 1 Diabetes Mellitus is based on basal-bolus insulin replacement, with dosing calculated from carbohydrate intake and corrected for hyperglycemia. The Type 2 Diabetes algorithm is a stepwise, patient-centered approach beginning with lifestyle modification and metformin. Subsequent therapy is stratified by high-risk comorbidities, such as ASCVD, HF, or CKD, which prioritize SGLT2 inhibitors or GLP-1 receptor agonists. Thyroid disorder algorithms are distinct: hypothyroidism is managed with weight-based levothyroxine replacement, titrating the dose to a target TSH. Hyperthyroidism management is bifurcated by etiology, with Graves' disease treated via a three-pronged algorithm (beta-blockers for symptoms, anti-thyroid drugs, or definitive ablation/surgery), while nodular disease often requires ablation. Adrenal disorder algorithms are also specific: Addison's disease (insufficiency) requires lifelong glucocorticoid and mineralocorticoid replacement, whereas Cushing's syndrome (excess) requires a surgical algorithm to resect the causative tumor. The algorithm for Metabolic Syndrome is a multi-faceted approach focused on aggressive risk factor reduction, including weight loss and management of dyslipidemia and hypertension.

Keywords: *Endocrine Algorithms, Diabetes Mellitus, Thyroid Disorders, Adrenal Disorders, Metabolic Syndrome, Glycemic Control*

Learning Objectives

After completion of the chapter, the learners should be able to:

- List the diagnostic criteria for Diabetes Mellitus and Metabolic Syndrome.
- Explain the therapeutic algorithm for managing Diabetic Ketoacidosis (DKA), including fluid, insulin, and electrolyte management.
- Develop a treatment plan for a patient with new-onset Type 2 Diabetes, selecting agents based on comorbidities (e.g., CKD, ASCVD).
- Compare and contrast the treatment algorithms for hyperthyroidism (Graves' disease) versus hypothyroidism (Hashimoto's thyroiditis).
- Prioritize the components of the management algorithm for a patient in adrenal crisis (Addisonian crisis).

DIABETES MELLITUS

Diabetes Mellitus (DM) is a group of metabolic disorders characterized by hyperglycemia resulting from defects in insulin secretion, insulin action, or both. Treatment algorithms differ fundamentally between Type 1 and Type 2 diabetes.

Pathophysiology

Diabetes Mellitus (DM) is characterized by hyperglycemia resulting from defects in insulin secretion, insulin action, or both.

Type 1 Diabetes (T1DM)

This is an autoimmune disease. The pathophysiology involves a T-cell-mediated destruction of the pancreatic beta cells, leading to absolute insulin deficiency. This autoimmune attack is triggered by a combination of genetic susceptibility (e.g., HLA-DR3/DR4) and environmental factors. Without insulin, glucose cannot enter peripheral tissues (muscle, fat), and the liver, unopposed by insulin, engages in rampant gluconeogenesis and glycogenolysis, releasing more glucose. Furthermore, the lack of insulin disinhibits hormone-sensitive lipase, leading to massive lipolysis. This releases free fatty acids, which are converted by the liver into ketone bodies, resulting in diabetic ketoacidosis (DKA).

Type 2 Diabetes (T2DM)

This is a progressive disorder that begins with insulin resistance. Peripheral tissues, particularly muscle, fat, and liver, fail to respond appropriately to normal levels of insulin. The pancreas compensates by producing *more* insulin (hyperinsulinemia) to maintain euglycemia. Over years to decades, this high demand exhausts the pancreatic beta cells, which begin to fail. This leads to a state of relative insulin deficiency, and hyperglycemia ensues. The pathophysiology is strongly linked to central obesity, which promotes a chronic, low-grade inflammatory state and ectopic fat deposition that directly impairs insulin signaling.

Diagnosis and Classification

Diagnosis is established by meeting one of several criteria: a fasting plasma glucose ≥ 126 mg/dL, a 2-hour plasma glucose ≥ 200 mg/dL during an oral glucose tolerance test (OGTT), a hemoglobin A1c (HbA1c) ≥ 6.5%, or random plasma glucose ≥ 200 mg/dL in a patient with classic symptoms of hyperglycemia.

Type 1 DM (T1DM)

Results from autoimmune beta-cell destruction, leading to absolute insulin deficiency. It is confirmed by positive autoantibodies (e.g., anti-GAD).

Type 2 DM (T2DM)

Results from a progressive loss of beta-cell insulin secretion, frequently on the background of insulin resistance.

Differential Diagnosis

The differential for hyperglycemia includes stress-induced hyperglycemia (in hospitalized patients), monogenic diabetes (MODY), latent autoimmune diabetes in adults (LADA, a slow-progressing form of T1DM), and secondary causes such as pancreatitis or drug-induced diabetes (e.g., from glucocorticoids or atypical antipsychotics).

Treatment Algorithm

Type 1 Diabetes Mellitus (T1DM)

The algorithm for T1DM is one of total insulin replacement. The standard-of-care is a basal-bolus regimen, often delivered via multiple daily injections (MDI) or an insulin pump.

- **Basal Insulin:** A long-acting (e.g., glargine, detemir, degludec) or intermediate-acting (NPH) insulin is used to provide a steady background level and suppress hepatic gluconeogenesis.
- **Bolus Insulin:** A rapid-acting (e.g., lispro, aspart, glulisine) or short-acting (Regular) insulin is used to cover meals (prandial coverage) and correct high blood glucose readings. The algorithm for dosing is patient-specific, based on an insulin-to-carbohydrate ratio (ICR) for meals and an insulin sensitivity factor (ISF) for corrections. Continuous glucose monitoring (CGM) is now a core part of the management algorithm to guide dosing and minimize hypoglycemia.

Type 2 Diabetes Mellitus (T2DM)

The T2DM algorithm is a stepwise, patient-centered approach based on glycemic targets (usually HbA1c < 7.0%) and, critically, cardiovascular and renal risk.

- **Step 1:** The algorithm begins universally with comprehensive lifestyle modifications (diet, exercise, weight loss) and initiation of metformin, assuming no contraindications.
- **Step 2 (Risk-Based Stratification):** If HbA1c remains above target, the choice of the second agent is based on comorbidities.
    - **High-Risk ASCVD:** The algorithm prioritizes a GLP-1 receptor agonist (GLP-1 RA) or an SGLT2 inhibitor, as these classes have proven cardiovascular outcome benefits.
    - **Heart Failure (HF) or CKD:** The algorithm mandates the use of an SGLT2 inhibitor due to proven benefits in reducing HF hospitalizations and slowing CKD progression.

- **Step 3 (Glycemic-Based Stratification):** In the absence of these high-risk conditions, the choice of a second agent is based on other factors:
  - **High Hypoglycemia Risk:** GLP-1 RAs, SGLT2 inhibitors, DPP-4 inhibitors, or thiazolidinediones (TZDs) are preferred. Sulfonylureas are avoided.
  - **Need for Weight Loss:** GLP-1 RAs or SGLT2 inhibitors are strongly preferred.
  - **Cost Concerns:** Sulfonylureas or TZDs may be considered.
- **Step 4 (Intensification):** The algorithm proceeds with the stepwise addition of agents from different classes. If glycemic targets are still not met, the final step is the initiation of insulin therapy, typically starting with basal insulin.

Table 4.1: Pharmacological Algorithm for Type 2 Diabetes

Step	Patient Profile	Recommended Therapy
Step 1 (All)	Newly Diagnosed T2DM	Metformin + Comprehensive Lifestyle Modification
Step 2 (ASCVD)	Established ASCVD or High Risk	Add GLP-1 RA or SGLT2i (with proven benefit)
Step 2 (HF or CKD)	Established HF or CKD	Add SGLT2i (proven benefit). (GLP-1 RA if SGLT2i not tolerated)
Step 2 (No Comorbidities)	Need to minimize hypoglycemia.	Add DPP-4i, GLP-1 RA, SGLT2i, or TZD.

Monitoring and Follow-Up

Monitoring for both types of diabetes is centered on glycemic control and complication screening. The primary metric for long-term control is the Hemoglobin A1c (HbA1c), which reflects average blood glucose over the prior 2-3 months and should be checked every 3-6 months. Daily self-monitoring of blood glucose (SMBG) is essential for T1DM and insulin-treated T2DM. For T2DM patients on oral agents, SMBG is used to guide lifestyle and medication adjustments. Continuous Glucose Monitors (CGMs) are increasingly becoming the standard of care, providing real-time data on glucose levels, trends, and "time-in-range."

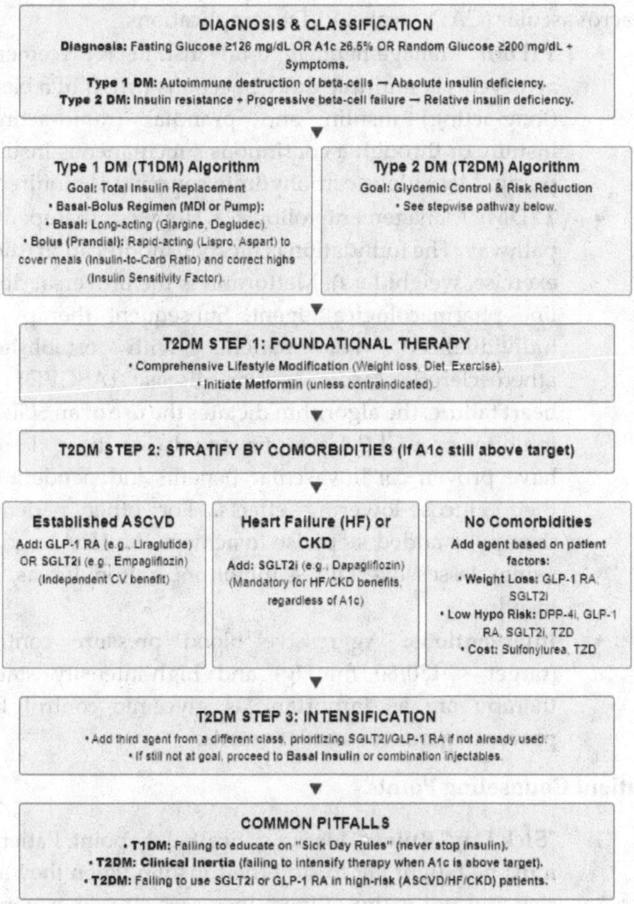

Figure 4.1: Diabetes Mellitus

Follow-up visits (every 3-6 months) must also include blood pressure checks and a foot exam (monofilament testing). Annual monitoring is critical for complications: a urine albumin-to-creatinine ratio (UACR) for nephropathy, a comprehensive dilated eye exam for retinopathy, and a fasting lipid panel.

Long-Term Management / Secondary Prevention

The goal of long-term management is to prevent microvascular (retinopathy, nephropathy, neuropathy) and macrovascular (CAD, stroke, PVD) complications.

- **T1DM:** Management is total insulin replacement, achieved via multiple daily injections (MDI) of a basal (long-acting) insulin and prandial (rapid-acting) insulin, or through a continuous subcutaneous insulin pump. Meticulous carbohydrate counting is required.
- **T2DM:** Management follows a stepwise therapeutic pathway. The foundation is lifestyle modification (diet, exercise, weight loss). Metformin is the universal first-line pharmacological agent. Subsequent therapy is individualized. For patients with established atherosclerotic cardiovascular disease (ASCVD) or heart failure, the algorithm dictates the use of an SGLT2 inhibitor or a GLP-1 receptor agonist, as these classes have proven cardiovascular benefits independent of their glucose-lowering effects. For other patients, therapy is added stepwise to achieve the HbA1c goal, using classes like DPP-4 inhibitors, sulfonylureas, or insulin.
- **Interventions:** Aggressive blood pressure control (target < 130/80 mmHg) and high-intensity statin therapy are as important as glycemic control for preventing macrovascular events.

Patient Counseling Points

1. **"Sick Day" Rules:** This is a critical safety point. Patients must be taught *not* to stop their insulin when they are sick and not eating. Illness increases stress hormones and hyperglycemia, so they often need *more* insulin. They should check their glucose more frequently and,

for T1DM, check for ketones.

2. **Hypoglycemia Recognition and Treatment:** Counsel on the "15-15 Rule." If glucose is < 70 mg/dL, consume 15 grams of fast-acting carbs (e.g., 4 oz juice, glucose tabs). Re-check in 15 minutes and repeat if still low. They must also recognize symptoms: shaking, sweating, anxiety (adrenergic) and confusion, slurred speech, seizure (neuroglycopenic).
3. **T2DM as a Progressive Disease:** Explain that T2DM is a progressive disease of beta-cell failure. Needing to add more medications, or eventually start insulin, is *not* a personal failure but a reflection of the natural history of the disease.
4. **Foot Care:** Teach patients to inspect their feet *daily* for any cuts, blisters, or redness. Counsel on proper footwear and against walking barefoot.
5. **Lifestyle:** Emphasize that for T2DM, lifestyle changes are not just advice but a cornerstone of therapy, as effective as any medication.

Common Pitfalls in Management

In T1DM, a common pitfall is failing to adjust insulin ratios for changes in diet, activity, or illness, leading to poor control. In T2DM, the most significant pitfall is clinical inertia, the failure to intensify therapy (add a second or third agent) when a patient's HbA1c is persistently above target. Another critical error is the failure to use SGLT2 inhibitors or GLP-1 RAs in high-risk patients (HF, CKD, ASCVD), instead "defaulting" to older agents like sulfonylureas, thereby missing an opportunity for organ protection.

Case Study

A 55-year-old male (Mr. Smith) with a 5-year history of Type 2 Diabetes Mellitus (T2DM) presents for follow-up. He is currently on Metformin 1000 mg BID. His BMI is 31. His recent labs show an **HbA1c of 8.5%** (goal is <7.0%). He has a history of a **myocardial infarction (MI)** 3 years ago.

Discussion

This patient has uncontrolled T2DM despite being on an optimal dose of Metformin. The modern T2DM algorithm dictates that the choice of the *second* agent is based on comorbidities. This patient has established atherosclerotic cardiovascular disease (ASCVD) from his prior MI.

Treatment Algorithm

1. **Diagnosis:** Uncontrolled T2DM with established ASCVD.
2. **Algorithm Step 1:** Lifestyle modification + Metformin (currently in place).
3. **Algorithm Step 2 (Risk-Based):** Because his HbA1c is above target and he has established ASCVD, the algorithm *mandates* adding an agent with proven cardiovascular benefit.
4. **Therapeutic Choice:** The two first-line classes in this scenario are **SGLT2 inhibitors** or **GLP-1 receptor agonists.**
    - You select an **SGLT2 inhibitor** for its dual cardiac and renal benefits. You prescribe **Empagliflozin 10 mg daily**.
5. **Follow-up:** You schedule a follow-up in 3 months to re-check his HbA1c and monitor renal function.

Outcome

Mr. Smith is started on Empagliflozin 10 mg daily in addition to his Metformin. This choice addresses his hyperglycemia while also providing critical secondary prevention for his cardiovascular disease.

THYROID DISORDERS

Thyroid disorders, resulting from an over- or under-production of thyroid hormone, are highly prevalent. Their treatment algorithms are aimed at restoring a euthyroid state.

Pathophysiology

Thyroid disorders result from the abnormal production of thyroid hormone (T4 and T3), which is regulated by the hypothalamic-pituitary-thyroid (HPT) axis. TSH (Thyroid-Stimulating Hormone) from the pituitary stimulates the thyroid to produce T4 and T3, which in turn negatively feedback to the pituitary.

Hypothyroidism (Primary)

The most common cause is Hashimoto's thyroiditis, an autoimmune disease. T-cells and autoantibodies (e.g., anti-TPO, anti-thyroglobulin) attack and destroy the thyroid gland. As the gland fails, T4/T3 levels fall. The loss of negative feedback causes the pituitary to secrete large amounts of TSH. The high TSH and low T4/T3 are the diagnostic hallmarks. The resulting low metabolic state causes symptoms of fatigue, cold intolerance, weight gain, and bradycardia.

Hyperthyroidism (Primary)

The most common cause is Graves' disease. This is also an autoimmune disease, but in this case, the body produces a stimulating autoantibody (Thyroid-Stimulating Immunoglobulin, or TSI). This TSI antibody *mimics* TSH and binds to the TSH receptor, "stepping on the gas" and causing the thyroid to grow and overproduce massive amounts of T4/T3. The high T4/T3 levels successfully suppress TSH, leading to the hallmark labs of a low TSH and high T4/T3. The resulting hypermetabolic state causes anxiety, tremor, palpitations, heat intolerance, and weight loss.

Diagnosis and Classification

The diagnostic algorithm begins with a single test: serum Thyroid-Stimulating Hormone (TSH).

High TSH

Indicates hypothyroidism. The algorithm proceeds to check a free T4 (thyroxine). A high TSH with a low free T4 confirms primary hypothyroidism. A high TSH with a normal free T4 is subclinical hypothyroidism.

Low TSH

Indicates hyperthyroidism (thyrotoxicosis). The algorithm proceeds to check a free T4 and T3. If elevated, the next step is a radioactive iodine uptake (RAIU) scan to determine etiology. A high, diffuse uptake indicates Graves' disease. A high, nodular uptake indicates a toxic adenoma or multinodular goiter. A low uptake indicates thyroiditis (release of pre-formed hormone) or exogenous hormone use.

Differential Diagnosis

The differential for hypothyroidism includes central hypothyroidism (pituitary failure, with a low TSH and low free T4) and euthyroid sick syndrome (abnormal thyroid function tests in a critically ill patient). The differential for hyperthyroidism symptoms (tachycardia, anxiety) includes anxiety disorders, pheochromocytoma, and stimulant use.

Treatment Algorithm

Hypothyroidism

The algorithm is one of hormone replacement. The drug of choice is levothyroxine (T4).

- **Step 1:** Initiate levothyroxine at a weight-based dose (approx. 1.6 mcg/kg/day in a young, healthy adult; lower doses in elderly or cardiac patients).
- **Step 2:** The patient must be instructed to take the medication on an empty stomach, 30-60 minutes before breakfast.
- **Step 3:** Re-check TSH in 6-8 weeks. The dose is titrated (increased or decreased by 12.5-25 mcg) to achieve a target TSH within the normal reference range. This process is repeated until the TSH is stable.

Table 4.2: Treatment Algorithms for Thyroid Dysfunction

Condition	Labs (TSH / Free T4)	Primary Treatment Algorithm
Overt Hypothyroidism	High TSH / Low T4	Levothyroxine (T4) replacement. Titrate dose based on TSH (target 0.4-4.0 mIU/L).
Subclinical Hypo	High TSH / Normal T4	Treat with Levothyroxine if TSH > 10, or if TSH 5-10 + symptoms/goiter/CV risk.
Hyperthyroidism (Graves')	Low TSH / High T4	**1.** Beta-blocker (symptom control). **2.** Antithyroid drugs (Methimazole) or Radioactive Iodine (RAI) or Surgery.

Hyperthyroidism (Graves' Disease)

The algorithm for Graves' disease (autoimmune hyperthyroidism) is three-step approach.

- **Symptom Control:** All symptomatic patients are started on a beta-blocker (e.g., propranolol, atenolol) to control tachycardia, tremor, and anxiety.
- **Definitive Therapy:** Patients are given a choice between three options:
  1. **Anti-thyroid Drugs (ATDs):** Methimazole (MMI) or propylthiouracil (PTU, preferred in 1st trimester of pregnancy). This algorithm aims for remission over 12-18 months.
  2. **Radioactive Iodine (RAI) Ablation:** A single dose of I-131 destroys the thyroid gland, leading to permanent hypothyroidism.
  3. **Thyroidectomy:** Surgical removal, reserved for patients with very large goiters, suspected malignancy, or contraindications to other therapies. The algorithm for toxic nodules or multinodular goiter is simpler, as these do not remit. The definitive treatment is RAI ablation or surgery.

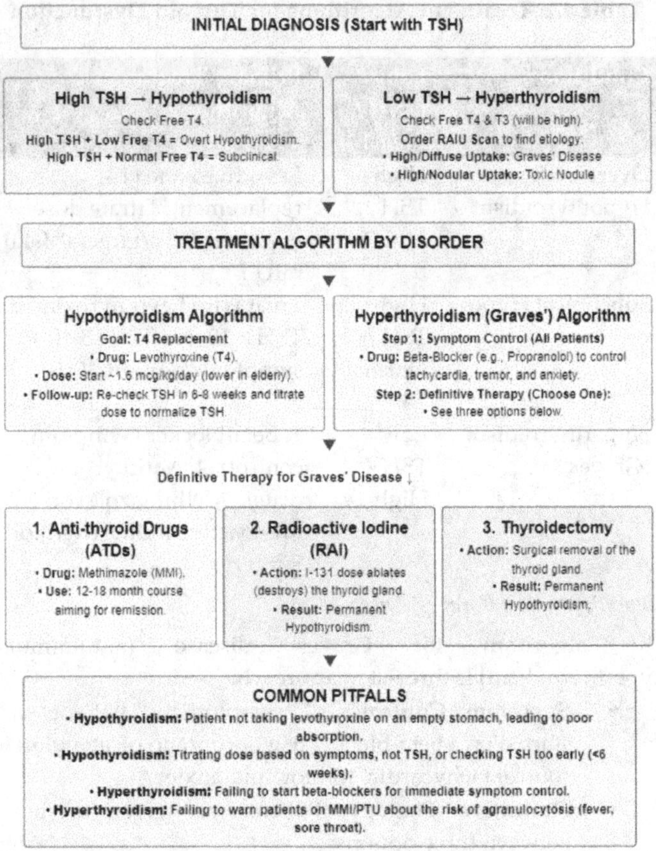

Figure 4.2: Thyroid Disorders

Monitoring and Follow-Up

For **hypothyroidism**, monitoring is simple. After initiating levothyroxine, the TSH should be re-checked in 6-8 weeks (the time it takes to reach a new steady state). The dose is then titrated (increased or decreased by 12.5-25 mcg) to achieve a TSH within the normal reference range (typically 0.5-4.5 mIU/L). Once stable, annual TSH monitoring is sufficient.

For **hyperthyroidism**, monitoring is more complex. If using anti-thyroid drugs (methimazole, PTU), TSH, free T4, and free T3 are monitored every 4-6 weeks to titrate the dose. LFTs and a

CBC must be monitored due to the rare but dangerous side effects of hepatotoxicity and agranulocytosis. If the patient undergoes radioactive iodine (RAI) ablation or surgery, they will become hypothyroid, and monitoring will then follow the hypothyroidism protocol (titrating levothyroxine to a normal TSH).

Long-Term Management / Secondary Prevention

For **hypothyroidism**, long-term management is lifelong replacement with levothyroxine, titrated to maintain a euthyroid state (normal TSH).

For **hyperthyroidism**, the long-term management involves choosing one of three definitive therapies: 1) **Anti-thyroid drugs (ATDs):** Methimazole (preferred) or PTU (used in 1st trimester of pregnancy). This is often used as a bridge to definitive therapy or for a 12-18 month trial in hopes of remission. 2) **Radioactive Iodine-131 (RAI):** The radioactive iodine is selectively absorbed by the overactive thyroid cells, destroying them. This is the most common definitive treatment in the US and leads to permanent hypothyroidism. 3. **Thyroidectomy:** Surgical removal of the gland, which also leads to permanent hypothyroidism. This is the preferred treatment for patients with very large goiters, co-existing cancer, or Graves' ophthalmopathy.

Patient Counseling Points

1. **Levothyroxine Timing (Hypo):** This is the most critical counseling point. Levothyroxine must be taken on an empty stomach, first thing in the morning, at least 30-60 minutes *before* any food, coffee, or other medications (especially calcium and iron, which block its absorption).
2. **Lifelong Therapy (Hypo):** Emphasize that this is a replacement hormone, not a "drug," and it will be required for life.
3. **Agranulocytosis (Hyper - ATDs):** This is a rare but life-threatening emergency. The patient must be counseled to *immediately stop* their methimazole or PTU and go to an ER for a CBC if they develop any fever or sore throat.
4. **RAI vs. Surgery (Hyper):** Explain that both definitive

treatments are excellent but will result in permanent hypothyroidism, which is easily managed with lifelong levothyroxine.

5. **Symptoms (Both):** Reassure the patient that their symptoms (fatigue, anxiety, etc.) are a direct result of the hormone imbalance and will resolve completely once a euthyroid state is achieved with treatment.

Common Pitfalls in Management

In hypothyroidism, a common pitfall is inconsistent absorption of levothyroxine due to co-administration with food, coffee, calcium, or iron. Another is titrating the dose based on symptoms rather than the TSH, or checking the TSH too soon (e.g., at 2 weeks) before a steady state is reached. In hyperthyroidism, a critical error is failing to initiate beta-blockers for symptom control while awaiting definitive therapy. A major safety pitfall is failing to warn patients on MMI or PTU about the rare but life-threatening side effect of agranulocytosis.

Case Study

A 42-year-old female (Ms. Brown) presents with a 6-month history of profound fatigue, 15-lb weight gain, constipation, and "always feeling cold." Her TSH is **14.2 mIU/L** (Ref: 0.4-4.0) and her Free T4 is **0.6 ng/dL** (Ref: 0.8-1.8).

Discussion

The clinical picture (fatigue, weight gain, cold intolerance) is classic for hypothyroidism. The labs—a **high TSH** (pituitary is "shouting") and a **low Free T4** (thyroid is not "listening")—confirm a diagnosis of **Primary Hypothyroidism**. The algorithm is hormone replacement.

Treatment Algorithm

1. **Diagnosis:** Primary Hypothyroidism.
2. **Algorithm (Replacement):** The drug of choice is **Levothyroxine (T4)**.
3. **Dosing:** The standard starting dose for a healthy adult is ~1.6 mcg/kg/day. The patient weighs 70 kg (154 lbs).
    - 70 kg * 1.6 mcg/kg = 112 mcg.

    - You select a common starting dose of **Levothyroxine 100 mcg daily**.
4. **Counseling:** You provide critical counseling: "Take this pill on an empty stomach, first thing in the morning, with only water. Wait at least 30-60 minutes before eating, drinking coffee, or taking other pills (especially calcium or iron)."
5. **Follow-up:** The algorithm dictates re-checking TSH in **6-8 weeks** (not sooner) to assess the dose.

Outcome

Ms. Brown starts Levothyroxine 100 mcg daily. You will titrate this dose (e.g., to 112 mcg or 125 mcg) based on her 6-week follow-up TSH, with the goal of normalizing her TSH level.

ADRENAL DISORDERS

Adrenal disorders involve dysfunction of the adrenal cortex, leading to imbalances in cortisol, aldosterone, and androgens. The primary algorithms concern adrenal insufficiency (Addison's) and cortisol excess (Cushing's).

Pathophysiology

Adrenal Insufficiency (Addison's Disease)

This is a state of cortisol deficiency. Primary insufficiency (Addison's) is the autoimmune destruction of the entire adrenal cortex. This leads to a deficiency of *both* cortisol and aldosterone. The lack of cortisol causes fatigue, weight loss, and hypoglycemia. The lack of aldosterone (which normally saves sodium and excretes potassium) leads to hyponatremia, hyperkalemia, and hypotension. The HPA axis is intact, so the pituitary secretes high levels of ACTH in a futile attempt to stimulate the dead gland.

Cushing's Syndrome

This is a state of chronic cortisol excess. The pathophysiology is divided by cause. It can be **ACTH-independent** (e.g., an adrenal adenoma autonomously secreting cortisol; ACTH is suppressed) or, more commonly, **ACTH-dependent**. This is usually caused by a pituitary adenoma secreting ACTH (Cushing's *disease*) or, rarely, an ectopic tumor (e.g., small cell lung cancer) secreting ACTH. Chronic high cortisol creates the classic phenotype: central obesity, muscle wasting, "moon facies," a "buffalo hump," skin atrophy (easy bruising, striae), hypertension, and diabetes

Diagnosis

Adrenal Insufficiency (AI)

The diagnostic algorithm for suspected primary AI (Addison's disease) begins with an 8 AM serum cortisol and a plasma ACTH. A low cortisol with a high ACTH is diagnostic. If equivocal, an ACTH stimulation test (cosyntropin test) is performed; a failure of cortisol to rise (e.g., < 18 mcg/dL) confirms the diagnosis.

Cushing's Syndrome (Cortisol Excess)

The screening algorithm requires one of several tests: a 24-hour urine free cortisol, a late-night salivary cortisol, or a 1 mg overnight dexamethasone suppression test. A positive (abnormal) result on two different tests confirms hypercortisolism. The algorithm then proceeds to an ACTH level to determine the etiology (ACTH-dependent [pituitary/ectopic] vs. ACTH-independent [adrenal tumor]).

Differential Diagnosis

The differential for symptoms of adrenal insufficiency (fatigue, weakness, hypotension) is vast but includes chronic fatigue syndrome and hypothyroidism. The differential for Cushing's syndrome includes metabolic syndrome, polycystic ovary syndrome (PCOS), and exogenous glucocorticoid use, which is the most common cause of cushingoid features.

Treatment Algorithm

Adrenal Insufficiency (Addison's Disease)

The algorithm is one of hormone replacement.

- **Glucocorticoid Replacement:** Hydrocortisone is the drug of choice, given in 2-3 divided doses (e.g., 15 mg in AM, 5 mg in PM) to mimic the natural diurnal rhythm.

- **Mineralocorticoid Replacement:** Fludrocortisone is given once daily to replace aldosterone, with the dose titrated to normalize blood pressure and serum potassium.
- **Stress Dosing:** This is a critical part of the algorithm. Patients must be educated to double or triple their glucocorticoid dose during times of illness (e.g., fever, infection). For severe stress (e.g., surgery, trauma, vomiting), parenteral hydrocortisone is required.

Table 4.3: Management of Adrenal Disorders

Disorder	Pathophysiology	Treatment Algorithm
Primary Adrenal Insufficiency (Addison's)	Adrenal gland destruction. (Low Cortisol, Low Aldosterone)	Glucocorticoid (Hydrocortisone) + Mineralocorticoid (Fludrocortisone) replacement.
Secondary Adrenal Insufficiency	Pituitary failure. (Low Cortisol, Normal Aldosterone)	Glucocorticoid (Hydrocortisone) replacement ONLY.
Cushing's Syndrome	Excess cortisol.	Surgical Resection (pituitary adenoma or adrenal tumor). (Medical therapy if surgery fails).

Cushing's Syndrome

The algorithm is almost always surgical. The goal is to remove the source of cortisol overproduction.

- **Cushing's Disease (Pituitary Adenoma):** The first-line algorithm is transsphenoidal surgery to resect the pituitary adenoma.
- **Adrenal Adenoma:** The algorithm is laparoscopic adrenalectomy.

- **Ectopic ACTH Syndrome:** The algorithm involves locating and resecting the neuroendocrine tumor (e.g., in the lung or pancreas) that is producing ACTH. Medical therapy (e.g., ketoconazole, metyrapone) is reserved as a bridging therapy to surgery or for unresectable cases.

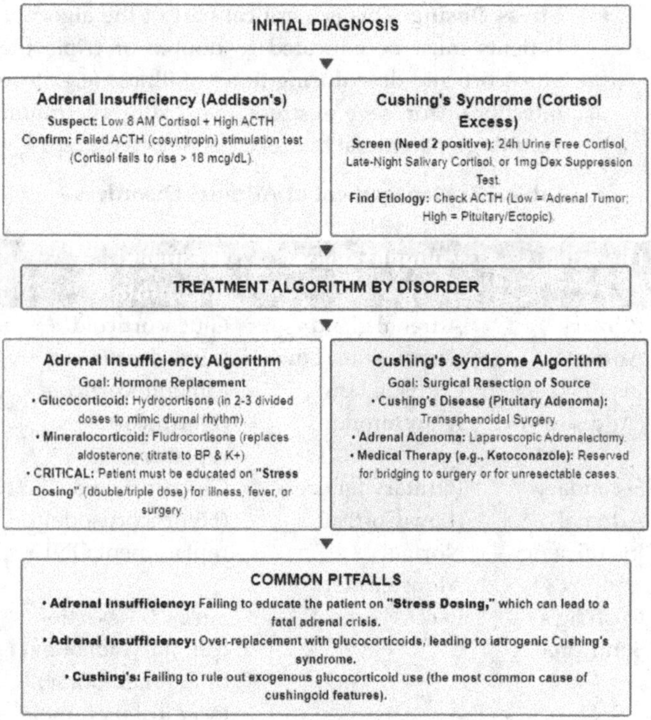
INITIAL DIAGNOSIS
Adrenal Insufficiency (Addison's)
Suspect: Low 8 AM Cortisol + High ACTH
Confirm: Failed ACTH (cosyntropin) stimulation test (Cortisol fails to rise > 18 mcg/dL).
Cushing's Syndrome (Cortisol Excess)
Screen (Need 2 positive): 24h Urine Free Cortisol, Late-Night Salivary Cortisol, or 1mg Dex Suppression Test.
Find Etiology: Check ACTH (Low = Adrenal Tumor; High = Pituitary/Ectopic).
TREATMENT ALGORITHM BY DISORDER
Adrenal Insufficiency Algorithm
Goal: Hormone Replacement
• Glucocorticoid: Hydrocortisone (in 2-3 divided doses to mimic diurnal rhythm).
• Mineralocorticoid: Fludrocortisone (replaces aldosterone; titrate to BP & K+).
• CRITICAL: Patient must be educated on "Stress Dosing" (double/triple dose) for illness, fever, or surgery.
Cushing's Syndrome Algorithm
Goal: Surgical Resection of Source
• Cushing's Disease (Pituitary Adenoma): Transsphenoidal Surgery.
• Adrenal Adenoma: Laparoscopic Adrenalectomy.
• Medical Therapy (e.g., Ketoconazole): Reserved for bridging to surgery or for unresectable cases.
COMMON PITFALLS
• Adrenal Insufficiency: Failing to educate the patient on "Stress Dosing," which can lead to a fatal adrenal crisis.
• Adrenal Insufficiency: Over-replacement with glucocorticoids, leading to iatrogenic Cushing's syndrome.
• Cushing's: Failing to rule out exogenous glucocorticoid use (the most common cause of cushingoid features).

Figure 4.3: Adrenal Disorders

Monitoring and Follow-Up

For **Adrenal Insufficiency**, monitoring is primarily clinical. Patients are monitored for symptoms of over-replacement (Cushingoid features) or under-replacement (fatigue, weight loss). Unlike thyroid disease, there is no simple lab test to monitor glucocorticoid replacement; doses are titrated to the lowest level that provides symptom relief. However, mineralocorticoid (fludrocortisone) replacement is monitored by checking blood pressure and electrolytes (sodium, potassium).

For **Cushing's Syndrome**, post-operative monitoring after removal of the adenoma is key. The patient will experience a period of temporary adrenal insufficiency (as the contralateral gland has atrophied) and will require replacement steroids for months to years. Long-term monitoring involves periodic (e.g., annual) 24-hour urine free cortisol or late-night salivary cortisol tests to screen for disease recurrence.

Long-Term Management / Secondary Prevention

For **Adrenal Insufficiency**, management is lifelong hormone replacement. This involves daily glucocorticoids (e.g., hydrocortisone, divided into 2-3 doses to mimic natural diurnal rhythm) and, for primary insufficiency, a mineralocorticoid (fludrocortisone). Secondary prevention is focused on preventing an "adrenal crisis" (see counseling points).

For **Cushing's Syndrome**, the primary management is surgical resection of the causative tumor (pituitary, adrenal, or ectopic). If surgery fails or is not possible, medical therapy (e.g., ketoconazole, metyrapone, pasireotide) may be used to block steroid production.

Patient Counseling Points

1. **Stress Dosing (Adrenal Insufficiency):** This is the single most important life-saving counseling point. The body normally makes extra cortisol during stress (e.g., fever, flu, surgery). These patients cannot. They must be taught to *double* or *triple* their oral glucocorticoid dose during minor illness.
2. **Emergency Injection (Adrenal Insufficiency):** Patients must have an emergency kit with an injectable form of hydrocortisone or dexamethasone. They and their family must be taught how to give this injection if the patient is vomiting and unable to take their oral "stress dose," or if they are found unresponsive.
3. **Medical Alert Bracelet (Adrenal Insufficiency):** All patients must wear a medical alert bracelet or necklace

stating "Adrenal Insufficiency - Needs Steroids."

4. **Steroid Replacement (Cushing's):** For post-operative Cushing's patients, they must understand why they now need to *take* steroids when their problem was *too many* steroids. Explain that their healthy adrenal glands are "asleep" and need time to wake up, so they are taking replacement doses, not suppressive doses.

Common Pitfalls in Management

In adrenal insufficiency, the most life-threatening pitfall is the failure to educate the patient on stress dosing, which can lead to a fatal adrenal crisis. Over-replacement with glucocorticoids, in an attempt to improve "well-being," is also common and leads to iatrogenic Cushing's syndrome. In Cushing's syndrome, the most common pitfall is a diagnostic one, failing to recognize the clinical features or performing screening tests incorrectly (e.g., a patient on an oral contraceptive having a false-positive dexamethasone suppression test).

Case Study

A 35-year-old male (Mr. Wale) presents with a 3-month history of progressive weakness, fatigue, 10-lb weight loss, salt cravings, and new, diffuse skin hyperpigmentation. His BP is 90/60 mmHg. Labs show: Na+ 128 (low), K+ 5.4 (high). An 8 AM cortisol level is **1.8 mcg/dL** (very low), and his plasma ACTH is **250 pg/mL** (very high).

Discussion

The clinical picture (hypotension, hyperpigmentation) and labs (hyponatremia, hyperkalemia, a very low cortisol with a very high ACTH) are the classic presentation for **Primary Adrenal Insufficiency (Addison's Disease)**. The high ACTH confirms the adrenal gland itself is the problem. He is deficient in both glucocorticoids (cortisol) and mineralocorticoids (aldosterone).

Treatment Algorithm

1. **Diagnosis:** Primary Adrenal Insufficiency (Addison's Disease).
2. **Algorithm (Hormone Replacement):**
   - **Glucocorticoid:** Start **Hydrocortisone 15 mg in the AM** and **5 mg in the PM** to mimic the body's natural diurnal rhythm.
   - **Mineralocorticoid:** Start **Fludrocortisone 0.1 mg daily** to replace aldosterone (this will correct his sodium, potassium, and BP).
3. **Critical Counseling ("Stress Dosing"):** You must provide life-saving education:
   - "You must **double or triple** your hydrocortisone dose if you have a fever, flu, or significant illness."
   - "You must have an emergency **hydrocortisone injection kit** and be trained to use it if you are vomiting and cannot take your pills."
   - He is given a medical alert bracelet.

Outcome

Mr. Wale is started on lifelong replacement therapy. His follow-up will focus on clinical symptoms (managing fatigue) and monitoring his BP and electrolytes (to titrate his fludrocortisone).

METABOLIC SYNDROME

Metabolic Syndrome is not a single disease but a clustering of at-risk cardiovascular risk factors: central obesity, dyslipidemia (high triglycerides, low HDL), elevated blood pressure, and hyperglycemia. The treatment algorithm is a multi-pronged, aggressive risk-reduction strategy.

Pathophysiology

The main pathophysiological driver is **insulin resistance**, which is promoted by central (visceral) adiposity. Visceral fat is metabolically active and pro-inflammatory, releasing adipokines and free fatty acids that impair insulin signaling in the liver and muscle. This insulin resistance directly causes hyperglycemia, and the liver's response to it (increased VLDL production) drives the characteristic dyslipidemia (high TGs, low HDL).

Diagnosis

Diagnosis is made by the presence of three or more of the five following criteria (NCEP-ATP III guidelines):

1. Abdominal Obesity (Waist circumference > 102 cm/40 in for men, > 88 cm/35 in for women)
2. High Triglycerides (≥ 150 mg/dL)
3. Low HDL Cholesterol (< 40 mg/dL for men, < 50 mg/dL for women)
4. Elevated Blood Pressure (≥ 130/85 mmHg or on antihypertensive medication)
5. Elevated Fasting Glucose (≥ 100 mg/dL or on diabetes medication)

Differential Diagnosis

The main differential is Cushing's syndrome, which can present with an identical cluster of findings. Polycystic ovary syndrome (PCOS) in women also has significant metabolic overlap. Exogenous obesity without the associated metabolic derangements must also be distinguished.

Treatment Algorithm

The algorithm is a simultaneous attack on all components.

- **Step 1 (Foundation):** The cornerstone of the algorithm is intensive therapeutic lifestyle change. This includes a 7-10% weight loss goal, a heart-healthy diet (e.g., Mediterranean diet), and at least 150 minutes of moderate-intensity exercise per week.
- **Step 2 (Pharmacological Algorithm):** Each component is treated to its respective guideline target.
    - **Hypertension:** Treated according to the hypertension algorithm (see Chapter 1), often with ACE inhibitors or ARBs, which may have metabolic benefits.
    - **Dyslipidemia:** High triglycerides are addressed first with lifestyle changes and, if severe, fibrates or high-dose omega-3 fatty acids. High LDL-C (often present, though not a diagnostic criterion) is treated with statins.
    - **Hyperglycemia/Insulin Resistance:** If the patient has pre-diabetes, metformin is the first-line agent. If they have overt T2DM, the algorithm follows T2DM guidelines (see 4.1.3.2), with GLP-1 RAs and SGLT2 inhibitors being highly effective as they also promote weight loss.
- **Step 3 (Bariatric Surgery):** For patients with refractory metabolic syndrome and significant obesity (e.g., BMI ≥ 35-40), bariatric surgery is a highly effective algorithm that can lead to remission of all components.

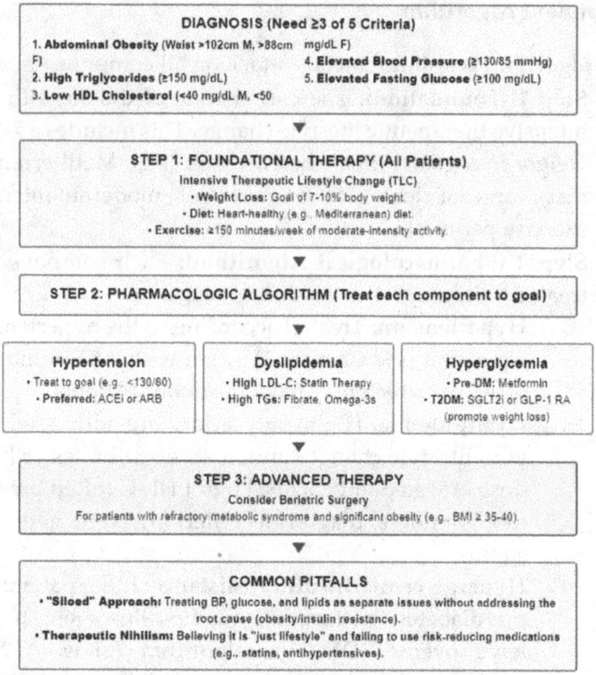

Figure 4.4: Metabolic Syndrome

Table 4.4: Clinical Algorithm for Metabolic Syndrome (NCEP ATP III)

Component	Diagnostic Threshold	Primary Management Goal
Abdominal Obesity	Waist > 102 cm (M), > 88 cm (F)	Weight loss (Diet, Exercise)
Triglycerides	≥ 150 mg/dL	Lifestyle, Fibrate, or Niacin
HDL-C	< 40 mg/dL (M), < 50 mg/dL (F)	Lifestyle, Niacin, or Fibrate
Blood Pressure	≥ 130/≥ 85 mmHg	Lifestyle, ACEi/ARB, CCB
Fasting Glucose	≥ 100 mg/dL (or T2DM)	Lifestyle, Metformin

Monitoring and Follow-Up

Monitoring is simply the periodic re-assessment of the five diagnostic components. This involves an annual check of waist circumference, blood pressure, fasting glucose, and a fasting lipid panel. Patients should also be screened for complications of the syndrome, such as non-alcoholic fatty liver disease (NAFLD/NASH) via LFTs or ultrasound, and obstructive sleep apnea.

Long-Term Management / Secondary Prevention

The primary goal is to prevent the two major outcomes: ASCVD and T2DM. The cornerstone of all management is **therapeutic lifestyle change (TLC)**.

1. **Lifestyle:** The primary intervention is weight loss (7-10% of body weight) through a combination of caloric restriction and regular moderate-intensity exercise (e.g., 150 minutes/week). This is the *only* intervention that addresses the root-cause pathophysiology.
2. **Pharmacological Management:** After lifestyle, the algorithm dictates treating each component individually and aggressively:
    - **Hypertension:** Treat to goal (e.g., with an ACEi/ARB).
    - **Hyperlipidemia:** Treat with a statin (as these patients are high-risk for ASCVD).
    - **Hyperglycemia:** Treat with Metformin, which is the first-line choice as it also targets insulin resistance.
    - **Low HDL / High TGs:** These are best treated by lifestyle, statins, and glycemic control.

Patient Counseling Points

1. **Not a "Disease," but a "Risk State":** Explain that Metabolic Syndrome is a "warning sign" from their body that they are at a very high risk for a future heart attack, stroke, or diabetes.
2. **Weight Loss is the "Cure":** Emphasize that this is not just a collection of five problems to be treated with five

pills. It is one central problem (insulin resistance from visceral fat) that can be reversed. Counsel that even a modest 5-10% weight loss can dramatically improve or even resolve all five components.

3. **Waist Circumference:** Teach them that this is not about "vanity" but about health. Explain that waist circumference is a vital sign, just like blood pressure, that measures the "unhealthy" internal fat.
4. **Focus on Diet and Exercise:** This is the primary prescription. All other medications are secondary. Counsel on a heart-healthy diet (e.g., Mediterranean style) and the importance of 30 minutes of activity most days of the week.

Common Pitfalls in Management

The most common pitfall is a "siloed" approach, where a clinician treats the blood pressure, another treats the glucose, and no one addresses the underlying driver, which is obesity and insulin resistance. Another error is therapeutic nihilism, believing the condition is "just lifestyle" and failing to be aggressive with pharmacological interventions (e.g., statins, antihypertensives) that are proven to reduce cardiovascular risk.

Case Study

A 50-year-old female (Mrs. Garcia) presents for a new patient visit. She has no specific complaints but feels "tired." Her vitals: BP **142/88 mmHg.** Her waist circumference is **38 inches**. Her fasting labs are: Glucose **115 mg/dL**, Triglycerides **210 mg/dL**, and HDL **42 mg/dL**.

Discussion

You must check the patient against the 5 criteria for **Metabolic Syndrome** (needs ≥3):

Abdominal Obesity (Waist > 35 in for women): **Yes (38 in)**
High TGs (≥150): **Yes (210)**
Low HDL (< 50 for women): **Yes (42)**
Elevated BP (≥130/85): **Yes (142/88)**
Elevated Fasting Glucose (≥100): **Yes (115)**

Result

5/5 criteria met. The algorithm is a multi-step approach founded on lifestyle, with pharmacological therapy for each component.

Treatment Algorithm

1. **Diagnosis:** Metabolic Syndrome with Stage 1 HTN and Pre-diabetes.
2. **Algorithm Step 1 (Foundation):** The primary prescription is **Intensive Therapeutic Lifestyle Change**. You counsel her on a 7-10% weight loss goal, a Mediterranean diet, and 150 minutes of weekly exercise.
3. **Algorithm Step 2 (Pharmacology):** You must also treat each component to its guideline target.
    - **Hypertension:** Start **Lisinopril 10 mg daily** (an ACEi is a good choice in a patient with pre-diabetes).
    - **Hyperglycemia/Insulin Resistance:** Her glucose is in the pre-diabetes range. **Metformin 500 mg daily** is the appropriate first-line agent.
    - **Dyslipidemia:** Although her TGs are high, her ASCVD risk is high, and a statin is indicated. You start a **moderate-intensity statin (e.g., Atorvastatin 20 mg)**.

Outcome

Mrs. Garcia is diagnosed with Metabolic Syndrome and started on Metformin, Lisinopril, and Atorvastatin. The most important part of her follow-up will be tracking her weight loss and lifestyle adherence.

Summary

Diabetes Mellitus: T1DM is managed with a basal-bolus insulin replacement algorithm. T2DM is a stepwise algorithm starting with lifestyle and metformin, with subsequent agents (SGLT2i, GLP-1 RA) chosen based on cardiovascular and renal risk.

Thyroid Disorders: Hypothyroidism is a simple replacement algorithm, titrating levothyroxine to a target TSH. Hyperthyroidism (Graves' disease) is a three-pronged algorithm: beta-blockers for symptoms, plus a definitive choice of anti-thyroid drugs, radioactive iodine, or surgery.

Adrenal Disorders: Adrenal insufficiency requires lifelong glucocorticoid and mineralocorticoid replacement, with a critical "stress-dosing" algorithm. Cushing's syndrome is a surgical algorithm to resect the source of cortisol excess.

Metabolic Syndrome: This is a multi-pronged algorithm focused on aggressive lifestyle intervention (weight loss) and simultaneous pharmacological treatment of all components (hypertension, dyslipidemia, hyperglycemia) to reduce cardiovascular risk.

Multiple Choice Questions

1. A 30-year-old male is diagnosed with T1DM. He is starting a basal-bolus regimen. What is the purpose of his prandial (bolus) rapid-acting insulin?

   A) To suppress hepatic gluconeogenesis overnight.

   B) To cover the carbohydrates consumed in a meal.

   C) To replace aldosterone.

   D) To be used only if his blood sugar is above 200 mg/dL.

2. A 62-year-old female with T2DM (HbA1c 8.2% on metformin) has a history of a myocardial infarction. According to risk-based algorithms, which is the most appropriate second-line agent?

   A) Glipizide (a sulfonylurea)

   B) Sitagliptin (a DPP-4 inhibitor)

   C) Pioglitazone (a TZD)

   D) Liraglutide (a GLP-1 receptor agonist)

3. A 50-year-old is diagnosed with primary hypothyroidism. After initiating levothyroxine, when is the earliest the TSH should be re-checked to assess the algorithm's steady state? A) 3-5 days

   B) 1-2 weeks

   C) 6-8 weeks

   D) 6-8 months

4. A 35-year-old female is diagnosed with Graves' disease and has severe palpitations and tremor. What is the most appropriate initial pharmacological agent to add to her algorithm?

   A) Methimazole

   B) Propranolol

   C) Levothyroxine

   D) Radioactive iodine (I-131)

5. The diagnostic algorithm for suspected primary adrenal insufficiency (Addison's) is confirmed by:

   A) A high 8 AM cortisol and a high ACTH.

   B) A low 8 AM cortisol and a low ACTH.

   C) A failed ACTH (cosyntropin) stimulation test.

D) A positive 1 mg dexamethasone suppression test.

6. A patient with Cushing's syndrome is found to have a high ACTH level. This finding in the algorithm points to what source?
   A) An adrenal adenoma
   B) Exogenous steroid use
   C) A pituitary adenoma or ectopic ACTH source
   D) Addison's disease
7. Which of the following is not one of the 5 criteria in the diagnostic algorithm for Metabolic Syndrome?
   A) Elevated fasting glucose
   B) High HDL cholesterol
   C) High triglycerides
   D) Abdominal obesity
8. A life-threatening pitfall in the management of adrenal insufficiency is:
   A) Failing to replace mineralocorticoids.
   B) Failing to educate the patient on stress dosing.
   C) Titrating hydrocortisone to the TSH level.
   D) Checking a late-night salivary cortisol.
9. A 60-year-old male with T2DM on metformin and glipizide is found to have new-onset HFrEF. Which agent in his regimen is now prioritized by the HF algorithm?
   A) Metformin
   B) Glipizide
   C) An SGLT2 inhibitor (e.g., dapagliflozin)
   D) Basal insulin
10. The first-line, foundational algorithm for all components of metabolic syndrome is:
    A) Initiation of metformin
    B) Initiation of a statin
    C) Bariatric surgery
    D) Intensive therapeutic lifestyle change

Self-Assessment Questions

1. Describe the basal-bolus insulin algorithm for T1DM, including the purpose of an insulin-to-carbohydrate ratio (ICR) and an insulin sensitivity factor (ISF).
2. A 55-year-old with T2DM and an HbA1c of 8.5% on metformin also has HFrEF (LVEF 30%). What is the mandatory next step in the pharmacological algorithm?
3. A 40-year-old female has a TSH of 15.0 mIU/L and a low free T4. Outline the 3-step algorithm for initiating and titrating her therapy.
4. What are the three definitive treatment algorithms for a patient with newly diagnosed Graves' disease, and what is the universal first-line symptomatic therapy?
5. A patient with known Addison's disease develops a fever of 102°F. What is the "stress-dosing" algorithm they must follow?
6. A patient has two positive screening tests for Cushing's syndrome. What is the next diagnostic test in the algorithm, and how does it bifurcate the subsequent workup?
7. Define the 5 diagnostic criteria for Metabolic Syndrome.
8. Why is it considered a pitfall to use a "siloed" approach in managing metabolic syndrome?
9. A patient's TSH is 0.01 mIU/L, and their free T4 is high. The radioactive iodine uptake scan shows 0% uptake. What are the two most likely diagnoses?
10. Identify two common pitfalls in the management of T2DM, one related to clinical inertia and one related to comorbidity management.

Bibliography

1. American Diabetes Association. 9. Pharmacological Approaches to Glycemic Treatment: Standards of Care in Diabetes—2024. Diabetes Care. 2024 Jan 1;47(Suppl 1):S158–S178.
2. American Diabetes Association. 6. Glycemic Targets: Standards of Care in Diabetes—2024. Diabetes Care. 2024 Jan 1;47(Suppl 1):S111–S125.
3. Zinman B, Wanner C, Lachin JM, Fitchett D, Bluhmki E, Hantel S, et al. Empagliflozin, Cardiovascular Outcomes, and Mortality in Type 2 Diabetes. N Engl J Med. 2015 Nov 26;373(22):2117–28.
4. Marso SP, Daniels GH, Brown-Frandsen K, Kristensen P, Mann JFE, Nauck MA, et al. Liraglutide and Cardiovascular Outcomes in Type 2 Diabetes. N Engl J Med. 2016 Jul 28;375(4):311–22.
5. Garber AJ, Handelsman Y, Grunberger G, Einhorn D, Abrahamson MJ, Barzilay JI, et al. Consensus Statement by the American Association of Clinical Endocrinologists and American College of Endocrinology on the Comprehensive Type 2 Diabetes Management Algorithm - 2020 Executive Summary. Endocr Pract. 2020 Jan;26(1):107–39.
6. Jonklaas J, Bianco AC, Bauer AJ, Burman KD, Cappola AR, Celi FS, et al. Guidelines for the Treatment of Hypothyroidism: Prepared by the American Thyroid Association Task Force on Thyroid Hormone Replacement. Thyroid. 2014 Dec;24(12):1670–751.
7. Ross DS, Burch HB, Cooper DS, Greenlee MC, Laurberg P, Maia AL, et al. 2016 American Thyroid Association Guidelines for Diagnosis and Management of Hyperthyroidism and Other Causes of Thyrotoxicosis. Thyroid. 2016 Oct;26(10):1343–1421.
8. Bornstein SR, Allolio B, Arlt W, Barthel A, Don-Wauchope A, Hammer GD, et al. Diagnosis and Treatment of Primary Adrenal Insufficiency: An Endocrine Society Clinical Practice Guideline. J Clin Endocrinol Metab. 2016 Feb;101(2):364–89.
9. Nieman LK, Biller BMK, Findling JW, Murad MH, Newell-Price J, Savage MO, et al. Treatment of Cushing's Syndrome: An Endocrine Society Clinical Practice Guideline. J Clin Endocrinol Metab. 2015 Aug;100(8):2807–31.
10. Grundy SM, Cleeman JI, Daniels SR, Donato KA, Eckel RH, Franklin BA, et al. Diagnosis and Management of the Metabolic Syndrome: An American Heart Association/National Heart, Lung, and Blood Institute Scientific Statement. Circulation. 2005 Oct 25;112(17):2735–52.
11. UK Prospective Diabetes Study (UKPDS) Group. Intensive blood-glucose control with sulphonylureas or insulin compared with conventional treatment and risk of complications in patients with type 2 diabetes (UKPDS 33). Lancet. 1998 Sep 12;352(9131):837–53.
12. Davies MJ, D'Alessio DA, Fradkin J, Kernan WN, Kunz M, Roslynn M, et al. Management of Hyperglycemia in Type 2 Diabetes, 2018. A Consensus Report by the American Diabetes Association (ADA) and the European Association for the Study of Diabetes (EASD). Diabetes Care. 2018 Dec;41(12):2669–2701.
13. McMurray JJV, Solomon SD, Inzucchi SE, Køber L, Kosiborod MN, Martinez FA, et al. Dapagliflozin in Patients with Heart Failure and

Reduced Ejection Fraction. N Engl J Med. 2019 Nov 21;381(21):1995–2008.

14. Funder JW, Carey RM, Mantero F, Murad MH, Reincke M, Shibata H, et al. The Management of Primary Aldosteronism: Case Detection, Diagnosis, and Treatment: An Endocrine Society Clinical Practice Guideline. J Clin Endocrinol Metab. 2016 May;101(5):1889–916.
15. Whitlock G, Lewington S, Sherliker P, Clarke R, Emberson J, Halsey J, et al. Body-mass index and cause-specific mortality in 900 000 adults: collaborative analyses of 57 prospective studies. Lancet. 2009 Mar 28;373(9669):1083–96.

CHAPTER 5

TREATMENT ALGORITHMS FOR NEUROLOGICAL DISORDERS

Author

Mrs. Nagalakshmi Konarachapalle, Associate Professor, Department of Pharmaceutical Chemistry, Annamacharya College of Pharmacy, Rajampet, Andhra Pradesh, India

Abstract

Neurological treatment algorithms are highly time-sensitive and etiology-specific, aimed at preventing neuronal death, controlling abnormal signaling, or slowing progressive degeneration. The algorithm for acute ischemic stroke is one of emergency reperfusion, stratified by time from onset, using intravenous thrombolysis (alteplase) within 4.5 hours or mechanical thrombectomy up to 24 hours for large vessel occlusions. The epilepsy algorithm is stratified by seizure type (focal vs. generalized), with the goal of achieving seizure freedom via first-line monotherapy (e.g., levetiracetam, valproate); failure leads to a stepwise trial of alternative or adjunctive agents. The status epilepticus algorithm is a rapid, timed protocol beginning with benzodiazepines. Multiple sclerosis management is bifurcated: acute relapses are treated with high-dose corticosteroids, while the long-term algorithm involves early initiation of disease-modifying therapies (DMTs), selected based on an "escalation" vs. "induction" strategy. Parkinson's disease follows a symptomatic algorithm, initiating therapy with MAO-B inhibitors or dopamine agonists in younger patients, and progressing to levodopa/carbidopa as the gold standard for motor control, with adjunctive therapies to manage motor fluctuations. Alzheimer's disease management is currently symptomatic, using cholinesterase inhibitors (e.g., donepezil) for mild-to-moderate stages and memantine for moderate-to-severe disease to modestly improve cognition and function.

Keywords: *Neurological Algorithms, Stroke, Epilepsy, Multiple Sclerosis, Parkinson's Disease, Alzheimer's Disease*

Learning Objectives

After completion of the chapter, the learners should be able to:

- Identify the critical time window for alteplase (tPA) administration in the treatment algorithm for acute ischemic stroke.
- Explain the rationale for selecting a first-line anti-epileptic drug based on seizure type (e.g., focal vs. generalized vs. absence).
- Select an appropriate therapeutic algorithm (e.g., abortive vs. prophylactic) for a patient with chronic migraines.
- Differentiate the treatment algorithms for acute multiple sclerosis relapses versus long-term disease-modifying therapy.
- Justify the sequencing of pharmacological agents (e.g., levodopa vs. dopamine agonists) in the management of Parkinson's disease based on patient age and symptoms

STROKE

A stroke is a medical emergency characterized by a sudden interruption of the blood supply to the brain, causing neurologic deficits. The treatment algorithm is one of the most time-sensitive in medicine, as "time is brain."

Pathophysiology

Stroke is a clinical syndrome of acute focal neurologic deficit caused by a vascular event. The pathophysiology is dichotomous, defining the two major types of stroke.

Ischemic Stroke (80-85%)

The core pathophysiology is the abrupt cessation of blood flow to a region of the brain, leading to infarction. This occlusion is typically thrombotic (an atherosclerotic plaque ruptures within a cerebral artery) or embolic (a clot, often from the heart in atrial fibrillation, travels to and lodges in a cerebral artery). The brain tissue at the center of the occlusion, the "ischemic core," dies within minutes. Surrounding this core is the "penumbra," a region of dysfunctional but viable tissue maintained by collateral circulation. The entire acute treatment algorithm is based on salvaging this penumbra before it, too, infarcts.

Hemorrhagic Stroke (15-20%)

The pathophysiology is not ischemia, but direct tissue damage from an expanding hematoma and the toxic effects of blood components. **Intracerebral Hemorrhage (ICH)** is most often caused by chronic hypertension leading to rupture of small, deep-penetrating arteries (e.g., lenticulostriate). **Subarachnoid Hemorrhage (SAH)** is typically due to the rupture of a saccular "berry" aneurysm at an arterial bifurcation in the Circle of Willis. In both, the expanding blood collection causes a toxic injury and increases intracranial pressure (ICP), which can lead to herniation and death.

Diagnosis and Classification

The diagnostic algorithm begins with rapid clinical recognition of symptoms (e.g., F.A.S.T. - Face, Arms, Speech, Time). Upon emergency department arrival, the algorithm mandates an immediate non-contrast head CT scan. This imaging is the critical first branch point, differentiating:

- **Ischemic Stroke (85%):** Caused by a thrombus or embolus. The CT scan is typically normal in the first few hours.
- **Hemorrhagic Stroke (15%):** Caused by bleeding into the brain (intracerebral) or surrounding space (subarachnoid). The CT scan immediately shows hyperdense (white) blood. A Transient Ischemic Attack (TIA) is a transient stroke syndrome without acute infarction; its algorithm is one of urgent secondary prevention.

Differential Diagnosis

Stroke "mimics" are common. The differential diagnosis includes seizure with post-ictal paralysis (Todd's paralysis), complex migraine (hemiplegic migraine), hypoglycemia, systemic infection with sepsis-associated encephalopathy, and Bell's palsy (for isolated facial droop). A non-contrast head CT and a point-of-care glucose test are the fastest tools to navigate this differential.

Treatment Algorithm

Acute Ischemic Stroke Algorithm

This algorithm is strictly time-dependent.

- **Intravenous Thrombolysis:** Patients presenting within a 4.5-hour window from "last known normal" who have no contraindications (e.g., active bleeding, recent major surgery, uncontrolled hypertension) are candidates for intravenous alteplase (tPA). The "door-to-needle" time goal is < 60 minutes.
- **Mechanical Thrombectomy:** Patients with a large vessel occlusion (LVO) in the proximal anterior circulation are candidates for endovascular thrombectomy. The algorithm allows for this intervention up to 24 hours from last known normal, based on advanced imaging (CT perfusion) that identifies a salvageable penumbra.
- **General Measures:** All patients require blood pressure management (permissive hypertension, e.g., < 185/110 mmHg for tPA, < 220/120 mmHg if no tPA) and supportive care.

Secondary Prevention Algorithm

After the acute phase, the algorithm shifts to preventing recurrence. This includes:

- **Antiplatelet Therapy:** Aspirin is given acutely. For minor strokes or TIA, dual antiplatelet therapy (DAPT) with aspirin and clopidogrel is given for 21-90 days, followed by antiplatelet monotherapy.
- **Anticoagulation:** If the stroke is determined to be cardioembolic (e.g., from atrial fibrillation), antiplatelet therapy is transitioned to long-term anticoagulation.
- **Statin Therapy:** All patients with ischemic stroke, regardless of baseline LDL, are started on high-intensity statin therapy (e.g., atorvastatin 80 mg).
- **Risk Factor Control:** Aggressive management of hypertension, diabetes, and lifestyle factors is initiated.

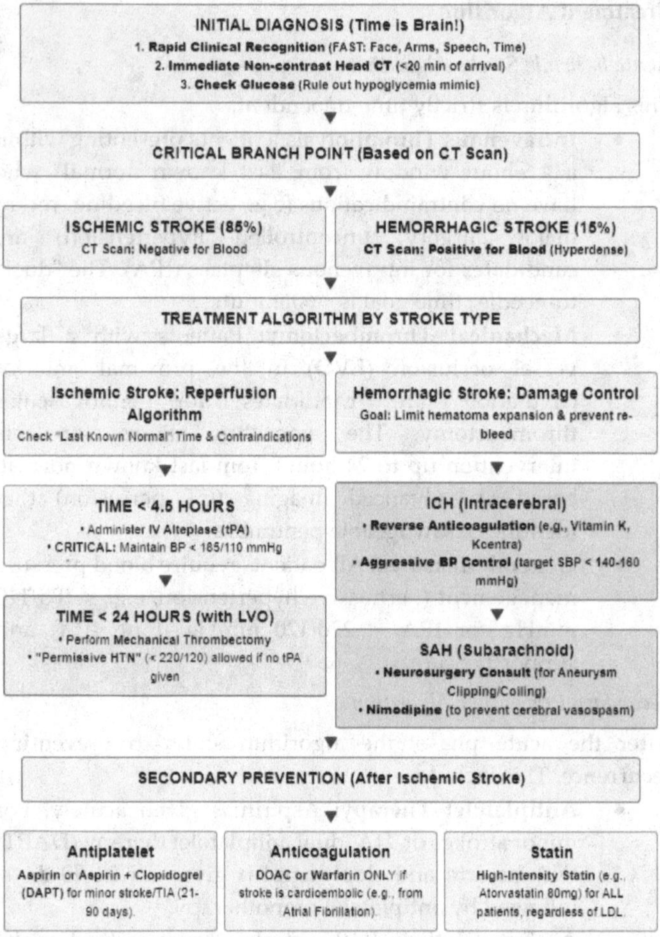

Figure 5.1: Stroke

Monitoring and Follow-Up

Ischemic Stroke

Post-reperfusion monitoring is critical.

- Post-tPA: The patient must be monitored in an ICU or stroke unit. Neurologic checks (using the NIHSS) and vital signs are required every 15 minutes for 2 hours, then every 30 minutes for 6 hours, then hourly for 16 hours. The primary focus is monitoring for hemorrhagic conversion (worsening NIHSS, severe headache, N/V), which requires an emergent head CT. Blood pressure must be meticulously kept below 180/105 mmHg.

- Post-Thrombectomy: Monitoring involves frequent neuro checks and vital signs, as well as puncture site (e.g., femoral) checks for bleeding or hematoma.

Table 5.1: Acute Stroke Management Algorithms

Stroke Type	Diagnostic Test	Immediate Treatment Algorithm
Ischemic (Acute)	Non-contrast Head CT (to exclude bleed)	**If < 4.5 hrs:** IV Alteplase (tPA). **If Large Vessel Occlusion (LVO):** Mechanical Thrombectomy (up to 24 hrs).
Hemorrhagic (ICH)	Non-contrast Head CT	**Reverse** anticoagulation. **Aggressive BP control** (e.g., target SBP < 140-160 mmHg). Surgical consultation.
TIA / Stroke (Secondary Prevention)	MRI, CTA/MRA, Echo	Antiplatelet (Aspirin + Clopidogrel x 21d then monotherapy), High-intensity Statin, BP control.

Hemorrhagic Stroke

Monitoring is focused on ICP and hematoma expansion. Patients are managed in a neuro-ICU with continuous ICP monitoring (if an external ventricular drain is placed), frequent neurologic exams (GCS), and serial head CT scans to ensure the hematoma is not expanding. Blood pressure must be aggressively controlled. For SAH, monitoring also involves screening for cerebral vasospasm (usually 4-14 days post-bleed) using transcranial dopplers.

Long-Term Management / Secondary Prevention

Secondary prevention is the cornerstone of long-term stroke care and is tailored to the stroke's etiology.

Ischemic Stroke

- Cardioembolic (e.g., Atrial Fibrillation): Long-term management is therapeutic anticoagulation (e.g., with a DOAC like apixaban or rivaroxaban).
- Large Artery Atherosclerosis (e.g., Carotid Stenosis): Management includes high-intensity statin therapy, antiplatelet therapy (e.g., aspirin + clopidogrel), and potential carotid endarterectomy or stenting for significant stenosis.
- Small Vessel (Lacunar): Management is strict blood pressure control and an antiplatelet agent.
- Universal: All ischemic stroke survivors require aggressive management of risk factors: hypertension (BP goal < 130/80), hyperlipidemia (high-intensity statin), diabetes, and smoking cessation.

Hemorrhagic Stroke

Management is focused on preventing re-bleeding. For SAH, this involves definitive neurosurgical (clipping) or endovascular (coiling) treatment of the ruptured aneurysm. For ICH, the focus is on aggressive, long-term blood pressure control (e.g., target < 130/80 mmHg).

Patient Counseling Points

1. **"Time is Brain":** This is the most critical counseling point for the patient and their family. They must be taught to recognize the F.A.S.T. (Face drooping, Arm weakness, Speech difficulty, Time to call emergency services) signs and to call emergency services *immediately*. Counsel them *not* to "wait and see" or "drive to the hospital."
2. **Risk Factor Modification:** "A stroke is a 'brain attack,' and it is a warning." Emphasize that the risk of a *second* stroke is extremely high and that controlling blood pressure, cholesterol, and blood sugar (and stopping

smoking) is not optional, but essential for survival.

3. **Anticoagulation vs. Antiplatelet:** For patients with AFib, explain the difference. "An aspirin is not enough. Your stroke came from a clot from your heart, which requires a 'blood thinner' (anticoagulant) to prevent. An antiplatelet is for clots from plaque in the arteries."
4. **Rehabilitation:** Frame rehabilitation (PT, OT, speech therapy) as the active, primary treatment for recovery. Emphasize that neurologic recovery is a long process that requires intensive work and participation.

Common Pitfalls in Management

The most critical pitfall is a delay in diagnosis or treatment, resulting in a missed tPA or thrombectomy window. Another is violating tPA contraindications, leading to hemorrhagic transformation. In secondary prevention, a common error is failing to screen for atrial fibrillation (e.g., with prolonged cardiac monitoring), thereby missing an indication for anticoagulation. Misdiagnosing a stroke mimic *as* a stroke can lead to unnecessary and harmful tPA administration.

Case Study

A 68-year-old female (Ms. Johnson) is at home when she suddenly develops slurred speech and a complete right-sided facial droop and arm weakness. Her husband calls emergency services immediately. She arrives at the ED **60 minutes after symptom onset**. Her BP is 175/98 mmHg.

Discussion

This is a classic acute stroke presentation, well within the "golden hour." The algorithm is "Time is Brain." The immediate priority is to get a non-contrast head CT to differentiate ischemic from hemorrhagic stroke, as this is the main branch point of the entire algorithm.

Treatment Algorithm

1. **Triage:** A "Stroke Alert" is called. The patient is taken directly to the CT scanner.
2. **Algorithm Step 1 (Imaging):** A **Non-Contrast Head**

CT is completed. It is **NEGATIVE for any bleeding.**

3. **Diagnosis:** This confirms an **Acute Ischemic Stroke.**
4. **Algorithm Step 2 (Reperfusion):**
   - **Time:** Her "last known normal" is 60 minutes ago, placing her well within the **4.5-hour window for thrombolysis.**
   - **Contraindications:** She has no contraindications. Her BP is <185/110 mmHg.
   - **Therapy:** The algorithm dictates immediate IV **Alteplase (tPA).**
5. **Monitoring:** She is admitted to the Stroke Unit for close neurologic and blood pressure monitoring.

Outcome

Ms. Johnson receives IV tPA at 75 minutes after symptom onset. Over the next 24 hours, her arm strength and speech begin to improve significantly

EPILEPSY

Epilepsy is a chronic neurological disorder characterized by an enduring predisposition to generate epileptic seizures. A diagnosis of epilepsy requires at least two unprovoked seizures occurring > 24 hours apart.

Pathophysiology

A seizure is a transient occurrence of signs/symptoms due to abnormal, excessive, or synchronous neuronal activity in the brain. The core pathophysiology is a state of **neuronal hyperexcitability**. This is caused by an imbalance between excitatory (glutamatergic) and inhibitory (GABAergic) neurotransmission. This imbalance can arise from many causes: genetic mutations in ion channels (channelopathies), structural brain lesions (e.g., tumors, scars from a prior stroke or trauma), or metabolic/autoimmune processes. A "seizure focus" is a region of the brain where this hyperexcitability begins. A focal seizure remains localized to one hemisphere, while a generalized seizure involves and spreads to both hemispheres from the onset.

Diagnosis and Classification

The diagnostic algorithm begins with a detailed clinical history of the seizure event (semiology) and a neurologic exam. An electroencephalogram (EEG) is used to look for interictal epileptiform discharges, and brain imaging (MRI) is used to search for a structural etiology. The algorithm then classifies the epilepsy type, which is the most critical step for treatment selection:

Focal Onset

Seizures originating in one hemisphere (e.g., focal aware, focal impaired awareness).

Generalized Onset

Seizures originating in and rapidly engaging bilateral networks (e.g., absence, tonic-clonic, myoclonic).

Unknown Onset

Insufficient evidence to classify.

Differential Diagnosis

The primary differential is syncope (cardiovascular vs. vasovagal), which is characterized by a brief loss of consciousness with a rapid recovery, unlike the typical post-ictal confusion of a seizure. Other main differentials include complex migraines, TIAs, and psychogenic non-epileptic seizures (PNES), a psychiatric condition that requires video-EEG monitoring to diagnose.

Treatment Algorithm

Chronic Epilepsy Algorithm

The goal is seizure freedom with minimal side effects.

- **Step 1: First-Line Monotherapy:** An anti-seizure medication (ASM) is chosen based on the epilepsy type.
    - **Focal Epilepsy:** First-line agents include levetiracetam, lamotrigine, or carbamazepine.
    - **Generalized Epilepsy:** Broad-spectrum agents are required. Valproic acid is highly

effective. Lamotrigine and levetiracetam are also options. Ethosuximide is first-line for absence seizures *only*.

- **Step 2: Second-Line Monotherapy:** If the first agent fails (either due to side effects or continued seizures), the algorithm dictates a switch to a different first-line monotherapy.
- **Step 3: Adjunctive "Polytherapy":** If the second monotherapy fails, the algorithm proceeds to add a second ASM from a different class, aiming for rational polytherapy.
- **Step 4: Refractory Epilepsy:** Failure of two appropriate ASMs defines refractory epilepsy. This triggers a referral to an epilepsy center for evaluation for epilepsy surgery, vagal nerve stimulation (VNS), or dietary therapies.

Status Epilepticus Algorithm

This is a neurologic emergency (seizure > 5 minutes). The algorithm is a timed protocol:

- **0-5 min (Stabilization):** ABCs, check glucose, obtain IV access.
- **5-20 min (Initial Therapy):** A benzodiazepine (e.g., IV lorazepam, IM midazolam).
- **20-40 min (Second-Line Therapy):** A non-benzodiazepine ASM (e.g., IV fosphenytoin, valproic acid, or levetiracetam).
- **> 40 min (Refractory SE):** The algorithm proceeds to anesthetic doses of midazolam, propofol, or pentobarbital with continuous EEG monitoring.

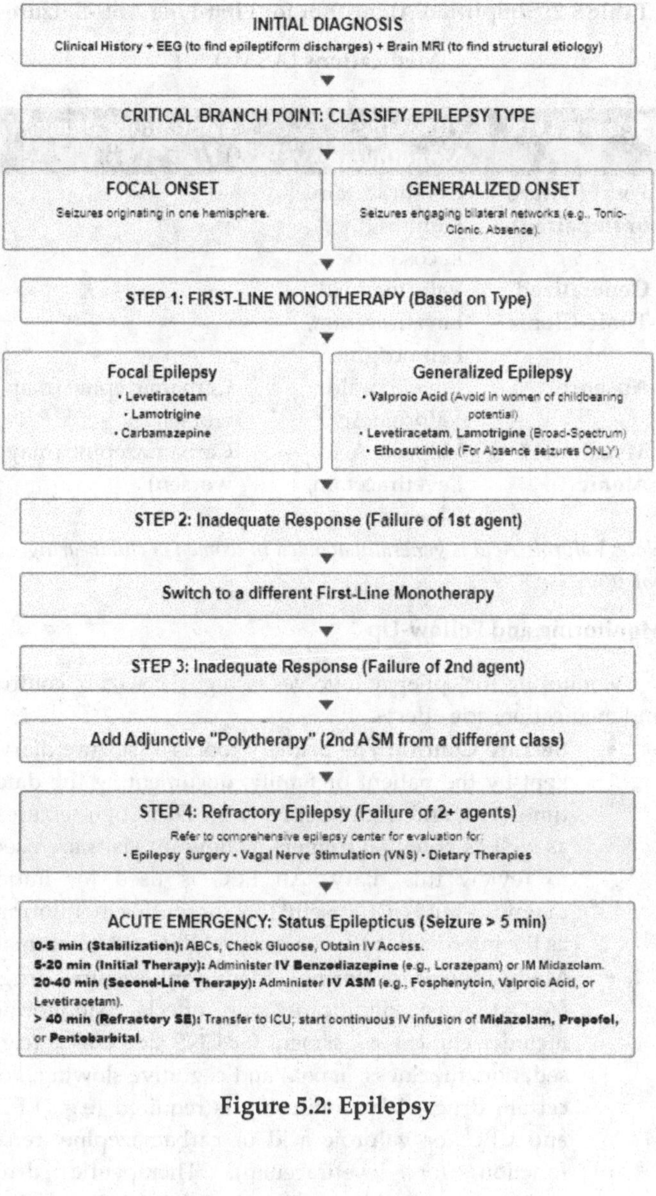

Figure 5.2: Epilepsy

Table 5.2: Simplified Algorithm for First-Line Anti-Seizure Medications (ASMs)

Seizure Type	First-Line Monotherapy	Contraindication(s)
Focal (Aware or Impaired)	Levetiracetam, Lamotrigine, Lacosamide	---
Generalized Tonic-Clonic	Valproic Acid, Levetiracetam, Lamotrigine	---
Absence	Ethosuximide, Valproic Acid	Carbamazepine (may worsen)
Myoclonic / Atonic	Valproic Acid, Levetiracetam, Clobazam	Carbamazepine (may worsen)

Note: Valproic Acid is generally avoided in women of childbearing potential.

Monitoring and Follow-Up

Monitoring for epilepsy involves two goals: seizure control and medication side effects.

- **Seizure Control:** The primary tool is a "seizure diary" kept by the patient or family, documenting the date, time, type, and duration of any breakthrough seizures, as well as potential triggers. Follow-up visits are used to review this diary. An EEG is used for initial diagnosis but is *not* a useful tool for routine monitoring, as the inter-ictal (between-seizure) EEG can be normal.
- **Medication Monitoring:** Many anti-seizure drugs (ASDs) have significant side effects. Monitoring includes clinical assessment for CNS side effects (e.g., sedation, dizziness, ataxia) and cognitive slowing. For certain drugs, lab monitoring is required (e.g., LFTs and CBC for valproic acid or carbamazepine; renal function for levetiracetam). Therapeutic drug monitoring (checking serum drug levels) is useful to confirm adherence or assess for toxicity, but treatment

should be guided by seizure control, not a specific number.

Long-Term Management / Secondary Prevention

The goal of long-term management is to achieve "no seizures, no side effects."

- **Pharmacological:** The algorithm begins with monotherapy with a first-line ASD selected based on the seizure type (focal vs. generalized), side effect profile, and patient-specific factors (e.g., pregnancy potential). Broad-spectrum agents (e.g., levetiracetam, lamotrigine, valproic acid) are effective for both focal and generalized seizures. If the first drug fails, the algorithm moves to a second monotherapy trial. If that fails, "rational polytherapy" (combining two drugs with different mechanisms of action) is used.
- **Non-Pharmacological:** For the ~30% of patients with "drug-resistant epilepsy" (failure of ≥2 appropriate ASDs), advanced management is considered. This includes referral to an epilepsy center for evaluation for epilepsy surgery (to resect the seizure focus), neurostimulation devices (e.g., Vagus Nerve Stimulator, VNS), or ketogenic diet therapy.

Patient Counseling Points

1. **Adherence is Everything:** "This is the most important part of your treatment. A single missed dose can be enough to break through your protection and cause a seizure." Emphasize using pillboxes and setting alarms.
2. **Safety and Driving:** This is a legal and safety mandate. "By law, you must be seizure-free for a specific period (e.g., 6 months) before you are cleared to drive." Counsel on seizure safety: do not swim or bathe alone, avoid heights.
3. **Side Effects vs. Seizures:** "Our goal is no seizures *and* no side effects. If the medicine is making you too tired or dizzy to function, that is not a success. We can often adjust the dose or try a different medicine."
4. **Teratogenicity (for women of childbearing potential):**

"This is a critical safety conversation. Some seizure medicines, especially Valproic Acid, can cause severe birth defects. We must have a reliable plan for contraception, and if you *ever* plan to become pregnant, we must plan this together *beforehand* to switch you to a safer medicine, like levetiracetam or lamotrigine." All women of childbearing potential should be on high-dose folic acid supplementation.

5. **No Abrupt Stoppage:** "You must *never* stop your seizure medication suddenly, even if you feel fine. Stopping abruptly can cause a severe, life-threatening cluster of seizures called status epilepticus."

Common Pitfalls in Management

A critical pitfall is using the wrong ASM for the epilepsy type. For example, prescribing carbamazepine (a narrow-spectrum agent) for generalized epilepsy can worsen absence or myoclonic seizures. Another error is non-adherence, often due to side effects or cost, which is a common cause of "breakthrough" seizures. Finally, failing to counsel women of childbearing potential on the teratogenicity of certain ASMs (especially valproic acid) is a major safety omission.

Case Study

A 22-year-old male (Mr. Chen) presents after having a seizure at work. His colleagues describe a 2-minute episode where he became rigid, fell to the ground, and had whole-body rhythmic shaking (a generalized tonic-clonic seizure). He was confused for 15 minutes afterward. He reports two "fainting spells" in the last year that were not witnessed.

Discussion

This patient has **Epilepsy**, defined as two or more unprovoked seizures (his unwitnessed "fainting spells" are presumed to be seizures in this context, now confirmed by a witnessed tonic-clonic event). The algorithm is to first classify the seizure type, then initiate first-line monotherapy.

Treatment Algorithm

1. **Diagnosis:** Epilepsy.
2. **Classification:** The witnessed event was a **Generalized Tonic-Clonic** seizure.
3. **Algorithm (First-Line Monotherapy):** The algorithm requires a "broad-spectrum" anti-seizure medication (ASM) that covers generalized seizures.
    - **Therapy:** You start **Levetiracetam 500 mg BID**. (Valproic Acid would also be a correct choice, but Levetiracetam is often chosen for its good side-effect profile and lack of teratogenicity).
    - *Pitfall:* You specifically AVOID a "narrow-spectrum" agent like Carbamazepine, which can worsen generalized epilepsy.
4. **Counseling:** You provide critical counseling on **adherence** (missing doses can cause a seizure) and **safety** (he must be seizure-free for a legally defined period, e.g., 6 months, before driving).

Outcome

Mr. Chen is started on Levetiracetam. An EEG and MRI are ordered to look for an underlying cause, and he is scheduled for follow-up in 3 months.

MULTIPLE SCLEROSIS

Multiple Sclerosis is a chronic, immune-mediated disease of the central nervous system characterized by inflammation, demyelination, and axonal degeneration. The management algorithm is focused on treating acute relapses and, more importantly, preventing long-term disability.

Pathophysiology

The pathophysiology involves an autoimmune attack against **myelin**, the protective sheath that insulates nerve axons. Autoreactive T-cells and B-cells cross the blood-brain barrier, enter the CNS, and mount an inflammatory response against myelin. This "demyelination" causes the formation of inflammatory plaques or lesions in the brain, spinal cord, and optic nerves. Demyelination disrupts or blocks neurotransmission, causing the characteristic neurologic symptoms (e.g., vision loss, weakness, numbness, ataxia). This process is "disseminated in time and space," meaning lesions occur in different parts of the CNS at different times, causing the classic relapsing-remitting course (RRMS). Over time, this chronic inflammation can lead to irreversible axonal loss and neurodegeneration, which drives the progressive (SPMS/PPMS) phase of the disease.

Diagnosis and Classification

Diagnosis is clinical, based on demonstrating "dissemination in space" (lesions in ≥ 2 CNS locations) and "dissemination in time" (lesions or clinical attacks occurring at different times). The McDonald Criteria use clinical findings and MRI results to formalize this. An MRI of the brain and spinal cord is the main diagnostic tool. The disease is classified into clinical phenotypes:

Relapsing-Remitting MS (RRMS)

The most common form, with discrete attacks (relapses) followed by remission.

Secondary Progressive MS (SPMS)

A progressive worsening of disability that follows an initial relapsing course.

Primary Progressive MS (PPMS)

Progressive accumulation of disability from onset.

Differential Diagnosis

The differential for neurologic symptoms disseminated in time and space is broad. The main "MS mimics" include neuromyelitis optica (NMO, identified by AQP4-IgG antibodies), MOG-antibody disease, sarcoidosis, CNS vasculitis, and infectious causes like Lyme disease or syphilis.

Treatment Algorithm

The MS algorithm is twofold: managing acute relapses and long-term disease modification.

Acute Relapse Algorithm

A new, objective neurologic deficit lasting > 24 hours is a relapse. The standard algorithm for moderate-to-severe relapses is a 3-5 day course of high-dose intravenous or oral corticosteroids (e.g., methylprednisolone 1000 mg/day). This shortens the relapse duration but does not affect long-term disability.

Table 5.3: Multiple Sclerosis (MS) Treatment Algorithm

MS Phase	Primary Goal	Treatment Algorithm
Acute Relapse (Flare)	Reduce inflammation, shorten relapse duration.	**High-Dose Corticosteroids** (e.g., IV Methylprednisolone). (Alt: ACTH gel, Plasmapheresis).
Relapsing-Remitting MS (RRMS)	Prevent new relapses & new MRI lesions.	**Disease-Modifying Therapy (DMT).** Start early. Choice based on efficacy, safety, route (e.g., Interferons, Fumarates, Monoclonal Abs).
Progressive MS (PPMS/SPMS)	Slow disability progression.	**Ocrelizumab** (PPMS, Active SPMS). (Siponimod for Active SPMS).
Symptom Mgmt	Improve quality of life.	e.g., Dalfampridine (gait), Baclofen (spasticity).

Disease-Modifying Therapy (DMT) Algorithm

This is the cornerstone of long-term management. The algorithm involves initiating a DMT as early as possible after diagnosis. The choice of DMT is complex and based on two main strategies:

1. **Escalation Approach:** Start with a "platform" injectable (e.g., interferons, glatiramer acetate) or a lower-efficacy

oral agent. If the patient has breakthrough disease (new relapses or lesions), the algorithm "escalates" to a higher-efficacy therapy.

2. **Induction (High-Efficacy) Approach:** Start with a high-efficacy therapy from the beginning (e.g., natalizumab, ocrelizumab, alemtuzumab), particularly in patients with high-risk disease. This choice is guided by disease severity, patient preference, and the safety profile of the agents, particularly the risk of progressive multifocal leukoencephalopathy (PML).

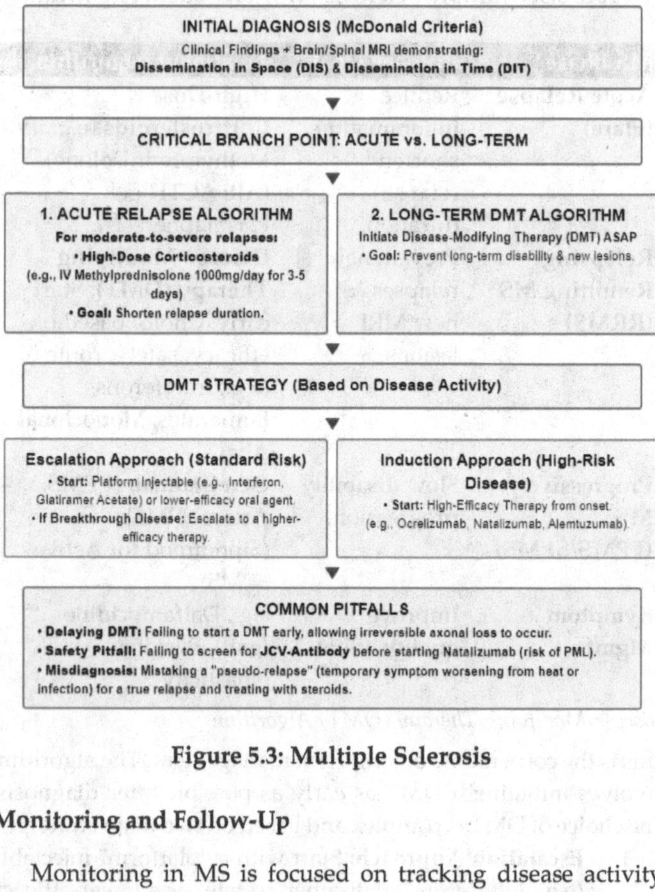

Figure 5.3: Multiple Sclerosis

Monitoring and Follow-Up

Monitoring in MS is focused on tracking disease activity, both clinical and subclinical.

- **Clinical:** Patients are monitored for new relapses (acute neurologic symptoms lasting > 24 hours). Functional status is tracked using the Expanded Disability Status Scale (EDSS) at clinic visits.
- **Radiologic:** This is the cornerstone of monitoring. A brain MRI (with and without gadolinium) is performed at baseline and then serially (e.g., every 6-12 months) to monitor for new or enhancing (active inflammation) lesions. The goal is to achieve "NEDA" (No Evidence of Disease Activity), which means no new relapses, no disability progression, and no new MRI lesions.
- **Safety Monitoring:** All disease-modifying therapies (DMTs) require safety monitoring (e.g., CBC for lymphopenia, LFTs, JCV virus antibody status for natalizumab due to PML risk).

Long-Term Management / Secondary Prevention

The goal of management is to prevent relapses and, more importantly, to prevent long-term disability accumulation.

- **Acute Relapse Management:** A severe, functionally disabling relapse is treated with a short course of high-dose intravenous corticosteroids (e.g., methylprednisolone) to shorten the duration of the relapse.
- **Disease-Modifying Therapy (DMT):** This is the foundation of long-term care. All patients with RRMS should be on a DMT. The therapeutic algorithm has shifted from an "escalation" approach (starting with safer, less effective drugs) to an "induction" approach (starting with high-efficacy therapies early). These include infusion therapies (e.g., ocrelizumab, natalizumab) or oral agents (e.g., S1P modulators like fingolimod, or fumarates). These drugs do not cure MS, but they significantly reduce the frequency of relapses and the accumulation of new MRI lesions, thereby preventing future disability.

Patient Counseling Points

1. **DMTs are a "Preventer," Not a "Symptom-Treater":** "This medication is an investment in your future. You will not *feel* it working on a daily basis. Its job is to stop the inflammation you *can't* feel (the MRI lesions) to prevent disability 10 or 20 years from now. You must take it even when you feel perfectly well."
2. **Infection Risk:** "Your medication works by modulating your immune system. This means you will be more susceptible to infections. You must be up-to-date on all your vaccines (especially flu and pneumonia) and call us if you develop a fever or signs of infection."
3. **PML Risk (for certain DMTs):** For drugs like natalizumab, a critical counseling point is the risk of Progressive Multifocal Leukoencephalopathy (PML), a rare but potentially fatal brain infection. "We monitor you for this with a blood test (JCV antibody) and by watching for any new, persistent neurologic symptoms."
4. **Managing Symptoms:** Differentiate DMTs from symptomatic treatment. "The DMT is for the disease, but we also have treatments for your *symptoms*." This includes medications for spasticity, fatigue, neuropathic pain, and bladder urgency.

Common Pitfalls in Management

The most significant pitfall is a delay in initiating DMT, as irreversible axonal loss occurs even in early, mild-appearing disease. Another major pitfall is failing to perform the required safety screening for high-efficacy DMTs, such as checking for JCV-antibody status before starting natalizumab (due to PML risk). Finally, a common error is "pseudo-relapse," misdiagnosing a temporary worsening of old symptoms due to heat or infection (Uhthoff's phenomenon) as a true relapse, leading to unnecessary steroid use.

Case Study

A 30-year-old female (Ms. Davis) presents with a 3-day history of complete vision loss in her right eye, associated with pain on eye movement. She also mentions an episode 6 months ago where her legs felt "numb and weak" for two weeks, which resolved on its own.

Discussion

This is a classic presentation for **Multiple Sclerosis (MS)**. She has symptoms (optic neuritis and a prior sensory deficit) that are "disseminated in time and space." The algorithm is two-pronged: 1) Treat the acute relapse. 2) Initiate long-term Disease-Modifying Therapy (DMT).

Treatment Algorithm

1. **Diagnosis:** Multiple Sclerosis (Relapsing-Remitting type). An MRI confirms demyelinating plaques in the optic nerve and thoracic spine.
2. **Algorithm (Part 1: Acute Relapse):** Her vision loss is a disabling relapse. The algorithm is to shorten the relapse with anti-inflammatory therapy.
   - **Therapy:** Start **High-Dose IV Methylprednisolone (Solu-Medrol) 1 gram daily for 3 days.**
3. **Algorithm (Part 2: Long-Term DMT):** The algorithm mandates starting a DMT as early as possible to prevent future relapses and long-term disability.
   - **Therapy:** You have a discussion about an "escalation" vs. "induction" approach. She prefers an oral agent and is started on **Dimethyl Fumarate (Tecfidera).**
4. **Safety Monitoring:** Baseline labs (CBC, LFTs) and an MRI are obtained before starting the DMT.

Outcome

The patient's vision improves after the steroid course. She is started on Dimethyl Fumarate for long-term disease modification and scheduled for a 6-month follow-up MRI.

PARKINSON'S DISEASE

Parkinson's Disease is a progressive neurodegenerative disorder characterized by the loss of dopaminergic neurons in the substantia nigra. This results in a classic motor syndrome of bradykinesia, rigidity, and resting tremor.

Pathophysiology

The cardinal pathophysiology is the selective death of **dopaminergic neurons** in the **substantia nigra pars compacta**, a structure in the midbrain. These neurons project to the striatum and are essential for initiating and controlling movement. The "dopamine hypothesis" states that the classic motor symptoms (bradykinesia, rigidity, resting tremor) do not appear until 60-80% of these dopaminergic neurons have already been lost. The underlying cause of this cell death is unknown, but the pathologic hallmark is the intracellular accumulation of a misfolded protein called **alpha-synuclein** into "Lewy bodies." This protein aggregation is believed to be toxic, spreading from cell to cell and leading to neuronal death.

Diagnosis

Diagnosis of PD is entirely clinical, based on the presence of the cardinal motor features (TRAP: Tremor at rest, Rigidity, Akinesia/Bradykinesia, Postural instability). A robust positive response to dopaminergic therapy (e.g., levodopa) is highly supportive of the diagnosis. There are no definitive diagnostic blood tests or imaging.

Differential Diagnosis

The main differential is Essential Tremor, which is typically an action tremor (not a rest tremor) and lacks bradykinesia or rigidity. It is also critical to differentiate PD from atypical "parkinsonian-plus" syndromes (e.g., Multiple System Atrophy [MSA], Progressive Supranuclear Palsy [PSP]), which have additional symptoms (e.g., early falls, autonomic failure) and respond poorly to levodopa. Drug-induced parkinsonism (e.g., from antipsychotics or antiemetics like metoclopramide) must always be ruled out.

Treatment Algorithm

The algorithm is purely symptomatic; no current therapy slows disease progression.

- **Step 1: Mild/Functionally Intact:** For mild symptoms that do not impact daily life, the algorithm may start with an MAO-B inhibitor (e.g., selegiline, rasagiline) to provide modest symptomatic benefit.
- **Step 2: Mild-Moderate Symptoms (Younger Patient < 65):** The algorithm often starts with a dopamine agonist (e.g., pramipexole, ropinirole) or an MAO-B inhibitor to delay the need for levodopa and its associated motor complications.
- **Step 3: Moderate-Severe Symptoms (Older Patient > 65 or Cognitive Impairment):** The gold-standard algorithm is to initiate levodopa/carbidopa. This is the most effective drug for motor symptoms.
- **Step 4: Managing Motor Complications:** As the disease progresses, patients on levodopa develop "off" periods (wearing-off of the drug) and dyskinesias (involuntary movements). The algorithm to manage this involves:
    - Adding a COMT inhibitor (e.g., entacapone) or an MAO-B inhibitor to prolong the effect of levodopa.
    - Adjusting levodopa dosing (e.g., smaller, more frequent doses).
    - For refractory motor fluctuations, the algorithm advances to deep brain stimulation (DBS) or an insulin-pump-like delivery of carbidopa/levodopa gel.

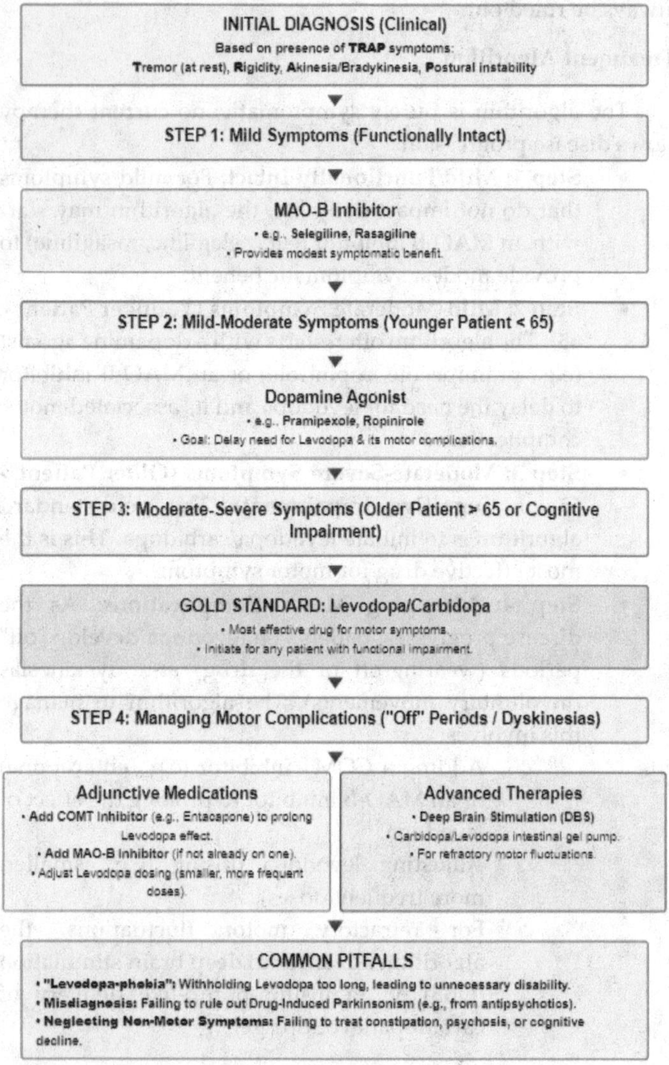

Figure 5.4: Parkinson's Disease

Table 5.4: Pharmacological Algorithm for Parkinson's Disease (PD)

Patient Profile	Primary Goal	First-Line Therapy
Mild Symptoms (No functional impairment)	Neuroprotection? (debated)	MAO-B Inhibitor (e.g., Rasagiline) or Amantadine.
Mod-Severe Symptoms (< 65 yrs or "Young")	Control motor symptoms, delay levodopa side effects.	Dopamine Agonist (e.g., Pramipexole, Ropinirole) or Levodopa/Carbidopa.
Mod-Severe Symptoms (> 65 yrs or "Older" / Cognitive impairment)	Robust symptom control.	**Levodopa/Carbidopa.** (Titrate to lowest effective dose).
"Off" Episodes (Motor fluctuations)	Reduce "off" time.	Add COMT Inhibitor (e.g., Entacapone) or MAO-B Inhibitor. Adjust Levodopa dosing.

Monitoring and Follow-Up

Monitoring for PD is entirely clinical. There are no blood tests or imaging scans to track progression. Disease staging and motor impairment are formally tracked in clinic using the Unified Parkinson's Disease Rating Scale (UPDRS). Follow-up visits (e.g., every 3-6 months) are used to assess:

1. **Motor Symptoms:** Is the patient's bradykinesia, tremor, or gait impaired?
2. **Dopaminergic Side Effects:** Is the patient experiencing medication-induced "dyskinesias" (writhing, involuntary movements from *too much* dopamine) or "off" periods (a wearing-off of the medication, where symptoms return before the next dose)?

3. **Non-Motor Symptoms:** These are just as important and include cognitive decline, depression/anxiety, sleep disturbance (RBD), and autonomic dysfunction (e.g., orthostatic hypotension, constipation).

Long-Term Management / Secondary Prevention

Management is purely symptomatic; no treatment stops or slows the underlying neurodegeneration.

- **Pharmacological:** The algorithm is based on symptom severity and patient age/goals.
    - **Mild Symptoms:** May start with an MAO-B inhibitor (e.g., rasagiline) to provide mild symptomatic benefit.
    - **Moderate/Severe Symptoms (Functionally Impaired):** The gold standard is **levodopa** (combined with carbidopa). This is a direct dopamine precursor and the most effective drug for motor symptoms. In younger patients, a dopamine agonist (e.g., pramipexole) may be used first to delay starting levodopa and its long-term complications (dyskinesias).
    - **Advanced Disease:** As the disease progresses, patients develop motor fluctuations. The algorithm involves "smoothing out" the levodopa response by adding a COMT inhibitor (e.g., entacapone) or using advanced therapies like a levodopa intestinal gel pump.
- **Surgical:** For patients with intractable tremor or severe motor fluctuations, **Deep Brain Stimulation (DBS)** is a highly effective option.

Patient Counseling Points

1. **Levodopa is the "Gold Standard":** "Levodopa is the most effective medicine we have. Many people are afraid to start it, but it is our best tool for improving your movement and quality of life."
2. **Dyskinesia vs. "Off" Time:** "As the disease progresses, you may notice two problems. One is 'off' time, where

the medicine wears off and your Parkinson's symptoms come back. The other is 'dyskinesia,' which is an extra, involuntary, wriggly movement *caused* by the medicine. Our job is to find the 'sweet spot' in between."

3. **Dopamine Agonist Side Effects:** "This medication (e.g., pramipexole) is very good, but we must watch for specific side effects like sudden sleepiness ('sleep attacks') and, importantly, **impulse control disorders**. This can include new or worsening problems with gambling, shopping, or hypersexuality. This is a *direct* effect of the drug, and you *must* tell us if this happens."
4. **Exercise is Neuroprotective:** "This is the one thing you can do that may slow the disease. Intensive exercise, like boxing, cycling, or Tai Chi, is a critical part of your treatment plan. 'Exercise is medicine.'"

Common Pitfalls in Management

A common historical pitfall is "levodopa-phobia," or withholding levodopa therapy for too long due to fears of dyskinesia, leading to unnecessary disability. A critical diagnostic pitfall is failing to recognize drug-induced parkinsonism and instead treating it with anti-PD medications. Finally, a major gap in care is the failure to address the non-motor symptoms (e.g., constipation, psychosis, cognitive decline), which are often more debilitating than the motor symptoms.

Case Study

A 72-year-old male (Mr. Lee) is brought in by his wife for "slowing down." She notes that for the past year, he has developed a "pill-rolling" tremor in his right hand *at rest*, a "mask-like" facial expression, and a slow, shuffling gait. He is having trouble buttoning his shirts and cutting his food.

Discussion

This clinical picture is the hallmark of **Parkinson's Disease (PD)**. He has the classic "TRAP" features (Tremor at rest, Rigidity, Akinesia/Bradykinesia). The algorithm is to start symptomatic therapy based on his age and degree of functional impairment.

Treatment Algorithm

1. **Diagnosis:** Clinical Parkinson's Disease.
2. **Algorithm (Symptomatic Therapy):**
   - **Patient Profile:** He is >65 years old and is **functionally impaired** (difficulty with ADLs like dressing and eating).
   - **Therapy:** The algorithm points directly to the most effective medication. You start **Carbidopa/Levodopa 25/100 mg TID**.
   - *Pitfall:* You do *not* start with a dopamine agonist, which is less effective and has a higher risk of side effects (e.g., hallucinations) in older adults.
3. **Follow-up:** You schedule a follow-up in 4 weeks.

Outcome

At his follow-up, Mr. Lee's wife reports a "night and day" improvement. His tremor is reduced, and his speed with dressing is significantly better. This positive response to Levodopa helps confirm the diagnosis

ALZHEIMER'S DISEASE

Alzheimer's Disease is the most common cause of dementia, a progressive neurodegenerative disorder characterized by the accumulation of amyloid-beta plaques and neurofibrillary (tau) tangles, leading to cognitive and functional decline.

Pathophysiology

The pathophysiology is defined by two hallmark protein aggregations.

Amyloid Plaques

Amyloid-beta (Aβ) protein, a fragment of a larger protein, accumulates *outside* the neurons into insoluble plaques. This process is thought to begin decades before symptoms appear and initiates a toxic cascade.

Neurofibrillary Tangles (NFTs)

The Aβ cascade is believed to trigger the hyperphosphorylation of **tau**, an intracellular protein that normally stabilizes microtubules. This "hyperphosphorylated tau" detaches from the microtubules and aggregates *inside* the neuron, forming tangles. These tangles are toxic and disrupt neuronal transport, leading to cell death. This pathologic process begins in the hippocampus (the memory center) and then spreads throughout the cortex, mirroring the clinical progression from memory loss to global cognitive failure.

Diagnosis

The algorithm for diagnosing AD is one of clinical exclusion and characterization. It requires a history of progressive cognitive decline (typically starting with short-term memory) from a patient and a reliable informant, confirmed by cognitive testing (e.g., MoCA, MMSE, or formal neuropsychological testing). The key part of the algorithm is to rule out reversible causes of dementia via lab work (e.g., TSH, B12, RPR) and brain imaging (MRI or CT) to exclude structural lesions (e.g., tumors, stroke, normal pressure hydrocephalus).

Differential Diagnosis

The differential for dementia is broad. The main distinctions include:

Vascular Dementia

Stepwise decline, prominent executive dysfunction, and significant cerebrovascular disease on imaging.

Lewy Body Dementia (LBD)

Early visual hallucinations, parkinsonism, and fluctuating cognition.

Frontotemporal Dementia (FTD)

Early, prominent changes in personality, behavior, or language, with relative sparing of memory.

Reversible Causes

Hypothyroidism, B12 deficiency, neurosyphilis, and depression (pseudodementia).

Treatment Algorithm

The current treatment algorithm is primarily symptomatic and supportive.

- **Step 1: Mild-to-Moderate AD:** The algorithm begins with a cholinesterase inhibitor (e.g., donepezil, rivastigmine, galantamine). These agents provide modest, temporary stabilization of cognitive and functional symptoms.
- **Step 2: Moderate-to-Severe AD:** The algorithm involves adding an NMDA-receptor antagonist, memantine, which can be used as monotherapy or in combination with a cholinesterase inhibitor.
- **Step 3: Behavioral Symptoms:** Non-pharmacological approaches (e.g., creating a safe environment, redirection) are first-line. For severe agitation or psychosis, the algorithm may require cautious use of atypical antipsychotics, balancing modest benefit with significant safety risks.
- **Newer Therapies:** Anti-amyloid monoclonal antibodies (e.g., lecanemab) represent a new, etiology-based algorithm for patients with early, confirmed-amyloid AD, but their use is complex and requires specialized monitoring for side effects (e.g., ARIA).

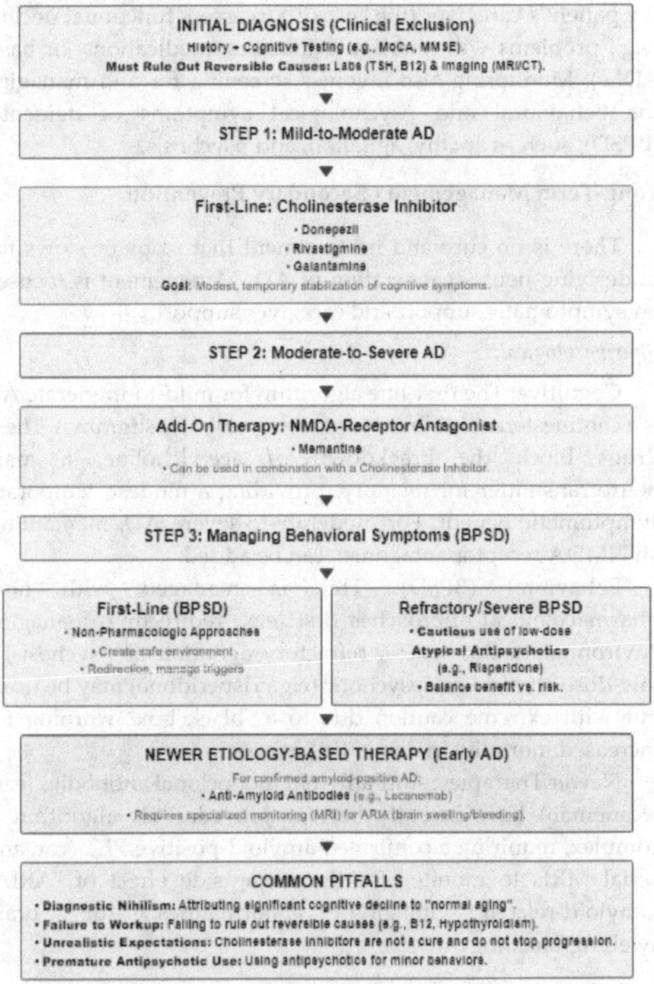

Figure 5.5: Alzheimer's Disease

Monitoring and Follow-Up

Monitoring is clinical, tracking the rate of cognitive and functional decline. This is done at follow-up visits (every 6-12 months) using cognitive screening tools (e.g., MoCA or MMSE) to objectively measure decline. Just as important is interviewing the patient's caregiver (the "proxy") to assess functional decline (e.g., problems with managing finances, medications, or basic ADLs). Monitoring also involves screening for and managing the behavioral and psychological symptoms of dementia (BPSD), such as apathy, agitation, and psychosis.

Long-Term Management / Secondary Prevention

There is no cure and no treatment that stops or slows the underlying neurodegeneration of AD. Management is focused on symptomatic support and caregiver support.

Pharmacological:

Cognitive: The first-line algorithm for mild-to-moderate AD is a cholinesterase inhibitor (e.g., donepezil, rivastigmine). These drugs block the breakdown of acetylcholine, a main neurotransmitter for memory, providing a modest, temporary symptomatic benefit. For moderate-to-severe AD, memantine, an NMDA receptor antagonist, can be added.

Behavioral (BPSD): This is managed with non-pharmacological approaches first (e.g., redirecting, managing environment). For severe, refractory agitation or psychosis, a low-dose atypical antipsychotic (e.g., risperidone) may be used, but with extreme caution due to a "black box" warning for increased mortality in dementia patients.

Newer Therapies: Anti-amyloid monoclonal antibodies (e.g., lecanemab) have recently been approved. This algorithm is complex, requiring a confirmed amyloid-positive PET scan and serial MRIs to monitor for the major side effect of "ARIA" (amyloid-related imaging abnormalities, or brain swelling/bleeding).

Patient Counseling Points

1. **Setting Expectations (Donepezil):** "This medicine (donepezil) is *not* a cure. It does not stop or slow the disease. The goal is to temporarily help with memory and thinking, but the disease will continue to progress. It is like a 'light-dimmer'—it may turn the lights up a bit, but it doesn't fix the wiring."
2. **Caregiver Support:** "The most important 'patient' in Alzheimer's disease is often the caregiver. This is a long

and difficult journey. We must make a plan for *your* support, including support groups, respite care, and education."

3. **Safety is Primary:** "As the disease progresses, our main goal shifts to safety." This includes discussions about driving cessation, kitchen/wandering safety, and preventing falls.
4. **Managing Agitation:** "If agitation or paranoia occurs, try not to argue or 'correct' them. Their reality is different. It is often better to 'join their reality,' validate their feeling, and then gently redirect their attention."

Common Pitfalls in Management

A common pitfall is diagnostic nihilism, attributing significant cognitive decline to "normal aging" and delaying diagnosis. Another is failing to perform the simple lab and imaging workup to rule out reversible causes of dementia. A therapeutic pitfall is having unrealistic expectations of cholinesterase inhibitors, which do not stop or reverse the disease. Finally, the premature or inappropriate use of antipsychotics for minor behavioral symptoms is a major safety concern.

Case Study

A 78-year-old female (Mrs. Jones) is brought to her PCP by her son, who is concerned about her memory. He reports that for the past 2 years, she has had progressive short-term memory loss (e.g., asks the same question multiple times, misplaces items). In the last 6 months, she has gotten lost while driving in her neighborhood and has had difficulty managing her finances.

Discussion

This is a classic, insidious onset of progressive cognitive decline, starting with short-term memory and now affecting instrumental activities of daily living (IADLs), consistent with **Alzheimer's Disease (AD)**. The algorithm is to first rule out reversible causes, then initiate symptomatic therapy.

Treatment Algorithm

1. **Diagnosis** (Step 1: Rule **out Reversibles):**
   - **Action:** You order labs (**TSH, Vitamin B12**) to rule out hypothyroidism or B12 deficiency. Both are normal.
   - **Action:** You order a **Non-Contrast Head CT** to rule out a stroke or tumor. It shows age-appropriate "cerebral atrophy."
   - **Action:** A MoCA test in the office scores 18/30, confirming cognitive impairment.
2. **Diagnosis (Confirmed):** Probable Alzheimer's Disease, Mild-to-Moderate stage.
3. **Algorithm (Symptomatic Therapy):**
   - **Therapy:** You start a first-line **Cholinesterase Inhibitor.**
   - **Regimen: Donepezil** 5 mg once **daily** at bedtime.
4. **Counseling:** You counsel the son that this is **not a cure** and will not stop the disease, but it may temporarily help stabilize her memory and function for 6-12 months. You also initiate a crucial discussion about driving safety.

Outcome

Mrs. Jones is started on Donepezil. Her son is given resources for caregiver support and long-term planning (e.g., power of attorney).

Summary

Acute Ischemic Stroke: A "time-is-brain" algorithm. Patients within 4.5 hours are assessed for IV thrombolysis (tPA). Patients with large vessel occlusions are assessed for mechanical thrombectomy up to 24 hours. Secondary prevention with antiplatelets, statins, and risk factor control is critical.

Epilepsy: The algorithm is stratified by seizure type (focal vs. generalized). It begins with first-line monotherapy, progressing to a second monotherapy trial, and then to rational polytherapy. Status epilepticus is a timed emergency algorithm starting with benzodiazepines.

Multiple Sclerosis: Management is twofold. Acute relapses are treated with high-dose corticosteroids. Long-term management involves early initiation of a Disease-Modifying Therapy (DMT) using either an "escalation" or "high-efficacy" (induction) strategy.

Parkinson's Disease: The algorithm is symptomatic. It begins with MAO-B inhibitors or dopamine agonists in younger patients and advances to levodopa/carbidopa, the most effective agent, for all patients with functional impairment. Motor complications are managed with adjunctive drugs or deep brain stimulation.

Alzheimer's Disease: The algorithm is symptomatic and supportive. Cholinesterase inhibitors (e.g., donepezil) are used for mild-to-moderate disease, and memantine is added for moderate-to-severe disease. Management of behavioral symptoms is a crucial challenge.

Multiple Choice Questions

1. A 68-year-old male presents to the ED 90 minutes after the onset of left-sided weakness. A non-contrast head CT is negative for hemorrhage. His blood pressure is 170/95 mmHg. What is the most appropriate next step?
   A) Administer IV alteplase (tPA).
   B) Administer IV labetalol to lower BP to < 140/90 mmHg. C) Perform CT angiography to look for a large vessel occlusion.
   D) Administer aspirin 325 mg and admit for observation.
2. Which anti-seizure medication is first-line for absence seizures but can worsen focal or tonic-clonic seizures?
   A) Levetiracetam
   B) Carbamazepine
   C) Ethosuximide
   D) Valproic Acid
3. A 30-year-old female is diagnosed with relapsing-remitting MS. She has high disease activity on her initial MRI. Which long-term treatment algorithm is increasingly favored?
   A) A high-efficacy or "induction" approach with a drug like ocrelizumab.
   B) An "escalation" approach, starting with interferon-beta. C) A 5-day course of high-dose IV methylprednisolone. D) Symptomatic management only until a second relapse occurs.
4. A 72-year-old male with Parkinson's Disease and functional impairment is "levodopa-naive." What is the most effective first-line symptomatic therapy?
   A) Pramipexole
   B) Selegiline
   C) Benztropine
   D) Carbidopa/Levodopa

5. A patient with known Parkinson's Disease on levodopa reports that his medication "wears off" 30 minutes before his next dose. What is an appropriate "add-on" to his algorithm?
   A) A cholinesterase inhibitor
   B) A COMT inhibitor (e.g., entacapone)
   C) A benzodiazepine
   D) An atypical antipsychotic
6. A patient with moderate Alzheimer's Disease is already taking donepezil. What is the appropriate next step in the pharmacological algorithm?
   A) Stop donepezil and switch to memantine.
   B) Add memantine in combination with donepezil.
   C) Increase the dose of donepezil.
   D) Add a high-dose statin.
7. A patient presents with a 10-minute tonic-clonic seizure and is still seizing in the ED. IV access is obtained. What is the first-line pharmacological agent to administer now?
   A) IV Lorazepam
   B) IV Fosphenytoin
   C) IV Valproic Acid
   D) IV Propofol
8. A 25-year-old female presents with a 3-day history of right-sided vision loss and pain with eye movement, consistent with optic neuritis. This is her first demyelinating event. What is the treatment algorithm?
   A) Initiate interferon-beta immediately.
   B) A 3-5 day course of high-dose corticosteroids.
   C) A 21-day course of DAPT (aspirin and clopidogrel).
   D) Observation only, as this is a "pseudo-relapse."
9. A 65-year-old male presents 6 hours after stroke symptom onset. A CT scan is negative. A CT

angiogram shows an M1 (middle cerebral artery) occlusion. What is the treatment?

A) IV Alteplase (tPA)

B) Mechanical thrombectomy

C) High-dose aspirin

D) IV Heparin infusion

10. A critical diagnostic pitfall is misdiagnosing Parkinson's Disease. Which of the following is not a primary differential?

A) Drug-induced parkinsonism (e.g., from metoclopramide)

B) Essential Tremor

C) Atypical parkinsonian syndrome (e.g., MSA, PSP)

D) Alzheimer's Disease

Self-Assessment Questions

1. Describe the acute "door-to-needle" and "door-to-device" algorithms for a patient presenting with an acute ischemic stroke.
2. What are the four key pillars of the secondary prevention algorithm after a TIA or minor ischemic stroke?
3. A patient is diagnosed with focal-onset epilepsy. What are two appropriate first-line monotherapies? How would this algorithm change if the diagnosis was generalized-onset epilepsy?
4. Outline the first three timed steps (0-40 minutes) of the algorithm for a patient in convulsive status epilepticus.
5. Differentiate the treatment algorithm for an acute MS relapse from the long-term algorithm for disease modification.
6. What is the key clinical "TRAP" mnemonic for diagnosing Parkinson's Disease, and why is "response to levodopa" a critical part of the diagnostic algorithm?
7. A younger patient (< 60) with mild Parkinson's is functionally intact. How does this differ from the algorithm for a 75-year-old with functionally limiting bradykinesia?
8. What is the first step in the diagnostic algorithm for a patient with suspected dementia, and why is this "ruling out" step so critical?
9. A patient is diagnosed with mild Alzheimer's disease. What is the first-line pharmacological algorithm? What agent would be added if their disease progresses to a severe stage?
10. Identify two "stroke mimics" and two "MS mimics" and explain why they are critical pitfalls.

Bibliography

1. Powers WJ, Rabinstein AA, Ackerson T, Adeoye OM, Bambakidis NC, Becker K, et al. Guidelines for the Early Management of Patients With Acute Ischemic Stroke: 2019 Update to the 2018 Guidelines for the Early Management of Acute Ischemic Stroke. Stroke. 2019 Dec;50(12):e344–e418.
2. Nogueira RG, Jadhav AP, Haussen DC, Bonafe A, Budzik RF, Bhuva P, et al. Thrombectomy 6 to 24 Hours after Stroke with a Mismatch between Deficit and Infarct. N Engl J Med. 2018 Jan 4;378(1):11–21.
3. Kleindorfer DO, Towfighi A, Chaturvedi S, Cockroft KM, Gutierrez J, Lombardi-Hill D, et al. 2021 Guideline for the Prevention of Stroke in Patients With Stroke and Transient Ischemic Attack: A Guideline From the American Heart Association/American Stroke Association. Stroke. 2021 Jul;52(7):e364–e467.
4. Fisher RS, Acevedo C, Arzimanoglou A, Bogacz A, Cross JH, Elger CE, et al. ILAE Official Report: A practical clinical definition of epilepsy. Epilepsia. 2014 Apr;55(4):475–82.
5. Glauser T, Shinnar S, Gloss D, Alldredge B, Arya R, Bainbridge J, et al. Evidence-Based Guideline: Treatment of Convulsive Status Epilepticus in Children and Adults: Report of the Guideline Committee of the American Epilepsy Society. Epilepsy Curr. 2016 Jan-Feb;16(1):48–61.
6. Kalia LV, Lang AE. Parkinson's disease. Lancet. 2015 Aug 29;386(9996):896–912.
7. Postuma RB, Berg D, Stern M, Poewe W, Olanow CW, Oertel W, et al. MDS clinical diagnostic criteria for Parkinson's disease. Mov Disord. 2015 Oct;30(12):1591–601.
8. Connolly BS, Lang AE. Pharmacological Treatment of Parkinson Disease: A Review. JAMA. 2014 Apr 23;311(16):1670–83.
9. Thompson AJ, Banwell BL, Barkhof F, Carroll WM, Coetzee T, Comi G, et al. Diagnosis of multiple sclerosis: 2017 revisions of the McDonald criteria. Lancet Neurol. 2018 Feb;17(2):162–73.
10. Hauser SL, Bar-Or A, Cohen JA, Comi G, Correale J, Coyle PK, et al. Ocrelizumab versus Interferon Beta-1a in Relapsing Multiple Sclerosis. N Engl J Med. 2017 Jan 19;376(3):221–34.
11. National Institute on Aging. Alzheimer's Disease Diagnostic Guidelines. [Accessed 2024 Oct 25]. Available from: https://www.nia.nih.gov/health/alzheimers-disease-diagnostic-guidelines

12. Atri A. The Diagnosis and Treatment of Alzheimer Disease. Continuum (Minneap Minn). 2019 Apr;25(2):318–44.
13. van Dyck CH, Swanson CJ, Aisen P, Bateman RJ, Chen C, Gee M, et al. Lecanemab in Early Alzheimer's Disease. N Engl J Med. 2023 Jan 5;388(1):9–21.
14. Kerty E, Mikkelsen C, Fure B, Stavem K. Differentiating stroke from stroke mimics: a prospective observational study. BMC Neurol. 2017 Jul 19;17(1):145.
15. Marson A, Burnside G, Appleton R, Smith D, Gamble C, Jacoby A, et al. The SANAD II study of the effectiveness and cost-effectiveness of valproate versus levetiracetam for newly diagnosed generalised and unclassifiable epilepsy: an open-label, non-inferiority, multicentre, phase 4, randomised controlled trial. Lancet. 2021 Apr 17;397(10283):1434–45

CHAPTER 6

TREATMENT ALGORITHMS FOR PSYCHIATRIC DISORDERS

Author

Mr. Sreedhar Sumalapu, Head of the Department, Department of Pharmacy Practice, Nirmala College of Pharmacy(Autonomous), Kadapa, Andhra Pradesh, India

Abstract

Psychiatric treatment algorithms are guideline-based, measurement-informed, and highly individualized, with a dual focus on symptom remission and functional recovery. The algorithm for Major Depressive Disorder (MDD) is a stepwise approach, beginning with first-line psychotherapy (e.g., CBT) or pharmacotherapy (e.g., SSRI/SNRI). Failure of an adequate trial (6-8 weeks) triggers a subsequent step, such as switching to a different agent or augmenting with a second medication (e.g., bupropion, aripiprazole). The algorithm for anxiety disorders (e.g., GAD) is similar, prioritizing CBT, SSRIs, or SNRIs, with agents like buspirone or pregabalin as second-line or adjunctive options; benzodiazepines are reserved for short-term, acute management. The algorithm for schizophrenia is stratified by treatment response. First-line therapy is a second-generation antipsychotic (SGA). Treatment resistance, defined by failure of two different antipsychotic trials, is a specific indication to advance the algorithm to clozapine. The algorithm for bipolar disorder is bifurcated by the patient's acute state. Mania is managed with mood stabilizers (e.g., lithium, valproate) or SGAs, whereas bipolar depression is treated with agents with specific efficacy for this phase (e.g., lurasidone, quetiapine), strictly avoiding antidepressant monotherapy.

Keywords: *Psychiatric Algorithms, Major Depressive Disorder, Anxiety Disorders, Schizophrenia, Bipolar Disorder, Pharmacotherapy*

Learning Objectives

After completion of the chapter, the learners should be able to:

- List first-line pharmacological classes (e.g., SSRIs, SNRIs) for Major Depressive Disorder and Generalized Anxiety Disorder.
- Explain the algorithm for managing an acute manic episode in a patient with Bipolar I Disorder, emphasizing the need for mood stabilization.
- Formulate a treatment augmentation plan for a patient with treatment-resistant depression.
- Differentiate the treatment algorithm for a positive-symptom-predominant schizophrenic episode versus a negative-symptom-predominant presentation.
- Justify the selection of a second-generation (atypical) antipsychotic over a first-generation (typical) agent for a newly diagnosed patient.

MAJOR DEPRESSIVE DISORDER

Major Depressive Disorder is a common and serious mood disorder characterized by a persistent low mood and/or anhedonia, causing significant impairment. The treatment algorithm is a stepwise, measurement-based approach aimed at achieving full remission.

Pathophysiology

The pathophysiology of Major Depressive Disorder (MDD) is complex and not fully elucidated, extending well beyond the traditional "monoamine hypothesis." While a deficiency in monoamine neurotransmitters (serotonin, norepinephrine, and dopamine) provides a framework for understanding antidepressant action, it is an incomplete explanation. Modern theories incorporate a neuro-circuitry and neurotrophic perspective. Chronic stress is known to dysregulate the hypothalamic-pituitary-adrenal (HPA) axis, leading to sustained high levels of cortisol. This hypercortisolemia is toxic to the hippocampus, a key brain region for mood regulation and memory. This leads to the "neurotrophic hypothesis," which posits that depression is associated with reduced brain-derived neurotrophic factor (BDNF), leading to atrophy and reduced neurogenesis in the hippocampus and prefrontal cortex. Antidepressants, in this model, may work by increasing BDNF, promoting synaptic plasticity, and restoring these crucial neural circuits.

Diagnosis

Diagnosis is made by fulfilling the DSM-5 criteria: at least five of nine symptoms (including depressed mood or anhedonia) for at least two weeks (often recalled by the mnemonic SIGECAPS: Sleep, Interest, Guilt, Energy, Concentration, Appetite, Psychomotor, Suicidality). The severity is assessed (mild, moderate, severe) to guide the initial algorithm.

Differential Diagnosis

The most critical differential is Bipolar-Disorder; diagnosing MDD and prescribing an antidepressant in a patient with bipolar disorder can induce mania or rapid cycling. This is the "MDD vs. Bipolar" pitfall. Medical differentials must be excluded, including hypothyroidism, anemia, vitamin deficiencies (B12, D), and neurological conditions (e.g., Parkinson's, stroke). Substance-induced depression (e.g., from alcohol, beta-blockers) and other psychiatric disorders (e.g., anxiety, adjustment disorder) must also be considered.

Treatment Algorithm

The algorithm is stratified by severity but generally follows a stepwise progression after an inadequate response to the prior step. An adequate trial is defined as 6-8 weeks at a therapeutic dose.

- **Step 1: First-Line Therapy:**
    - **Mild-Moderate MDD:** Psychotherapy (e.g., Cognitive Behavioral Therapy [CBT], Interpersonal Therapy [IPT]) OR a first-line antidepressant is appropriate.
    - **Moderate-Severe MDD:** Pharmacotherapy is the cornerstone, often in combination with psychotherapy. First-line agents include Selective Serotonin Reuptake Inhibitors

(SSRIs) or Serotonin-Norepinephrine Reuptake Inhibitors (SNRIs). Bupropion or mirtazapine may also be first-line, chosen based on symptom profile (e.g., bupropion for low energy, mirtazapine for insomnia/anorexia).

- **Step 2: First Treatment Failure:** If an adequate trial of an SSRI fails:
  - **Switch:** Change to a different agent within the same class (another SSRI) or to a different class (e.g., an SNRI, bupropion).
  - **Augment:** Add a second agent. Common evidence-based augmentation algorithms include adding bupropion to an SSRI, or adding an atypical (second-generation) antipsychotic (e.g., aripiprazole, quetiapine XR, olanzapine).
- **Step 3: Second Treatment Failure:** If a second trial (either switch or augmentation) fails, the algorithm proceeds to:
  - **Switch:** Change to a less common class, such as a tricyclic antidepressant (TCA), requires more monitoring.
  - **Augment:** Add lithium or thyroid hormone (T3, liothyronine).
- **Step 4: Treatment-Resistant Depression (TRD):** Failure of ≥ 2-3 adequate trials defines TRD. This triggers consideration of neurostimulation techniques, including Electroconvulsive Therapy (ECT), which is the most effective algorithm for severe or catatonic depression. Transcranial Magnetic Stimulation (TMS) or intranasal esketamine are other options.

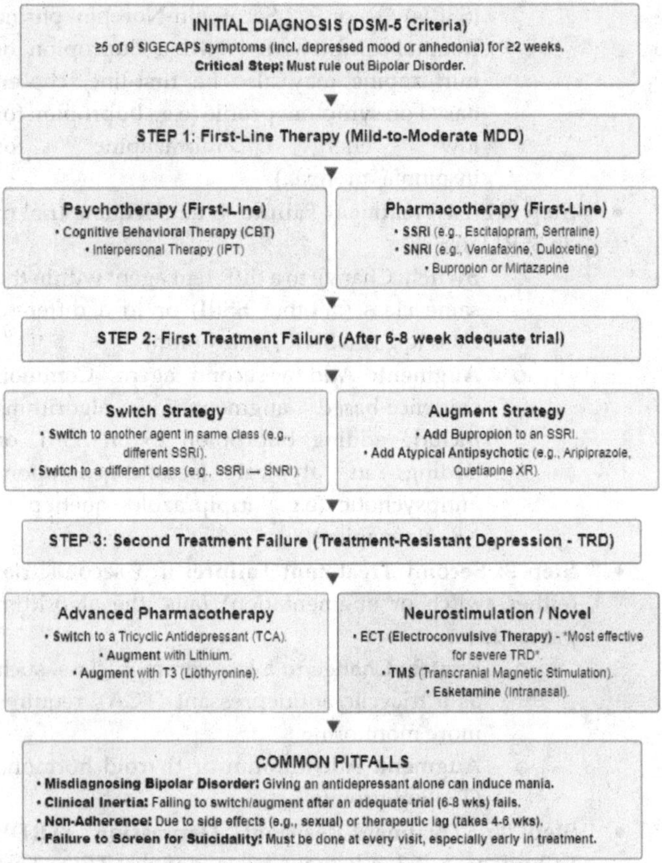

Figure 6.1: Major Depressive Disorder (MDD)

Monitoring and Follow-Up

Monitoring in MDD is primarily clinical and symptom-based. The first follow-up visit should occur within 2-4 weeks of initiating pharmacotherapy to assess for tolerability, side effects, and, critically, suicide risk. A "response" (a 50% reduction in symptoms) may not be evident for 4-6 weeks, while "remission" (the goal of treatment, where symptoms are absent) may take 8-12 weeks. Validated rating scales, such as the Patient Health Questionnaire-9 (PHQ-9), should be used at baseline and at regular intervals (e.g., every 4-8 weeks) to objectively track symptom burden. Monitoring must also include a specific assessment for the emergence of agitation, anxiety, or suicidal ideation, which can (rarely) be an early activating effect of SSRIs, particularly in younger patients. Once a patient achieves remission, follow-up can be extended to every 3-6 months

Table 6.1: Stepwise Algorithm for Major Depressive Disorder (MDD)

Step	Intervention	Rationale / Goal
Step 1	First-Line Agent (e.g., SSRI, SNRI, Bupropion)	Initiate monotherapy. (SSRI e.g., Escitalopram is common first choice).
Step 2 (Inadequate Response)	**Switch** to a different first-line agent OR **Augment** with a second agent (e.g., Bupropion, Mirtazapine, or Atypical Antipsychotic).	Optimize response.
Step 3 (Inadequate Response)	Switch or Augment again. (Consider different classes).	Achieve remission.
Step 4 (Treatment-Resistant)	Refer for specialist consult. Consider options like ECT, TMS	Manage complex/refractory illness.

Long-Term Management / Secondary Prevention

The management of MDD is divided into three phases. The *Acute Phase* (6-12 weeks) aims to achieve remission. The *Continuation Phase* lasts for 4-9 *months after* remission is achieved; continuing the antidepressant at the full therapeutic dose during this time is the single most important factor in preventing a short-term relapse. For patients with a high risk of recurrence (e.g., three or more lifetime episodes, early age of onset, severe episodes), *Maintenance Phase* therapy (lifelong antidepressant treatment) is the standard of care to prevent future episodes. Psychotherapy, particularly Cognitive Behavioral Therapy (CBT) or Interpersonal Therapy (IPT), is a first-line treatment and is highly effective for secondary prevention. The combination of pharmacotherapy and psychotherapy ("pills and skills") is considered the most effective long-term strategy.

Patient Counseling Points

1. **Therapeutic Lag:** This is the most important counseling point. The patient must understand that the antidepressant is not an "as-needed" pill and will take 4-6 weeks to exert its full effect, even though side effects may appear earlier.
2. **Adherence and Discontinuation:** Emphasize that the medication must be taken every day, even when they start to feel better, to prevent relapse. They must *never* stop the medication abruptly, as this can cause a "discontinuation syndrome" (flu-like symptoms, "brain zaps," anxiety).
3. **Side Effects:** Discuss common, transient side effects (e.g., nausea, headache) which often resolve in 1-2 weeks. Also discuss long-term side effects like sexual dysfunction or weight gain and encourage the patient to report them.
4. **Suicide Risk (Black Box Warning):** Patients under 25 (and their families) must be warned of the small, but real, risk of increased suicidal ideation or agitation in the first few weeks of treatment and told to report this immediately.
5. **Role of Psychotherapy:** Frame psychotherapy (CBT) as an active part of treatment that provides long-term skills to manage negative thought patterns and prevent future episodes.

Common Pitfalls in Management

The most critical pitfall is misdiagnosing Bipolar Disorder as unipolar MDD. Another is clinical inertia, failing to advance the algorithm after an inadequate trial, often due to insufficient dose or duration. A major safety pitfall is the failure to repeatedly and directly screen for suicidal ideation. Finally, overlooking medical or substance-induced causes can lead to treating the wrong condition.

Case Study

A 32-year-old female (Ms. Allen) presents with a 2-month history of a persistent sad mood, loss of interest in her hobbies (anhedonia), low energy, difficulty concentrating, and feelings of worthlessness. Her PHQ-9 score is 18 (moderately severe). She has no personal or family history of mania or hypomania.

Discussion

This is a classic presentation of a first episode of **Major Depressive Disorder**. Given the moderately-severe symptoms impacting her function, the algorithm supports initiating first-line therapy (pharmacotherapy, psychotherapy, or both). The critical first step is to rule out Bipolar Disorder.

Treatment Algorithm

1. **Diagnosis:** Moderately-severe Major Depressive Disorder.
2. **Critical Pitfall Check:** You screen for any history of mania (e.g., "Have you ever had a period of days where you had so much energy you didn't need to sleep?"). She denies any, making an SSRI safe to prescribe.
3. **Algorithm Step 1 (First-Line):** You offer both psychotherapy (CBT) and pharmacotherapy. She agrees to both.
    - **Pharmacotherapy:** Start a first-line SSRI, **Sertraline 50 mg daily**.
4. **Counseling:** You counsel her on the "therapeutic lag" (it may take 4-6 weeks to feel the full effect) and common, transient side effects (e.g., nausea).
5. **Follow-up:** You schedule a follow-up in 2-4 weeks to assess for side effects and monitor for any (rare) increase in suicidal ideation, and another at 8 weeks to assess for a full response.

Outcome

Ms. Allen is started on Sertraline 50 mg daily and given a referral for Cognitive Behavioral Therapy (CBT).

ANXIETY DISORDERS

This category includes Generalized Anxiety Disorder (GAD), Panic Disorder (PD), and Social Anxiety Disorder (SAD). The treatment algorithms share a common foundation.

Pathophysiology

Anxiety disorders are believed to arise from dysregulation in the brain's "fear circuit." The amygdala, a central processing hub for fear and threat, becomes hyper-responsive, sending false alarms to the rest of the brain. This activity is normally modulated and "turned off" by the prefrontal cortex, but in anxiety, this top-down control is deficient. Neurochemically, this maps onto a dysregulation of several systems. The inhibitory neurotransmitter GABA is a key player; benzodiazepines work by enhancing GABA's "braking" effect on this circuit. Furthermore, the serotonin and norepinephrine systems, which originate in the brainstem and project widely, are believed to be dysregulated, which is why SSRIs and SNRIs (the first-line agents) are effective in "re-tuning" this circuit over time.

Diagnosis

Diagnosis is based on DSM-5 criteria, characterized by excessive, persistent, and debilitating worry (GAD), discrete, recurrent, and unexpected panic attacks (PD), or marked fear of social situations (SAD).

Differential Diagnosis

Medical conditions that mimic anxiety ("anxiety mimics") must be ruled out. The main differentials include hyperthyroidism, cardiac arrhythmias (e.g., SVT), pheochromocytoma, pulmonary embolism, and vestibular dysfunction. Substance/medication-induced anxiety (e.g., caffeine, albuterol, stimulants, withdrawal syndromes) is also extremely common.

Treatment Algorithm

The algorithm for GAD is a representative model.

- **Step 1: First-Line Therapy:** Psychotherapy (CBT) is highly effective and considered first-line, equivalent to pharmacotherapy. First-line medications are SSRIs or SNRIs (e.g., venlafaxine XR, duloxetine). These agents may initially worsen anxiety, requiring a "start low, go slow" titration algorithm.
- **Step 2: Second-Line Therapy:** If an adequate SSRI/SNRI trial fails, the algorithm suggests:
    - **Switch:** Change to a different first-line agent (another SSRI or SNRI).
    - **Switch:** Change to a second-line agent, such as buspirone (GAD-specific, often better as augmentation) or pregabalin.
- **Step 3: Augmentation/Refractory:** For partial response, augmentation with buspirone or pregabalin is a common algorithm. Hydroxyzine can be used as a short-term, "as-needed" anxiolytic.
- **Algorithm for Acute/Panic Symptoms:** For acute panic attacks or severe, short-term anxiety, benzodiazepines (e.g., lorazepam, alprazolam) are highly effective. However, their algorithm is for short-term (< 2-4 weeks) or "as-needed" use only, to bridge the patient until long-term therapies (like SSRIs) take effect.

Monitoring and Follow-Up

Monitoring is clinical, tracking the frequency and severity of anxiety, panic attacks, and avoidance behaviors. The GAD-7 (for Generalized Anxiety Disorder) or Panic Disorder Severity Scale (PDSS) are useful objective tools. Follow-up should be scheduled 2-4 weeks after initiating an SSRI/SNRI to monitor for side effects, particularly the "jitteriness" or "activation syndrome," a common early side effect where anxiety transiently worsens. This is managed by "starting low and going slow." If benzodiazepines are used as a short-term bridge, monitoring must include assessing for frequency of use, tolerance, and any signs of dependence or misuse.

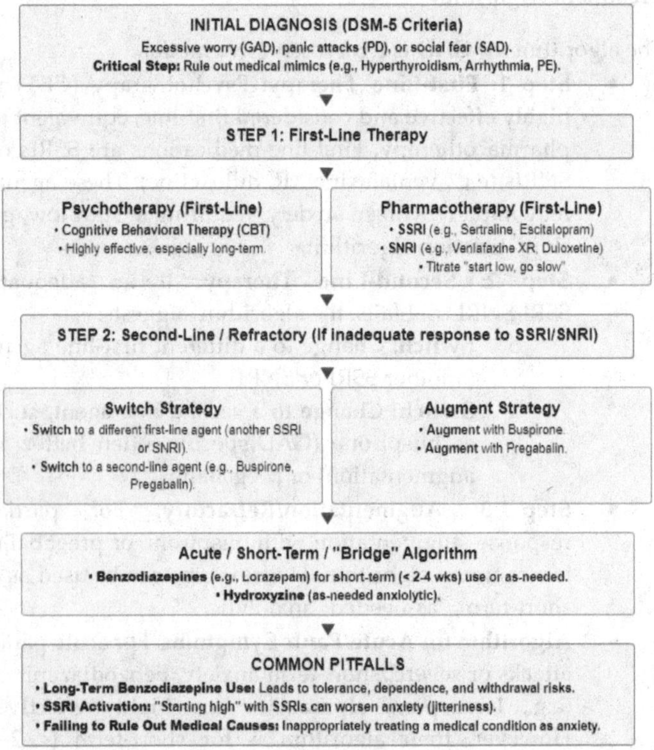

Figure 6.2: Anxiety Disorders (GAD, PD, SAD)

Long-Term Management / Secondary Prevention

The long-term management strategy for all anxiety disorders rests on two pillars: pharmacotherapy and psychotherapy. First-line pharmacotherapy is an SSRI or SNRI, which, unlike benzodiazepines, treats the underlying disorder and is not associated with dependence. Cognitive Behavioral Therapy (CBT) is equally first-line and is arguably the most effective long-term strategy for prevention. CBT for anxiety, particularly "Exposure and Response Prevention" (ERP), works by teaching the patient to gradually confront feared situations *without* engaging in avoidance or safety behaviors, thereby re-training the brain to extinguish the fear response. Benzodiazepines are explicitly *not* for long-term management; their use should be limited to 2-4 weeks or for infrequent, as-needed rescue.

Table 6.2: First-Line Pharmacological Algorithm for Anxiety Disorders

Disorder	First-Line Therapy (Long-Term)	Second-Line / Adjunct
Generalized Anxiety (GAD)	SSRI (e.g., Sertraline) or SNRI (e.g., Venlafaxine). Buspirone is an alt.	Pregabalin/Gabapentin. Hydroxyzine (PRN). (Short-term Benzodiazepine bridge).
Panic Disorder	SSRI or SNRI (at higher doses than GAD).	Benzodiazepines (risk of dependence).
Social Anxiety (SAD)	SSRI or SNRI. Propranolol (for performance-only type).	---
OCD	High-Dose SSRI (e.g., Fluvoxamine, Fluoxetine).	Clomipramine (TCA). Augment with Atypical Antipsychotic.

Patient Counseling Points

1. **CBT as a "Cure":** Explain that while medication can control symptoms, psychotherapy (CBT) provides the skills to overcome the anxiety itself and is the most effective tool for long-term prevention.
2. **SSRI Jitteriness:** Warn the patient that when starting an SSRI/SNRI, their anxiety might feel slightly *worse* for the first 1-2 weeks. This is a normal, temporary

"activation" and a sign the medicine is starting to work.

3. **Benzodiazepine Risk (e.g., Alprazolam, Lorazepam):** This is a critical safety point. Explain that these are "rescue" or "emergency" pills, not "controller" pills. They are highly effective but are habit-forming (addictive) and should *not* be taken every day for long periods.
4. **The "Trap" of Avoidance:** Counsel that the anxiety disorder is *maintained* by avoidance. While it feels better in the short term to avoid a feared situation (e.g., a social event, a public space), this avoidance only makes the anxiety stronger over time. The goal of treatment is to reverse this.

Common Pitfalls in Management

The most significant pitfall is the long-term, chronic prescribing of benzodiazepines, which leads to tolerance, dependence, and significant withdrawal risks. Another is the "start high, go fast" titration of SSRIs, which can cause activating side effects and lead to premature discontinuation. Finally, failing to rule out medical "anxiety mimics" can result in inappropriate psychiatric treatment for a medical condition.

Case Study

A 28-year-old male (Mr. Khan) presents with 8 months of "constant, uncontrollable" worry. He feels "on edge" all the time, restless, and has significant muscle tension in his neck and shoulders. He worries excessively about his job performance, his finances, and his health, even when there is no specific reason. His GAD-7 score is 16 (severe).

Discussion

This presentation (chronic, excessive, multi-domain worry with physical symptoms) is the hallmark of **Generalized Anxiety Disorder (GAD)**. The algorithm prioritizes first-line SSRIs/SNRIs and/or CBT.

Treatment Algorithm

1. **Diagnosis:** Generalized Anxiety Disorder (GAD).

2. **Rule out Medical Mimics:** You order a TSH to rule out hyperthyroidism, which is normal.
3. **Algorithm Step 1 (First-Line):** You start a first-line agent, an SNRI.
    - **Pharmacotherapy:** Start **Venlafaxine XR 37.5 mg daily.**
4. **Titration & Counseling:** You counsel him to "start low and go slow," as these medications can sometimes briefly increase anxiety (activation/jitteriness). You explain the plan to titrate up to a therapeutic dose (e.g., 75-150 mg).
5. **Adjunct (Optional):** To manage his severe initial symptoms, you prescribe a 2-week "as-needed" course of **Hydroxyzine 25 mg** to use for severe anxiety while the Venlafaxine takes effect. You specifically avoid benzodiazepines for long-term use.

Outcome

Mr. Khan is started on Venlafaxine XR with a plan to titrate the dose. He is also referred for CBT, which is highly effective for GAD

SCHIZOPHRENIA

Schizophrenia is a chronic, severe mental disorder affecting cognition, emotion, and perception. The algorithm is focused on symptom control, relapse prevention, and functional recovery.

Pathophysiology

Schizophrenia is a severe neurodevelopmental disorder of brain connectivity and information processing. The classic "dopamine hypothesis" remains central to its pathophysiology. It posits that *hyperactivity* of the dopamine D2 system in the mesolimbic pathway causes the "positive" symptoms (hallucinations, delusions, disorganized thought). Conversely, *hypoactivity* of the dopamine D1 system in the mesocortical pathway is thought to contribute to the "negative" symptoms (flat affect, amotivation, anhedonia) and cognitive deficits.

Glutamate dysregulation, specifically NMDA receptor hypofunction, is also a main area of research, as it may be the "upstream" cause of the dopamine dysregulation. All antipsychotic medications work by blocking the D2 receptor, which is effective for positive symptoms but less so for negative symptoms.

Diagnosis

Diagnosis is made via DSM-5 criteria, requiring ≥ 2 symptoms for at least one month (with continuous signs of disturbance for ≥ 6 months). Symptoms include positive symptoms (delusions, hallucinations, disorganized speech), negative symptoms (e.g., avolition, alogia, anhedonia), and cognitive dysfunction.

Differential Diagnosis

The differential is critical. It includes substance-induced psychotic disorders (especially from methamphetamine or cannabis), brief psychotic disorder (< 1 mo), schizophreniform disorder (1-6 mo), and schizoaffective disorder (which includes a prominent, co-occurring mood episode). Medical causes of psychosis (e.g., delirium, autoimmune encephalitis, complex partial seizures) must be excluded.

Treatment Algorithm

The algorithm is pharmacological, with psychosocial interventions (e.g., assertive community treatment [ACT]) as a mandatory adjunct.

- **Step 1: First Episode of Psychosis:** The algorithm begins with a Second-Generation Antipsychotic (SGA), also known as an atypical antipsychotic (e.g., risperidone, aripiprazole, olanzapine, quetiapine, ziprasidone). The choice is based on the patient's side-effect vulnerability (e.g., avoid olanzapine in a patient with diabetes; avoid ziprasidone in a patient with QTc prolongation).
- **Step 2: Inadequate Response:** After an adequate trial (4-6 weeks) of a first-line SGA, the algorithm dictates switching to a different SGA or, less commonly, a First-

Generation Antipsychotic (FGA) like haloperidol.

- **Step 3: Treatment-Resistant Schizophrenia (TRS):** This is specifically defined as a failure to respond to ≥ 2 adequate trials of different antipsychotics. This is a critical branch point in the algorithm. The *only* evidence-based medication for TRS is **clozapine.**
- **Algorithm for Non-Adherence:** Non-adherence is the primary driver of relapse. For patients with poor adherence, the algorithm moves to a long-acting injectable (LAI) formulation of an antipsychotic (e.g., paliperidone palmitate, aripiprazole lauroxil).

Table 6.3: Schizophrenia Treatment Algorithm by Phase

Phase	Primary Goal	Treatment Algorithm
Acute Psychosis	Reduce agitation, hostility, and positive symptoms (hallucinations, delusions).	**Second-Generation Antipsychotic (SGA)** (e.g., Risperidone, Olanzapine). (IM injection for agitation).
Stabilization	Consolidate gains, minimize side effects, ensure adherence.	Continue SGA. Titrate to optimal dose. Monitor metabolic effects (lipids, glucose, weight).
Maintenance	Prevent relapse.	Continue antipsychotic at lowest effective dose. **Clozapine** for Treatment-Resistant Schizophrenia.

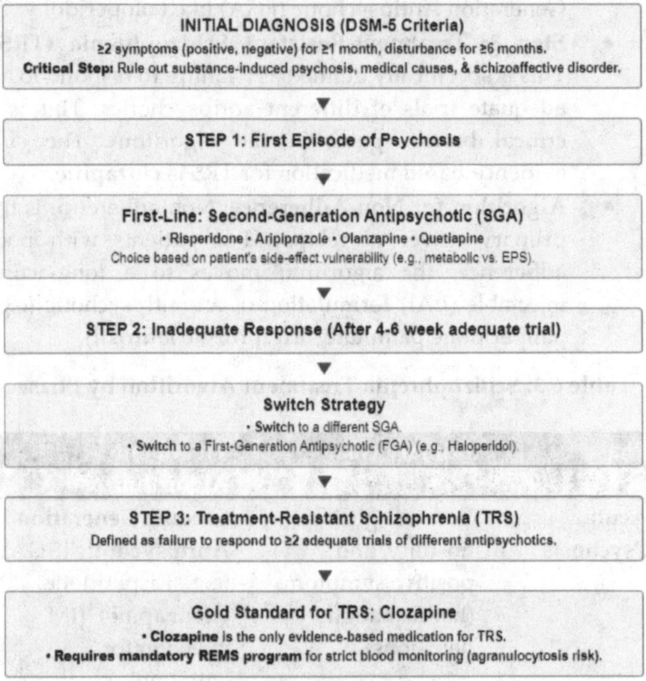

Figure 6.3: Schizophrenia

Monitoring and Follow-Up

Monitoring for schizophrenia is twofold: managing psychotic symptoms and, just as importantly, managing the severe side effects of antipsychotic medications.

1. **Psychiatric:** Monitor for positive/negative symptoms (e.g., using the PANSS or BPRS scales) and, critically, assess for adherence, as non-adherence is the #1 predictor of relapse. Also monitor for extrapyramidal symptoms (EPS: parkinsonism, dystonia), akathisia (an intense inner restlessness), and tardive dyskinesia (TD: involuntary, often irreversible, oro-facial movements).
2. **Metabolic:** Second-generation antipsychotics (SGAs) are notorious for causing metabolic syndrome. Monitoring must include a baseline and follow-up (e.g., 3 months, then annually) of: weight/BMI, waist

circumference, fasting glucose/HbA1c, and a fasting lipid panel.

3. **Clozapine:** For treatment-resistant schizophrenia, clozapine requires a mandatory REMS program with a weekly (then bi-weekly) CBC to monitor for agranulocytosis.

Long-Term Management / Secondary Prevention

The cornerstone of long-term management is lifelong adherence to antipsychotic medication. Second-generation antipsychotics (e.g., aripiprazole, risperidone, olanzapine, quetiapine) are first-line. Given the high rates of non-adherence, Long-Acting Injectable (LAI) formulations are a key strategy for secondary prevention and relapse reduction. For patients who fail two trials of standard antipsychotics (Treatment-Resistant Schizophrenia), clozapine is the gold-standard. Pharmacotherapy must be combined with psychosocial interventions, such as Assertive Community Treatment (ACT), supported employment, and family therapy, to improve functional outcomes.

Patient Counseling Points

1. **Adherence and Relapse:** This is a lifelong illness. Stopping medication, even when feeling 100% "cured," will lead to a psychotic relapse. A LAI (injection) is not a punishment but a tool to prevent relapse and remove the burden of taking a daily pill.
2. **Metabolic Syndrome:** This is a critical safety issue. "These medications are very effective for psychosis, but they can cause significant weight gain and increase your risk for diabetes and high cholesterol." This is why diet, exercise, and regular blood tests are a mandatory part of treatment.
3. **Movement Side Effects (EPS/TD):** Counsel the patient to immediately report any new, involuntary movements (like tongue-thrusting, pill-rolling tremors, or severe restlessness).
4. **Clozapine Safety:** If on clozapine, the patient must understand the absolute, non-negotiable need for their

regular bloodwork. Missing these appointments means they cannot get their medication refill.

5. **Substance Use:** Strongly counsel that substances, especially cannabis and stimulants (methamphetamine, cocaine), can directly cause psychosis and will make their illness much harder to treat.

Common Pitfalls in Management

The most common pitfall is non-adherence to medication. A critical therapeutic pitfall is delaying the initiation of clozapine in a patient with confirmed treatment resistance, as "time-to-clozapine" correlates with long-term outcomes. A major safety pitfall with clozapine is the failure to adhere to the strict blood monitoring algorithm (REMS program) for agranulocytosis. Finally, neglecting to monitor for and manage the severe metabolic side effects (e.g., weight gain, diabetes, dyslipidemia) of many SGAs is a common error.

Case Study

A 21-year-old male (Mr. Clark) is brought to the ED by his family. His parents report a 6-month history of social withdrawal, bizarre behavior, and a decline in his college grades. For the past month, he has been expressing paranoid beliefs that his professors are "spies" (paranoid delusions) and he is heard muttering to himself (auditory hallucinations).

Discussion

This is a classic presentation of a **First Episode of Psychosis (FEP)**, consistent with **Schizophrenia**. The algorithm for FEP is to rule out substance-induced or medical causes and initiate a Second-Generation Antipsychotic (SGA).

Treatment Algorithm

1. **Diagnosis:** Schizophrenia.
2. **Rule out Mimics:** A urine toxicology screen is negative for stimulants or cannabis.
3. **Algorithm Step 1 (First-Line):** Start a **Second-Generation Antipsychotic (SGA)**.

  - **Therapeutic Choice:** You select **Aripiprazole 10 mg daily**. This is often a good first choice as it has a lower risk of metabolic side effects (like weight gain) and sedation compared to other agents like Olanzapine.

4. **Safety Monitoring:** You order baseline labs (fasting glucose, lipid panel, CBC) and a baseline weight/BMI, as all SGAs carry metabolic risks.
5. **Psychosocial:** You refer the patient and his family to an Assertive Community Treatment (ACT) or FEP specialty program for psychosocial support.

Outcome

Mr. Clark is started on Aripiprazole 10 mg daily and admitted to an inpatient unit for stabilization and to connect him with long-term outpatient resources.

BIPOLAR DISORDER

Bipolar Disorder (BD) is a chronic mood disorder characterized by recurrent episodes of mania or hypomania and depression. The treatment algorithm is phase-dependent: acute mania, acute depression, or maintenance.

Pathophysiology

The pathophysiology is not fully known but involves a "bridge" between depressive disorders and schizophrenia, with shared genetic vulnerabilities. The core issue is a failure of emotional regulation circuits. During mania, this is thought to be related to excessive monoamine (norepinephrine, dopamine) activity, while depression involves a relative deficit. More deeply, the disorder is linked to dysregulation of intracellular signaling cascades (the proposed target of mood stabilizers like lithium and valproate) and severe disruption of circadian rhythms, which is a crucial trigger for new episodes.

Diagnosis and Classification

Diagnosis is based on DSM-5 criteria.

Bipolar I Disorder: Requires at least one full manic episode (a distinct period of abnormally elevated/irritable mood and energy lasting ≥ 1 week).

Bipolar II Disorder: Requires at least one hypomanic episode (similar symptoms, ≥ 4 days, but no severe functional impairment) AND at least one major depressive episode.

Cyclothymic Disorder: Chronic, fluctuating hypomanic and depressive symptoms that do not meet full criteria for an episode.

Differential Diagnosis

The primary differential is unipolar MDD. Other main differentials include schizoaffective disorder (psychosis outside of mood episodes), ADHD (chronic, not episodic, hyperactivity), borderline personality disorder (moment-to-moment instability vs. sustained episodes), and substance-induced mania (e.g., from stimulants, steroids, or antidepressant-induced).

Treatment Algorithm

The algorithm is based on the patient's current mood state.

- **Algorithm 1: Acute Mania (Bipolar I)**
    - **Step 1 (Severe):** The algorithm is often combination therapy with a mood stabilizer (Lithium or Valproate) *plus* an SGA (e.g., olanzapine, risperidone).
    - **Step 1 (Mild-Moderate):** Monotherapy with lithium, valproate, or an SGA may be sufficient.
    - **CRITICAL STEP:** Any antidepressant medication must be discontinued.
- **Algorithm 2: Bipolar Depression (Bipolar I or II)**
    - **CRITICAL STEP:** Antidepressant monotherapy is contraindicated as it can induce mania or rapid cycling.
    - **Step 1:** Optimize the current maintenance mood stabilizer.
    - **Step 2:** Add a medication with specific FDA approval for bipolar depression. The algorithm includes quetiapine, lurasidone, cariprazine, or the olanzapine-fluoxetine

combination. Lamotrigine can be initiated but is too slow for acute depression; it is better for maintenance.

- **Algorithm 3: Maintenance Phase**
    - **Step 1:** The goal is to prevent recurrence of *both* poles (mania and depression).
    - **First-line:** Lithium (strongest anti-suicidal and anti-manic data) or valproate.
    - **Other options:** Lamotrigine (stronger for preventing depression), or an SGA (especially if it was used to treat the acute episode, e.g., aripiprazole, quetiapine).

Table 6.4: Bipolar Disorder Management Algorithm (Pharmacology)

Episode Type	Primary Goal	First-Line Monotherapy / Combo
Acute Mania / Hypomania	Control symptoms, prevent harm.	**Mood Stabilizer** (Lithium, Valproic Acid) OR **SGA** (e.g., Olanzapine, Risperidone). (Often use in combination).
Acute Bipolar Depression	Treat depression without inducing mania.	**Quetiapine** or **Lurasidone** or Olanzapine/Fluoxetine combo. (Lamotrigine-titration).
Maintenance	Prevent recurrence of any mood episode.	**Lithium** or **Valproic Acid** or Lamotrigine or an SGA (e.g., Aripiprazole). (Monotherapy or combo).

Note: Antidepressant monotherapy is contraindicated as it can induce mania.

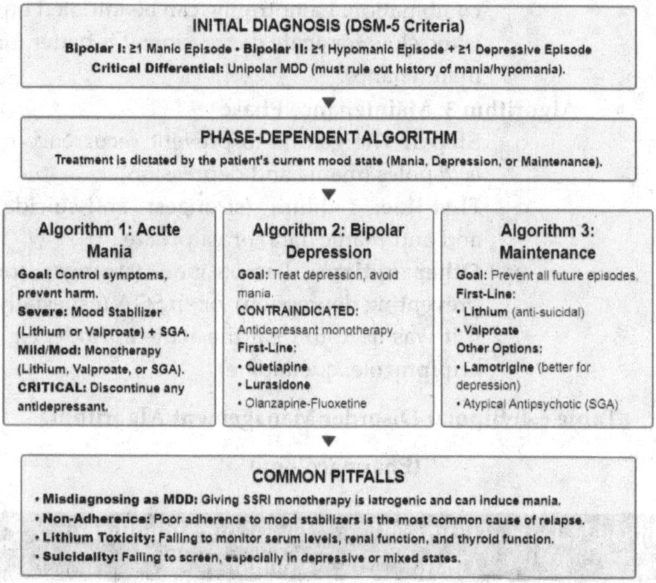

Figure 6.4: Bipolar Disorder

Monitoring and Follow-Up

Monitoring in bipolar disorder is focused on identifying and treating acute mood episodes (mania or depression) while preventing future ones. Mood charts are invaluable tools. The Young Mania Rating Scale (YMRS) can be used to track mania. The most critical aspect of monitoring is **Therapeutic Drug Monitoring (TDM)** for mood stabilizers.

- **Lithium:** Has a very narrow therapeutic index (target 0.6-1.0 mEq/L). Levels must be checked 5 days after every dose change and every 3-6 months once stable. Renal (BUN/Cr) and thyroid (TSH) function must be checked every 6-12 months.
- **Valproic Acid:** Requires TDM (target 50-125 mcg/mL) and monitoring of LFTs and a CBC (for rare but serious hepatotoxicity and thrombocytopenia).
- **Lamotrigine:** Does not require TDM but requires clinical monitoring for rash.

Long-Term Management / Secondary Prevention

The goal of long-term management is to prevent *mania* (and secondarily, depression). The foundation of all therapy is a **mood stabilizer**. This can be lithium (the gold standard), an anticonvulsant (valproic acid, lamotrigine), or an atypical antipsychotic (quetiapine, olanzapine). The single most important principle is that **antidepressants should not be used as monotherapy**, as this can induce mania or rapid-cycling. If an antidepressant is *required* for a severe depressive episode, it must be used in combination with a primary mood stabilizer. Psychotherapy, particularly psychoeducation and Interpersonal and Social Rhythm Therapy (IPSRT) which focuses on stabilizing routines, is a crucial component of preventing relapse.

Patient Counseling Points

1. **Antidepressant-Induced Mania:** This is the most critical counseling point. "Your illness is different from regular depression. If you take an antidepressant *alone,* it can be dangerous and trigger a manic episode. We must *always* use a mood stabilizer first."
2. **Lifelong Mood Stabilizer:** This is a lifelong illness. The mood stabilizer is the foundation of your health and must be taken every day, even when your mood is perfectly stable, to prevent future episodes.
3. **Lithium Safety:** "Lithium is an excellent medication, but we must respect it." Counsel on the narrow therapeutic window. "You *must* stay well-hydrated. You *must* tell us immediately if you have severe vomiting or diarrhea, or if you start a new blood pressure pill or an NSAID like ibuprofen, as these can make your level toxic." Teach signs of toxicity (coarse tremor, confusion, ataxia).
4. **Lamotrigine and "The Rash":** When starting lamotrigine, explain the "low and slow" titration. "We must increase this medicine very slowly. If you develop *any* new rash, especially with a fever or blisters, you must stop the medication and call us immediately, as it can be a rare but life-threatening allergic reaction (SJS)."

5. **Sleep, Routine, and Substances:** Emphasize that regular sleep and daily routines are a form of medicine for this illness. "A single all-nighter or substance use can be enough to trigger a full manic episode."

Common Pitfalls in Management

The single most critical pitfall is misdiagnosing Bipolar Disorder as unipolar MDD and initiating antidepressant monotherapy, which can be iatrogenic. In maintenance, a common error is poor adherence to mood stabilizers. With lithium, a major safety pitfall is the failure to monitor serum levels (narrow therapeutic index) and long-term renal and thyroid function. Finally, failing to screen for suicidality, which is extremely high in bipolar depression, is a critical omission.

Case Study

A 26-year-old female (Ms. Rios) is brought to the ED by her roommate. The roommate reports that for the past 5 days, Ms. Rios has not slept, has been talking "a mile a minute," and just spent $5,000 on a credit card for clothes she doesn't need. The patient is euphoric, irritable when questioned, and has pressured speech. Her roommate notes she had a "bad depression" 6 months ago.

Discussion

This is a classic **Acute Manic Episode**. The presence of one clear-cut manic episode (with a prior depressive episode) confirms the diagnosis of **Bipolar I Disorder**. The algorithm for acute mania is to prioritize mood stabilization and *stop* any antidepressants.

Treatment Algorithm:

1. **Diagnosis:** Bipolar I Disorder, current episode manic.
2. **Critical Pitfall Check:** You ask if she is on any medication. She states she was given Citalopram for her depression. The algorithm **mandates you discontinue the Citalopram (SSRI) immediately**, as it is fueling the mania.
3. **Algorithm Step 1 (Acute Mania):** Initiate a first-line mood stabilizer and/or an SGA.

  - **Therapeutic Choice:** You start **Valproic Acid** (loading dose) as a primary mood stabilizer. Due to her agitation and euphoria, you also start **Olanzapine** for its rapid anti-manic and sedative effects.

4. **Disposition:** The patient is admitted to an inpatient psychiatric unit for stabilization and safety.

Outcome

Ms. Rios's Citalopram is stopped. She is started on combination therapy with Valproic Acid and Olanzapine to control the acute manic episode. The long-term plan will be to transition her to a maintenance mood stabilizer (e.g., Valproic Acid or Lithium).

Summary

Major Depressive Disorder: The algorithm is a "step-up" approach, starting with first-line SSRIs/SNRIs or CBT. Non-response to an adequate trial leads to switching or augmenting (e.g., with bupropion or an atypical antipsychotic). ECT is reserved for treatment-resistant or severe cases.

Anxiety Disorders: The algorithm prioritizes first-line SSRIs, SNRIs, and CBT. Benzodiazepines are restricted to short-term, acute management to avoid dependence.

Schizophrenia: The algorithm begins with an SGA, with the choice guided by side-effect profiles. Non-adherence is managed with long-acting injectables (LAIs). Treatment resistance (failure of 2 agents) is a specific, critical indication to start clozapine.

Bipolar Disorder: The algorithm is phase-dependent. Acute mania is treated with mood stabilizers or SGAs, and antidepressants are stopped. Bipolar depression is treated with agents like lurasidone or quetiapine, not antidepressant monotherapy. Maintenance therapy aims to prevent both manic and depressive episodes.

Multiple Choice Questions

1. A 30-year-old female is diagnosed with moderate MDD. She prefers to start a medication. Which of the following is an appropriate first-line agent?
   A) Lithium
   B) Lurasidone
   C) Lorazepam
   D) Escitalopram
2. A 45-year-old male with MDD has a partial response to 8 weeks of fluoxetine 40 mg. Which of the following is an evidence-based "augmentation" algorithm?
   A) Add aripiprazole
   B) Add lorazepam
   C) Switch to valproic acid
   D) Switch to citalopram
3. The most critical pitfall in managing a patient with GAD is:
   A) Chronic prescribing of benzodiazepines
   B) Starting an SSRI at too high a dose
   C) Failing to rule out hyperthyroidism
   D) Using CBT as a first-line therapy
4. A 25-year-old male is admitted for a first episode of psychosis. After medical causes are ruled out, what is the first-line pharmacological algorithm?
   A) A trial of clozapine
   B) A trial of a second-generation antipsychotic (e.g., risperidone)
   C) A combination of haloperidol and benztropine
   D) Electroconvulsive Therapy (ECT)
5. A patient with schizophrenia has failed adequate trials of olanzapine and aripiprazole. What is the next step in the algorithm?
   A) Switch to haloperidol
   B) Switch to clozapine
   C) Augment with lithium

D) Add a long-acting injectable

6. A 28-year-old presents with 10 days of euphoria, grandiosity, 2 hours of sleep per night, and pressured speech. He is diagnosed with acute mania. What is the most appropriate initial algorithm?
   A) Initiate valproate and discontinue his paroxetine
   B) Initiate lamotrigine
   C) Initiate citalopram
   D) Initiate buspirone
7. Which medication is contraindicated as monotherapy in the treatment of bipolar depression?
   A) Quetiapine
   B) Lurasidone
   C) Sertraline
   D) Lamotrigine
8. What is the primary role of long-acting injectable (LAI) antipsychotics in the schizophrenia treatment algorithm? A) To treat treatment-resistant schizophrenia
   B) To manage acute psychosis in the ED
   C) To improve adherence and prevent relapse
   D) To minimize metabolic side effects
9. A patient with Bipolar I Disorder is stable and in remission. Which medication is FDA-approved for maintenance and has the strongest evidence for reducing suicidality?
   A) Lithium
   B) Lamotrigine
   C) Valproic Acid
   D) Aripiprazole
10. A 60-year-old female with severe, melancholic MDD and catatonic features is refusing to eat. What is the most effective and appropriate treatment algorithm?

A) Electroconvulsive Therapy (ECT)

B) High-dose intravenous lorazepam

C) Augmentation with aripiprazole

D) Initiation of intranasal ketamine

Self-Assessment Questions

1. What is the most critical differential diagnosis to rule out before initiating an SSRI for suspected MDD, and what is the risk of missing it?
2. An MDD patient fails an 8-week trial of sertraline 150 mg. Describe two distinct algorithm options for "Step 2" of therapy.
3. A patient with GAD is given a 30-day "bridge" prescription for lorazepam. What is the primary long-term therapy that should be initiated concurrently, and why is this bridging algorithm used?
4. A patient with schizophrenia has failed adequate trials of both risperidone and olanzapine. What is this condition called, and what is the specific next step in the pharmacological algorithm?
5. What is the main algorithm for managing a patient with schizophrenia who has persistent medication non-adherence?
6. Describe the main differences in the treatment algorithm for acute mania versus acute bipolar depression.
7. Why is antidepressant monotherapy contraindicated in the treatment of Bipolar Disorder?
8. A patient is started on clozapine. What is the most severe hematologic side effect, and what monitoring algorithm is required?
9. A patient with GAD complains that her new sertraline prescription is "making her more anxious." What is the likely cause, and how should the algorithm be adjusted?
10. Differentiate the role of lithium from the role of lamotrigine in the maintenance algorithm for Bipolar Disorder

Bibliography

1. American Psychiatric Association. Diagnostic and Statistical Manual of Mental Disorders. 5th ed. (DSM-5). Washington, DC: American Psychiatric Association; 2013.
2. Qaseem A, Barry M, Kansagara D. Nonpharmacological Versus Pharmacological Treatment of Adult Patients With Major Depressive Disorder: A Clinical Practice Guideline From the American College of Physicians. Ann Intern Med. 2016 Mar 1;164(5):350–9.
3. Gartlehner G, Wagner G, Matyas N, Titscher V, Greimel J, Kien C, et al. Pharmacological and non-pharmacological treatments for major depressive disorder: review of systematic reviews. BMJ Open. 2021 Jun 28;11(6):e048083.
4. Bauer M, Pfennig A, Severus E, Whybrow PC, Angst J, Möller HJ. World Federation of Societies of Biological Psychiatry (WFSBP) guidelines for biological treatment of unipolar depressive disorders, part 1: update 2013 on the acute and continuation treatment of unipolar depressive disorders. World J Biol Psychiatry. 2013 Jul;14(5):334–85.
5. Rush AJ, Trivedi MH, Wisniewski SR, Nierenberg AA, Fava M, Thase ME, et al. Bupropion-SR, sertraline, or venlafaxine-XR after failure of SSRIs for depression. N Engl J Med. 2006 Mar 23;354(12):1231–42.
6. Bandelow B, Michaelis S, Wedekind D. Treatment of anxiety disorders. Dialogues Clin Neurosci. 2017 Jun;19(2):93–107.
7. Stein MB, Craske MG. Treating Anxiety in 2017: Optimizing Care for Patients With Anxiety Disorders. JAMA. 2017 Jul 18;318(3):235–6.
8. Keepers GA, Fochtmann LJ, Anzia JM, Benjamin S, Lyness JM, Mojtabai R, et al. The American Psychiatric Association Practice Guideline for the Treatment of Patients With Schizophrenia. 3rd ed. Am J Psychiatry. 2020 Sep 1;177(9):868–72.
9. Buchanan RW, Kreyenbuhl J, Kelly DL, Noel JM, Boggs DL, Fischer BA, et al. The 2009 Schizophrenia PORT Psychopharmacological Treatment Recommendations and Summary Statements. Schizophr Bull. 2010 Jan;36(1):71–93.
10. Kane JM, Agid O, Baldwin M, Kern S, Correll CU, Lindenmayer JP, et al. Clinical guidance on the identification and management of treatment-resistant schizophrenia. J Clin Psychiatry. 2019 Mar 19;80(2).
11. Yatham LN, Kennedy SH, Parikh SV, Schaffer A, Bond DJ, Frey BN, et al. Canadian Network for Mood and Anxiety

Treatments (CANMAT) and International Society for Bipolar Disorders (ISBD) 2018 guidelines for the management of patients with bipolar disorder. Bipolar Disord. 2018 Mar;20(2):97–170.

12. Parker G, Graham R. Clinical features of bipolar depression: implications for treatment. CNS Drugs. 2010 Jun;24(6):459–70.
13. Taylor DM, Barnes TRE, Young AH. The Maudsley prescribing guidelines in psychiatry. 14th ed. Wiley-Blackwell; 2021.
14. Goodwin GM, Haddad PM, Ferrier IN, Aronson JK, Barnes T, Cipriani A, et al. Evidence-based guidelines for treating bipolar disorder: Revised third edition recommendations from the British Association for Psychopharmacology. J Psychopharmacol. 2016 Jun;30(6):495–553.
15. Tondo L, Baldessarini RJ. Long-term lithium treatment in the prevention of suicidal behavior in bipolar disorder patients. Epidemiol Psichiatr Soc. 2018 Jul;27(3):209–15.

CHAPTER 7

TREATMENT ALGORITHMS FOR MUSCULOSKELETAL DISORDERS

Author

Mrs. Anitha K, Assistant Professor,
Dept. of Pharmaceutical Chemistry, Dr M.G.R Educational and Research Institute, Vellappanchavadi, Chennai, Tamil Nadu, India

Abstract

Musculoskeletal disorder management requires distinct algorithms that differentiate between inflammatory, degenerative, metabolic, and crystal-driven pathologies. The algorithm for Rheumatoid Arthritis (RA) is a proactive "treat-to-target" strategy, initiating disease-modifying antirheumatic drugs (DMARDs), primarily methotrexate, immediately upon diagnosis. Failure to achieve low disease activity within 3-6 months triggers a stepwise escalation to combination DMARDs, biologic agents (e.g., TNF-inhibitors), or JAK inhibitors. In contrast, the algorithm for Osteoarthritis (OA) is a stepwise, symptom-focused approach beginning with non-pharmacological interventions like weight loss and physical therapy. The algorithm then progresses through analgesics, from topical and oral NSAIDs to intra-articular injections, culminating in surgical arthroplasty for refractory cases. The algorithm for Osteoporosis is one of risk prevention, using FRAX and DXA scores to identify high-risk individuals. First-line therapy is an antiresorptive agent, typically an oral bisphosphonate, with anabolic agents reserved for very high-risk patients. Gout management is bifurcated: acute attacks are treated with anti-inflammatories (NSAIDs, colchicine, or steroids), while the chronic algorithm involves urate-lowering therapy (e.g., allopurinol) titrated to a serum uric acid target of < 6 mg/dL

Keywords: *Musculoskeletal Algorithms, Rheumatoid Arthritis, Osteoarthritis, Osteoporosis, Gout, Treat-to-Target*

Learning Objectives

After completion of the chapter, the learners should be able to:

- Identify the first-line pharmacological agents for an acute gout flare.
- Explain the "treat-to-target" algorithm in Rheumatoid Arthritis (RA) and the role of DMARDs.
- Select an appropriate treatment algorithm for a postmenopausal woman with osteoporosis based on her T-score and FRAX risk.
- Compare and contrast the pharmacological algorithms for Rheumatoid Arthritis (immunomodulatory) versus Osteoarthritis (symptom-based).
- Justify the initiation of urate-lowering therapy (e.g., allopurinol) in a patient with recurrent gout.

RHEUMATOID ARTHRITIS

Rheumatoid Arthritis is a chronic, systemic, autoimmune inflammatory disease that primarily attacks the synovial joints, leading to progressive cartilage and bone erosion and, if untreated, severe disability.

Pathophysiology

The pathophysiology is that of a complex, sustained autoimmune attack. In a genetically susceptible individual (e.g., carrying the HLA-DR "shared epitope"), an unknown trigger initiates an autoimmune response. T-cells and B-cells are activated, leading to the production of autoantibodies, including Rheumatoid Factor (RF) and, more specifically, anti-citrullinated protein antibodies (ACPA). These immune cells and antibodies infiltrate the synovium (the lining of the joint capsule), causing it to become inflamed and hypertrophied. This inflamed, boggy synovium is known as a "pannus." The pannus is an invasive, tumor-like tissue that actively produces pro-inflammatory cytokines (especially TNF-α, IL-1, and IL-6) and enzymes (matrix metalloproteinases) that directly invade and destroy adjacent cartilage and bone, leading to the characteristic marginal erosions and joint destruction.

Diagnosis

The diagnostic algorithm relies on the 2010 ACR/EULAR

classification criteria. These criteria are based on a scoring system involving four domains: joint involvement (number and size of joints), serology (Rheumatoid Factor [RF] and anti-citrullinated protein antibodies [ACPA]), acute-phase reactants (CRP and ESR), and duration of symptoms. A score of ≥ 6/10 confirms the diagnosis. The diagnosis is clinical, supported by serology and imaging showing joint-space narrowing and marginal erosions.

Differential Diagnosis

The primary differential is other inflammatory polyarthritides. The main differentials include psoriatic arthritis (look for nail pitting, dactylitis), systemic lupus erythematosus (SLE, look for systemic non-joint features), viral arthritis (e.g., Parvovirus B19, which is acute and self-limiting), and pseudogout (CPPD, involves different joints). Differentiating RA from osteoarthritis can be difficult, but RA is "inflammatory" (morning stiffness > 1 hour, soft tissue swelling) while OA is "degenerative" (stiffness < 30 min, bony swelling).

Treatment Algorithm

The modern RA algorithm is a proactive "Treat-to-Target" (T2T) strategy. The goal is to achieve clinical remission or low disease activity (LDAS) as quickly as possible.

Step 1: Initiate DMARD Therapy

As soon as the diagnosis is made, a conventional synthetic Disease-Modifying Antirheumatic Drug (csDMARD) is initiated. Methotrexate (MTX) is the universal first-line "anchor" drug.

Bridging Therapy

NSAIDs and/or low-dose corticosteroids (e.g., prednisone ≤ 10 mg/day) are used for rapid symptom control but only as a "bridge" while waiting for the DMARD (which takes weeks to months) to take effect. They are not appropriate as monotherapy.

Step 2: T2T Assessment (3-6 Months)

The patient's disease activity is formally measured (e.g., DAS28, CDAI score).

Target Achieved: Continue current therapy.
Target Not Achieved: The algorithm escalates. Options include:

- Combination csDMARDs: Add another csDMARD, typically sulfasalazine and/or hydroxychloroquine (Triple Therapy).
- Add Biologic/Targeted Synthetic: For moderate-high disease activity, the algorithm advances to adding a biologic DMARD (bDMARD) or a targeted synthetic DMARD (tsDMARD). This includes TNF-inhibitors (e.g., adalimumab, etanercept), IL-6 inhibitors, or JAK inhibitors (e.g., tofacitinib). The choice is based on comorbidities, cost, and patient preference.

Step 3: Subsequent Failure

If the first biologic or tsDMARD fails, the algorithm dictates switching to another agent, often one with a different mechanism of action.

Table 7.1: Differential Features of Rheumatoid vs. Osteoarthritis

Feature	Rheumatoid Arthritis (RA)	Osteoarthritis (OA)
Pathology	Autoimmune / Inflammatory	Degenerative / "Wear & Tear"
Joints	Small joints (MCP, PIP), symmetric, wrists, ankles	Weight-bearing (knees, hips), DIP, PIP, 1st CMC
Stiffness	Morning stiffness > 60 min, improves with activity	Morning stiffness < 30 min, worsens with activity
Labs	RF / anti-CCP (+), High ESR/CRP	RF / anti-CCP (-), Normal ESR/CRP

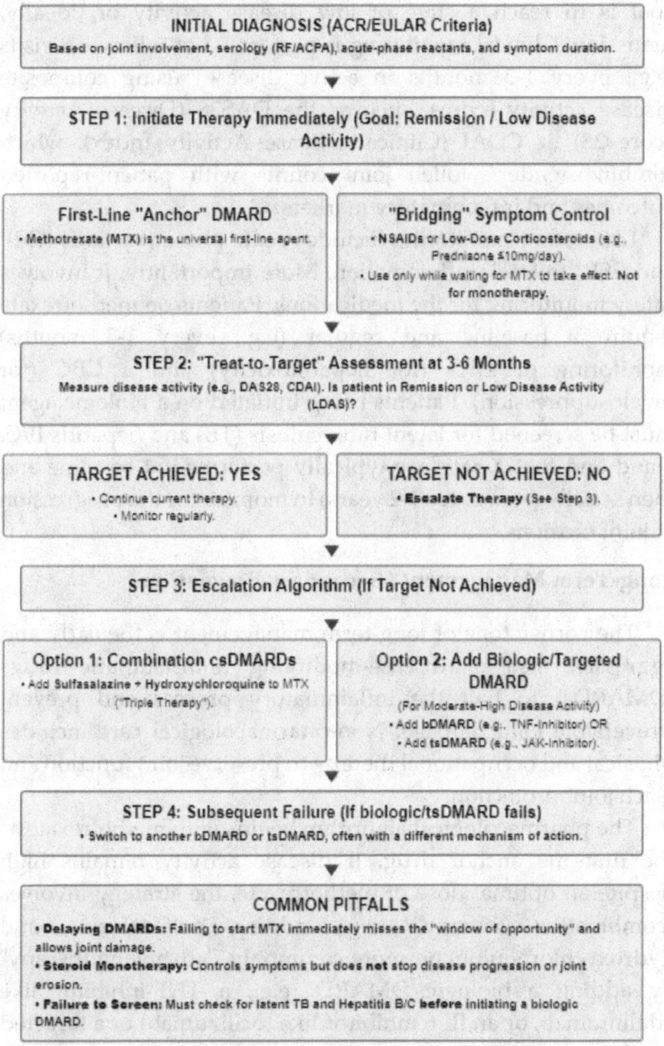

Figure 7.1: Rheumatoid Arthritis - "Treat-to-Target" (T2T)

Monitoring and Follow-Up

The modern management of RA follows a "Treat-to-Target" strategy, which requires frequent and objective monitoring. The goal is to reach a state of low disease activity or, ideally, remission. Clinical monitoring is performed at follow-up visits (e.g., every 1-3 months in active disease) using composite disease activity scores, such as the DAS28 (Disease Activity Score 28) or CDAI (Clinical Disease Activity Index), which combine tender/swollen joint counts with patient-reported outcomes and inflammatory markers.

Laboratory monitoring includes acute phase reactants (CRP and ESR) to track inflammation. More importantly, it involves safety monitoring for the medications. Patients on methotrexate require a baseline and regular (e.g., every 1-3 months) monitoring of LFTs (for hepatotoxicity) and a CBC (for myelosuppression). Patients being initiated on a biologic agent must be screened for latent tuberculosis (TB) and hepatitis B/C. Hand and foot X-rays are typically performed at baseline and then serially (e.g., every 1-2 years) to monitor for the progression of joint erosions.

Long-Term Management / Secondary Prevention

The cornerstone of long-term management is the early and aggressive use of disease-modifying antirheumatic drugs (DMARDs) to halt the inflammatory process and prevent irreversible joint damage. Non-pharmacological care includes physical and occupational therapy to preserve joint function and teach joint protection.

The pharmacological algorithm begins with methotrexate as the first-line anchor drug. If disease activity remains high despite an optimal dose of methotrexate, the strategy involves "combination therapy" (e.g., adding sulfasalazine and hydroxychloroquine) or, more commonly, "advancing therapy" by adding a biologic DMARD (e.g., a TNF-inhibitor like adalimumab, or an IL-6 inhibitor like tocilizumab) or a targeted synthetic DMARD (a JAK inhibitor like tofacitinib). Glucocorticoids (e.g., low-dose prednisone) may be used as a "bridge" therapy to control inflammation while waiting for DMARDs to take effect. Secondary prevention is focused on managing the systemic nature of RA, which includes aggressive cardiovascular risk reduction (as RA is a major risk factor for CAD), screening for osteoporosis, and managing extra-articular manifestations (e.g., interstitial lung disease).

Patient Counseling Points

1. **DMARDs vs. NSAIDs:** This is a crucial concept. "NSAIDs (like ibuprofen) are for *symptoms* (pain), while DMARDs (like methotrexate) are for the *disease*." Emphasize that the DMARD is the essential medication to prevent joint destruction, even if it doesn't relieve pain immediately.
2. **Therapeutic Lag:** Counsel that methotrexate and other DMARDs are "slow-acting." They are not painkillers and may take 6-12 weeks to exert their full effect.
3. **Infection Risk:** For patients on biologics or JAK inhibitors, this is a crucial safety point. "These medicines work by turning *down* parts of your immune system, which puts you at a higher risk for infections. You must call us immediately if you develop a fever, cough, or any sign of infection."
4. **MTX Safety:** Counsel on the importance of folic acid supplementation to reduce side effects. Emphasize that methotrexate is a once-a-*week* dose, and that it is an absolute teratogen (must not be used in pregnancy).
5. **Smoking Cessation:** Smoking is one of the strongest environmental risk factors for developing RA and makes the disease more severe and less responsive to treatment. Cessation is a primary therapeutic goal.

Common Pitfalls in Management

The most critical pitfall is a delay in diagnosis and DMARD initiation, as this "window of opportunity" is when intervention can prevent irreversible joint damage. A second pitfall is using corticosteroids or NSAIDs as long-term monotherapy, which controls symptoms but does not stop disease progression. A major safety pitfall is failing to screen for latent tuberculosis (TB) and viral hepatitis (B and C) *before* initiating a biologic DMARD. Finally, under-dosing methotrexate or failing to supplement with folic acid (which reduces side effects) is a common error.

Case Study

A 45-year-old female (Ms. Brier) presents with a 4-month history of symmetric, "boggy" swelling and pain in her hands (MCPs and PIPs) and wrists. She reports morning stiffness that lasts for over an hour. Her labs are positive for **Rheumatoid Factor (RF)** and **anti-CCP antibodies**.

Discussion

This is a classic presentation for **Rheumatoid Arthritis**. The symmetric, inflammatory polyarthritis of small joints, prolonged morning stiffness, and positive, specific autoantibodies (anti-CCP) confirm the diagnosis. The modern algorithm is "Treat-to-Target" (T2T), which mandates starting a DMARD immediately.

Treatment Algorithm

1. **Diagnosis:** Seropositive Rheumatoid Arthritis.
2. **Algorithm Strategy:** Initiate "Treat-to-Target" (T2T). The goal is rapid remission or low disease activity.
3. **Step 1 (Anchor Drug):** Start a conventional synthetic DMARD (csDMARD) immediately.
    - **Therapy: Methotrexate (MTX) 15 mg once weekly**.
    - **Adjunct:** Start **Folic Acid 1 mg daily** to reduce MTX side effects.
4. **Step 2 (Bridging):** To control her severe symptoms *now* (while the MTX takes weeks to work), start a "bridge" therapy.
    - **Therapy: Prednisone 10 mg daily** with a plan to taper off as soon as the MTX takes effect.
5. **Safety Monitoring:** Order baseline CBC, LFTs, and Hepatitis B/C screening before starting MTX.
6. **Follow-up:** Schedule follow-up in 3 months to assess disease activity (e.g., DAS28 score). If she is not at target, the algorithm would escalate (e.g., add a biologic).

Outcome

Ms. Brier is started on weekly Methotrexate for long-term disease control and a short-term prednisone taper for immediate symptom relief.

OSTEOARTHRITIS

Osteoarthritis is the most common form of arthritis, characterized by the mechanical breakdown of joint cartilage and underlying bone. It is a degenerative, "wear and tear" disease driven by mechanical stress, aging, and inflammation.

Pathophysiology

The pathophysiology involves a complex interplay of mechanical stress and low-grade inflammation. Repetitive micro-trauma or abnormal joint loading (e.g., from obesity or injury) leads to chondrocyte (cartilage cell) stress. These stressed chondrocytes release enzymes (matrix metalloproteinases) that break down the cartilage matrix faster than it can be repaired. The subchondral bone stiffens and develops microfractures, and bony outgrowths, or "osteophytes," form at the joint margins. Debris from the degrading cartilage sheds into the joint, triggering a secondary synovial inflammatory response, which in turn releases more pro-inflammatory cytokines that accelerate cartilage breakdown, creating a vicious cycle.

Diagnosis

Diagnosis is primarily clinical. It is based on a history of use-related joint pain (worse with activity, better with rest), morning stiffness lasting < 30 minutes, older age, and common joint involvement (hands [DIPs, PIPs], knees, hips, spine). Radiographs (X-rays) confirm the diagnosis by showing characteristic findings: joint space narrowing, osteophytes (bone spurs), subchondral sclerosis, and cysts.

Differential Diagnosis

The main differential is an inflammatory arthritis like RA,

which is distinguished by its prolonged morning stiffness, "boggy" synovial swelling, and positive serologies. Other differentials include gout or pseudogout (acute, episodic, crystal-proven), psoriatic arthritis (check skin/nails), and soft-tissue conditions like bursitis or tendonitis, which are localized to peri-articular structures rather than the joint itself.

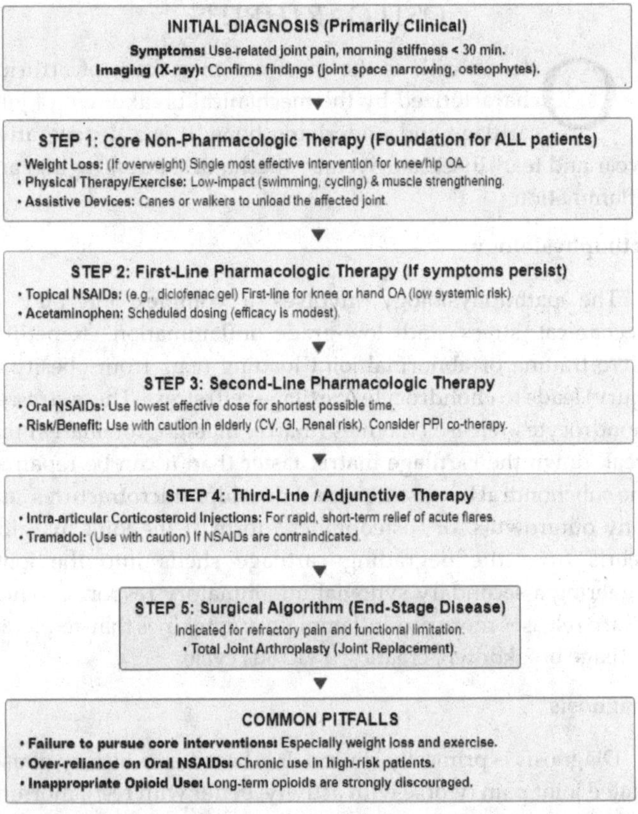

Figure 7.2: Osteoarthritis - Symptom-Based Algorithm

Treatment Algorithm

The OA algorithm is a stepwise, patient-centered approach focused on symptom management and functional improvement.

- **Step 1: Core Non-Pharmacological Therapy:** This is the foundation of the algorithm for all patients. It includes:
    1. **Weight Loss:** For overweight patients with knee/hip OA, this is the single most effective intervention.
    2. **Physical Therapy/Exercise:** Low-impact exercise (e.g., swimming, cycling) and specific muscle-strengthening exercises (e.g., for quadriceps) are critical.
    3. **Assistive Devices:** Canes or walkers can unload the affected joint.
- **Step 2: First-Line Pharmacological Therapy:** If core interventions are insufficient.
    - **Topical NSAIDs:** For knee or hand OA, these are first-line due to their high efficacy and low systemic risk.
    - **Acetaminophen (Paracetamol):** Scheduled, not "as needed," is an option, though its efficacy is now considered modest.
- **Step 3: Second-Line Pharmacological Therapy:** For moderate-severe pain.
    - **Oral NSAIDs:** The lowest effective dose for the shortest possible time. This requires a risk/benefit calculation, especially in elderly patients with renal, GI, or cardiovascular risk. Use with a proton-pump inhibitor (PPI) is often warranted.
- **Step 4: Third-Line/Adjunctive Therapy:**
    - **Intra-articular Corticosteroid Injections:** Provide rapid, short-term (weeks to months) pain relief, particularly for acute flares.
    - **Tramadol:** An option if NSAIDs are contraindicated, but carries risk of opiate dependence and other side effects.

- **Step 5: Surgical Algorithm:** For end-stage disease with refractory pain, functional limitation, and radiographic evidence. The algorithm proceeds to **total joint arthroplasty** (joint replacement), which is a highly effective procedure for pain relief and functional restoration.

Table 7.2: Simplified RA Treatment Algorithm (Treat-to-Target)

Step	Intervention	Rationale / Goal
Step 1	**Methotrexate (MTX)** monotherapy (± bridge w/ NSAID or low-dose steroid)	First-line csDMARD (Conventional Synthetic DMARD).
Step 2 (Mod-High Activity)	**Add bDMARD** (e.g., TNF-inhibitor) or tsDMARD (e.g., JAK-inhibitor)	Dual therapy for inadequate response to MTX.
Step 3 (Mod-High Activity)	**Switch b/tsDMARD** (e.g., different mechanism of action)	Target refractory disease.

Monitoring and Follow-Up

Monitoring for OA is almost entirely clinical, focused on the patient's symptoms (pain, stiffness) and functional status. Validated questionnaires, such as the WOMAC (Western Ontario and McMaster Universities Osteoarthritis Index) or KOOS/HOOS (Knee/Hip Disability and Osteoarthritis Outcome Score), can be used to objectively track pain and function over time. Weight should be monitored at every visit. Radiographic monitoring (X-rays) is used for initial diagnosis (to show joint space narrowing, osteophytes, and subchondral sclerosis) but is *not* useful for routine follow-up, as radiographic findings correlate very poorly with a patient's pain level.

Long-Term Management / Secondary Prevention

The long-term management of OA is a multimodal, non-curative approach aimed at controlling pain and improving function.

- **Non-Pharmacological:** This is the cornerstone of all OA management. It includes: 1) **Weight Loss:** For overweight patients, this is the single most effective intervention for knee/hip OA. 2) **Physical Therapy:** Strengthening exercises (especially for the quadriceps in knee OA) and range-of-motion exercises are critical. 3) **Assistive Devices:** Canes or walkers to offload the affected joint.
- **Pharmacological:** The algorithm is stepwise:
    1. **Topical NSAIDs:** (e.g., diclofenac gel) are first-line for knee OA, offering good efficacy with minimal systemic risk.
    2. **Oral NSAIDs:** (e.g., naproxen, ibuprofen) are used for moderate-to-severe pain, using the lowest effective dose for the shortest duration.
    3. **Intra-articular Injections:** Corticosteroid injections can provide rapid, temporary (weeks to months) relief for acute flares.
    4. **Surgical:** For end-stage, refractory OA, total joint replacement (arthroplasty) is the definitive management.

Patient Counseling Points

1. **Weight Loss as Therapy:** "For every 1 pound of weight you lose, it takes 4-6 pounds of pressure off your knees." This is the most powerful "drug" for knee and hip OA.
2. **Exercise is Medicine:** "Motion is lotion." Patients often fear exercise will "wear out" the joint faster. The opposite is true. Low-impact exercise (walking, swimming, cycling) and physical therapy strengthen the muscles that support the joint, which *reduces* pain and improves stability.
3. **Pain vs. Damage:** Reassure the patient that their X-ray does not define them. "We treat the *patient*, not the X-ray." A person with "bone-on-bone" X-rays can be functional, while another with "mild" X-rays can have severe pain.

4. **Topical NSAIDs:** Counsel on correct use—it is not an "as-needed" rub. It must be applied 3-4 times *daily* for 1-2 weeks to build up a therapeutic level in the joint tissue.

Common Pitfalls in Management

The most common pitfall is a failure to aggressively pursue the core non-pharmacological interventions, especially weight loss. Another major error is the over-reliance on and chronic prescribing of oral NSAIDs in high-risk patients. A critical pitfall is the inappropriate use of long-term opioids for OA, which is strongly discouraged due to high risks and poor long-term efficacy. Finally, misdiagnosing an inflammatory arthritis as OA leads to undertreatment and joint destruction.

Case Study

A 68-year-old male (Mr. Frank) with a BMI of 32 presents with a 2-year history of right knee pain. The pain is a "deep ache" that is *worse* at the end of the day or after walking. His morning stiffness is minimal, lasting only 5-10 minutes. An X-ray shows joint space narrowing and osteophytes.

Discussion

This presentation is the hallmark of **Osteoarthritis (OA)**: a degenerative (not inflammatory) process. The pain is "mechanical" (worse with use), stiffness is brief, and it affects a large, weight-bearing joint. The algorithm is a stepwise approach focused on symptoms and function.

Treatment Algorithm

1. **Diagnosis:** Clinical and radiographic Osteoarthritis of the knee.
2. **Algorithm Step 1 (Core Non-Pharmacological):** This is the foundation of therapy.
    - **Counseling:** Emphasize **weight loss** (the single most effective intervention) and **Physical Therapy** (for quadriceps strengthening).
3. **Step 2 (First-Line Pharm):** He has already tried

acetaminophen with minimal relief.

   - **Therapy:** Start **Topical NSAID (e.g., Diclofenac gel 1%)** applied to the knee 3-4 times daily. This has high efficacy and low systemic risk.

4. **Step 3 (Second-Line):** If topical therapy is insufficient, you would move to oral NSAIDs.
   - **Therapy: Naproxen 500 mg BID** *with* a PPI (e.g., Omeprazole) for gastroprotection, given his age.
5. **Step 4 (Refractory):** If he has a severe flare, an **intra-articular corticosteroid injection** is an option. If he has end-stage, disabling pain, the final step is referral for **total knee arthroplasty**.

Outcome

Mr. Frank is referred to physical therapy, a weight-loss program, and started on topical diclofenac gel, with a plan to try oral NSAIDs if this fails.

OSTEOPOROSIS

Osteoporosis is a metabolic bone disease characterized by low bone mass and microarchitectural deterioration of bone tissue, leading to enhanced bone fragility and a consequent increase in fracture risk.

Pathophysiology

The pathophysiology is a fundamental imbalance in the normal bone remodeling cycle, where bone resorption (by osteoclasts) outpaces bone formation (by osteoblasts). The most common cause is **post-menopausal osteoporosis**. The sharp decline in estrogen at menopause removes estrogen's "braking" effect on osteoclasts, leading to a period of rapid bone resorption and bone loss. Senile osteoporosis occurs later in life from age-related factors. A major secondary cause is **glucocorticoid-induced osteoporosis**, as steroids are directly toxic to osteoblasts and promote osteoclast activity.

Diagnosis

The diagnostic algorithm has two entry points:

1. **Fragility Fracture:** A fracture from a fall from standing height or less (e.g., hip, vertebral, wrist). This is diagnostic of osteoporosis regardless of bone density.
2. **DXA Scan:** Bone mineral density (BMD) measured by dual-energy X-ray absorptiometry (DXA). A T-score of ≤ -2.5 at the lumbar spine, femoral neck, or total hip is diagnostic. A T-score between -1.0 and -2.5 is defined as osteopenia. The algorithm also includes risk assessment, using the **FRAX score** to calculate the 10-year probability of a major osteoporotic fracture, which helps guide treatment decisions in patients with osteopenia.

Differential Diagnosis

The main step is to differentiate primary osteoporosis (age-related or postmenopausal) from secondary causes. The algorithm must include a workup to rule out hyperparathyroidism, vitamin D deficiency, multiple myeloma (in the setting of vertebral fractures), glucocorticoid-induced osteoporosis, hyperthyroidism, and hypogonadism. Osteomalacia (impaired bone mineralization, often from severe vitamin D deficiency) can also mimic osteoporosis.

Treatment Algorithm

The algorithm is stratified by fracture risk.

- **Step 1: Universal Measures (All Patients):**
    - Adequate calcium (1200 mg/day) and vitamin D (800-1000 IU/day) intake.
    - Weight-bearing exercise and fall prevention strategies.
    - Smoking cessation and alcohol moderation.
- **Step 2: Initiate Pharmacotherapy (High-Risk Patients):**
    - **High Risk:** T-score ≤ -2.5 OR history of fragility fracture OR high-risk FRAX score.
    - **First-Line Therapy:** Oral bisphosphonates

(e.g., alendronate, risedronate). These are the first-line antiresorptive agents.
  - **Alternatives:** For patients who cannot tolerate oral bisphosphonates (e.g., GERD, esophageal issues) or have adherence issues, the algorithm moves to IV bisphosphonates (zoledronic acid, once yearly) or subcutaneous denosumab (every 6 months).
- **Step 3: Very High-Risk Patients:**
  - **Very High Risk:** Recent fragility fracture (< 12 months), multiple fractures, or extremely low T-score (e.g., < -3.0).
  - **Algorithm:** Initiate an anabolic agent *first* (e.g., teriparatide, abaloparatide) for 1-2 years to rapidly build bone. This is *always* followed by an antiresorptive agent (bisphosphonate or denosumab) to "lock in" the gains.
- **Step 4: Duration and Monitoring:**
  - The algorithm for oral bisphosphonates includes a "drug holiday" re-evaluation after 5 years (3 years for IV) in low-moderate risk patients.

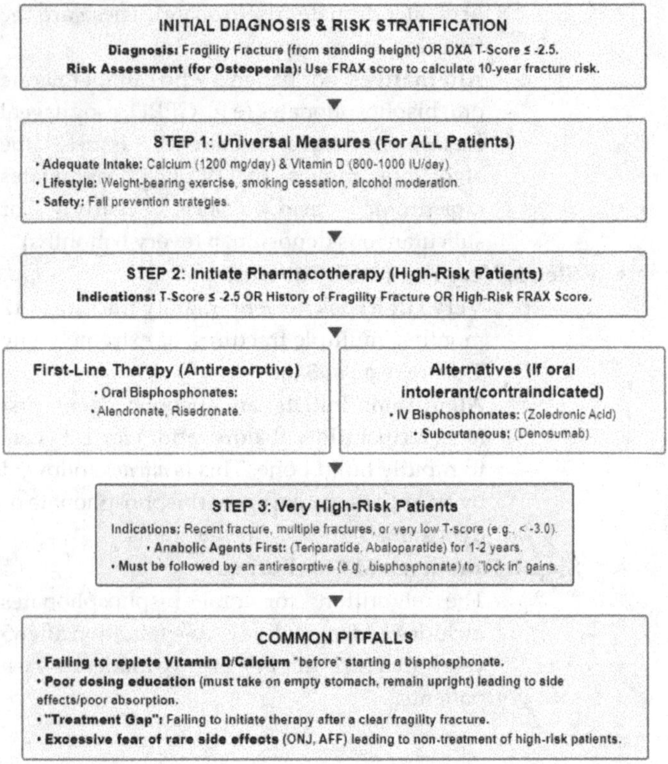

Figure 7.3: Osteoporosis - Risk-Prevention Algorithm

Monitoring and Follow-Up

The diagnosis is made by a central DEXA (Dual-energy X-ray Absorptiometry) scan, which defines osteoporosis as a T-score of ≤ -2.5. The 10-year fracture risk is calculated using the FRAX score. After initiating pharmacological therapy, a follow-up DEXA scan is typically performed in 1-2 years to ensure the BMD is stable or increasing; this confirms adherence and therapeutic response. Routine lab work (e.g., calcium, 25-hydroxyvitamin D, renal function) should be monitored annually. Patients should also be monitored for height loss (a sign of vertebral fracture) at each visit.

Table 7.3: Osteoporosis Treatment Algorithm

Patient Profile	Diagnostic Criteria	Treatment Algorithm
Low Bone Mass (Osteopenia)	T-score -1.0 to -2.5	Lifestyle (Vit D/Calcium, exercise). (Pharmacological therapy if high FRAX score).
Osteoporosis	T-score ≤ -2.5 OR Fragility Fracture	**1. Lifestyle** (Vit D/Calcium). **2. First-Line:** Oral Bisphosphonate (e.g., Alendronate). **3. Alt:** IV Bisphosphonate, Denosumab.
Severe / High-Risk	Very low T-score or multiple fractures.	Anabolic Agents (e.g., Teriparatide) followed by antiresorptive.

Long-Term Management / Secondary Prevention

The primary goal is the prevention of fragility fractures.

- **Non-Pharmacological:** This is a universal requirement for all patients. It includes adequate intake of **Calcium** (1200 mg/day total) and **Vitamin D** (800-1000 IU/day), participation in **weight-bearing exercise** (like walking), and rigorous **fall prevention** (e.g., home safety evaluation).
- **Pharmacological:** Indicated for patients with a T-score ≤ -2.5 or a history of a fragility fracture.
    1. **First-line:** Anti-resorptive agents, specifically oral **bisphosphonates** (e.g., alendronate, risedronate). IV bisphosphonates (e.g., zoledronic acid) are an option for intolerance. Denosumab (a biologic) is another potent anti-resorptive first-line option.
    2. **Anabolic Agents:** For very severe osteoporosis (e.g., T-score < -3.0 or multiple fractures), anabolic agents (e.g., teriparatide) that *build* new bone are used.

3. **Drug Holiday:** For patients on oral bisphosphonates, a "drug holiday" (a 1-2 year pause in therapy) may be considered after 5 years (3 for IV) to reduce the risk of rare side effects.

Patient Counseling Points

1. **Bisphosphonate Dosing:** This is a critical counseling point to ensure absorption and prevent esophagitis. "You must take this pill *first thing* in the morning, on a *completely empty stomach,* with a *full glass of plain water* (no coffee/juice). You must then remain *sitting or standing upright* for at least 30 minutes (60 for ibandronate)."
2. **Osteonecrosis of the Jaw (ONJ):** Patients are often scared of this. Put it in perspective: "This is a very *rare* side effect, most often seen in cancer patients on high-dose IV versions. The risk for you is extremely low. The risk of a hip fracture from *not* treating your osteoporosis is *far, far higher*."
3. **Fall Prevention:** "The medicine makes your bones stronger, but your job is to not fall." Counsel on removing tripping hazards (rugs), ensuring good lighting, and getting vision checked.
4. **"Silent Disease":** "You cannot *feel* your bones getting weaker." This is why they must take their medication even though they feel fine.

Common Pitfalls in Management

A critical pitfall is initiating a bisphosphonate *before* checking and repleting a patient's vitamin D and calcium levels, which can worsen hypocalcemia. A second is poor patient education on oral bisphosphonate administration (must be taken with a full glass of water, on an empty stomach, and remain upright for 30-60 min), which leads to poor absorption and esophageal irritation. A major gap in care is the "treatment gap": failing to initiate therapy in a patient who has just sustained a clear fragility fracture. Finally, excessive fear of rare side effects (atypical femur fracture, osteonecrosis of the jaw) often leads to non-treatment of high-risk patients who have a much higher risk of fracture.

Case Study

A 70-year-old female (Mrs. Lee) sustained a **wrist fracture** after tripping on a rug (a "fragility fracture"). She has a history of smoking. A DEXA scan is ordered and shows a T-score of -2.2 at the femoral neck (consistent with *osteopenia*).

Discussion

This is a critical concept. Even though her DEXA scan only shows osteopenia, her **fragility fracture (a fracture from a fall from standing height or less)** ***is*** **a clinical diagnosis of severe osteoporosis**. She is at very high risk for a future, more devastating hip fracture. The algorithm mandates treatment.

Treatment Algorithm

1. **Diagnosis:** Severe Osteoporosis (clinically defined by fragility fracture).
2. **Step 1 (Labs):** You order baseline labs, including serum calcium, renal function, and **25-hydroxy Vitamin D**. Her Vitamin D level is 18 ng/mL (deficient).
3. **Step 2 (Repletion):** The algorithm dictates you must **replete Vitamin D** ***before*** **starting a bisphosphonate** to prevent hypocalcemia.
    - **Therapy:** Start **Vitamin D3 50,000 IU once weekly for 8 weeks**, followed by 2000 IU daily.
4. **Step 3 (First-Line Pharm):** Once her Vitamin D level is sufficient, you initiate a first-line antiresorptive agent.
    - **Therapy: Alendronate 70 mg once weekly**.
5. **Counseling:** You provide critical counseling on how to take Alendronate (first thing in the morning, empty stomach, full glass of water, remain upright for 30 min) and on fall prevention.

Outcome

Mrs. Lee is started on high-dose Vitamin D repletion, to be followed by Alendronate 70 mg weekly for long-term fracture prevention.

GOUT

Gout is a crystal-deposition disease characterized by recurrent episodes of acute, intensely painful inflammatory arthritis (gout flare) and, in chronic cases, tophi formation, resulting from hyperuricemia and the deposition of monosodium urate (MSU) crystals in and around joints.

Pathophysiology

Gout is a severe inflammatory arthritis caused by the deposition of monosodium urate (MSU) crystals in and around the joints. This deposition is a direct consequence of chronic hyperuricemia (serum uric acid > 6.8 mg/dL), the level at which urate saturates in the blood. Hyperuricemia is most commonly (in 90% of cases) due to inefficient **renal under-excretion** of uric acid, not overproduction. When MSU crystals precipitate in the joint, they are seen as "foreign" by the innate immune system. Macrophages attempt to phagocytose the crystals, triggering the NALP3 inflammasome. This leads to a massive release of IL-1β, a potent pro-inflammatory cytokine that drives a catastrophic influx of neutrophils into the joint, resulting in the classic, exquisitely painful, erythematous, and swollen joint (often the big toe, or "podagra").

Diagnosis

The gold standard for diagnosis is **synovial fluid analysis** (arthrocentesis) of an affected joint, which shows needle-shaped, negatively birefringent MSU crystals under polarized light. This also definitively rules out septic arthritis. A clinical diagnosis is often made in classic cases (e.g., podagra [1st MTP joint] with acute onset, erythema, and hyperuricemia). A serum uric acid (sUA) level supports the diagnosis, but it can be falsely normal or low during an acute flare.

Differential Diagnosis

The most critical, "cannot-miss" differential for a hot, swollen, monoarticular joint is **septic arthritis**. This is an orthopedic emergency. Other differentials include pseudogout

(CPPD, different crystals [rhomboid, positively birefringent]), cellulitis (which has diffuse erythema *without* primary joint pain), and psoriatic arthritis.

Treatment Algorithm

The management algorithm is bifurcated into treating the acute attack and long-term urate-lowering therapy.

Acute Gout Attack Algorithm

The goal is rapid anti-inflammatory relief. This is *not* the time to start urate-lowering therapy.

First-Line Options

- **NSAIDs:** High-dose, full-strength (e.g., naproxen 500 mg BID, indomethacin 50 mg TID) are highly effective.
- **Colchicine:** Must be started within 24-36 hours of onset. The algorithm uses a low-dose regimen (1.2 mg STAT, then 0.6 mg one hour later, followed by 0.6 mg BID) which is as effective and less toxic than older regimens.
- **Corticosteroids:** Oral prednisone (e.g., 30-40 mg daily for 5 days) or an intra-articular steroid injection (if one joint is involved and sepsis is ruled out). The choice is based on comorbidities (e.g., avoid NSAIDs in CKD; avoid steroids in uncontrolled diabetes).

Table 7.4: Gout Management Algorithms (Acute vs. Chronic)

Phase	Primary Goal	First-Line Therapy
Acute Flare (Attack)	Pain relief, resolve inflammation.	**1. NSAIDs** (e.g., Naproxen) OR **2. Colchicine** OR **3. Corticosteroids** (Oral or Intra-articular).
Chronic (Prevention)	Lower serum urate (< 6 mg/dL) to prevent flares.	**Urate-Lowering Therapy (ULT): 1. Allopurinol** (first-line). **2. Febuxostat.** (Probenecid as alternative).

Chronic Urate-Lowering Therapy (ULT) Algorithm

The goal is to lower sUA to a target of < 6 mg/dL (< 5 mg/dL in tophaceous gout) to dissolve crystals and prevent future flares.

- **Indications:** ULT is *not* for everyone. Indications include ≥ 2 gout flares per year, presence of tophi, or radiographic evidence of gouty arthropathy.
- **Step 1: Initiate ULT:** The first-line agent is **allopurinol**, a xanthine oxidase inhibitor. The algorithm is to "start low, go slow." Start at 100 mg daily (50 mg in CKD) and titrate the dose upwards every 2-5 weeks until the sUA target (< 6 mg/dL) is reached.
- **Step 2: Prophylaxis:** When starting ULT, mobilization flares are common. The algorithm requires co-administration of prophylactic anti-inflammatory therapy (e.g., colchicine 0.6 mg daily or a low-dose NSAID) for the first 3-6 months.
- **Step 3: Second-Line:** If allopurinol fails to reach target (often due to under-dosing) or is not tolerated, the algorithm moves to **febuxostat** (another xanthine oxidase inhibitor).

Monitoring and Follow-Up

Monitoring for gout is two-fold:

1. **Acute Flare:** Monitoring is clinical, assessing for resolution of pain and inflammation.
2. **Long-Term (Prophylaxis):** The primary goal is monitoring the serum uric acid (sUA). After initiating urate-lowering therapy (ULT), the sUA is checked every 2-5 weeks while titrating the dose. The goal is to achieve and maintain a sUA < 6.0 mg/dL (or < 5.0 mg/dL if tophi are present). Once the target is reached, sUA can be monitored every 6-12 months.

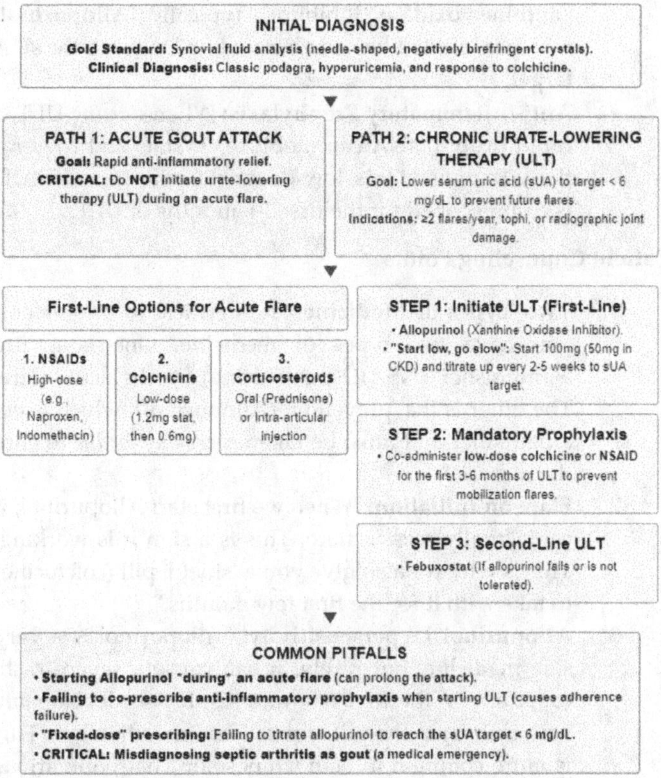

Figure 7.4: Gout - Bifurcated Management Algorithm

Long-Term Management / Secondary Prevention

The management algorithm is divided into treating the acute flare and preventing future flares (which is the long-term cure).

- **Acute Flare Treatment:** The goal is rapid inflammation control. First-line options are high-dose **NSAIDs** (e.g., naproxen, indomethacin), oral **colchicine** (low-dose protocol: 1.2 mg, then 0.6 mg one hour later), or **corticosteroids** (oral prednisone or intra-articular injection).
- **Long-Term Prophylaxis (ULT):** This is the definitive treatment to *cure* the disease by lowering sUA. It is *not* started during an acute flare. First-line ULT is a

xanthine oxidase inhibitor, typically **Allopurinol**, which is "started low and titrated up" to reach the sUA target.

- **Anti-inflammatory Prophylaxis:** When *starting* ULT, a rapid drop in sUA can mobilize crystals and *trigger* a flare. To prevent this, low-dose colchicine or an NSAID is co-prescribed for the first 3-6 months of ULT.

Patient Counseling Points

1. **Two Types of Medicine:** "It is critical to understand you have two types of medicine. One is a 'fire extinguisher' (NSAIDs, colchicine) for the acute flare. The other is the 'preventer' (Allopurinol), which is *not* a painkiller and must be taken *every day for life* to cure the disease."
2. **Flare on Initiation:** "When we first start Allopurinol, it can actually *cause* a flare. This is a sign it is working. This is why we also give you a 'shield' pill (colchicine) to take with it for the first few months."
3. **Allopurinol Hypersensitivity:** "Allopurinol is a very safe medicine, but rarely, it can cause a severe rash, especially in the first few months. If you develop *any* new rash, stop the pill and call us immediately." (This is more common in Han Chinese or Thai populations with the HLA-B*5801 allele).
4. **Lifestyle:** "While diet is not the main *cause*, it is a *trigger*." Counsel to limit alcohol (especially beer), high-purine meats (e.g., organ meats, shellfish), and high-fructose corn syrup (sugary sodas).

Common Pitfalls in Management

The most common pitfall is starting allopurinol *during* an acute gout flare, which can prolong the attack. A second is "fixed-dose" allopurinol prescribing, typically starting and leaving the patient on 300 mg without titrating to the sUA target, leading to treatment failure. A third major error is failing to provide prophylactic colchicine or NSAIDs when initiating ULT, resulting in a painful "mobilization flare" and non-adherence.

Finally, the most dangerous pitfall is misdiagnosing septic arthritis as a gout flare, which can lead to joint destruction.

Case Study

A 52-year-old male (Mr. Davis) with a history of hypertension (treated with HCTZ) and obesity wakes at 2 AM with a **10/10, exquisite pain in his left great toe**. The joint is swollen, red, hot, and he cannot even tolerate a bedsheet on it (podagra). This is his third such attack in the last year.

Discussion

This is a classic presentation of an **Acute Gouty Attack**. The management algorithm is bifurcated: 1) Treat the acute, painful inflammation *now*. 2) Address the long-term hyperuricemia *later* to prevent future attacks.

Treatment Algorithm

1. **Diagnosis:** Acute Gout (Podagra).
2. **Algorithm (Part 1: Acute Flare):** The goal is rapid anti-inflammation.
    - **Therapy:** Start **Indomethacin 50 mg TID** (a high-dose NSAID) for 3-5 days. (Oral prednisone or colchicine would also be correct).
    - **Critical Pitfall:** You do **NOT** start Allopurinol during the acute flare. You also review his HCTZ, a medication known to trigger gout.
3. **Algorithm (Part 2: Chronic ULT):** The patient has recurrent gout (≥2 flares/year), which is an indication for Urate-Lowering Therapy (ULT).
    - **Therapy (to start *after* flare resolves):** Start **Allopurinol 100 mg daily** (a "start low, go slow" approach).
    - **Prophylaxis (Critical Step):** *Concurrently* with the Allopurinol, you must start **Colchicine 0.6 mg daily** for 3-6 months. This prevents the "mobilization flare" that occurs when starting ULT.
    - **Target:** You will titrate the Alloplurinol dose

every 4-6 weeks to achieve a target serum uric acid of **< 6 mg/dL**.

Outcome

Mr. Davis is given Indomethacin for his acute pain. You schedule a follow-up in 1 week to start his long-term Allopurinol and colchicine prophylaxis

Summary

Rheumatoid Arthritis: The algorithm is a "Treat-to-Target" (T2T) strategy. It begins with immediate initiation of methotrexate (MTX) and uses bridging steroids/NSAIDs. Failure to reach low disease activity by 3-6 months triggers escalation to combination DMARDs, biologics, or JAK inhibitors.

Osteoarthritis: The algorithm is a stepwise, symptom-based approach. It starts with foundational non-pharmacological interventions (weight loss, exercise). It then progresses pharmacologically from topical NSAIDs, to oral NSAIDs, to intra-articular injections. End-stage disease is managed with surgical joint replacement.

Osteoporosis: The algorithm is risk-based, using FRAX and DXA. High-risk patients are started on first-line antiresorptives (oral bisphosphonates). Very high-risk patients may be started on an anabolic agent (e.g., teriparatide) first, followed by an antiresorptive.

Gout: The algorithm is bifurcated. Acute attacks are managed with anti-inflammatories (NSAIDs, colchicine, or steroids). Chronic management (ULT) is indicated for recurrent attacks or tophi, using a "start low, go slow" titration of allopurinol to a serum uric acid target of < 6 mg/dL, with co-prescribed prophylaxis.

Multiple Choice Questions

1. A 45-year-old female is newly diagnosed with seropositive Rheumatoid Arthritis. What is the most appropriate initial step in the long-term treatment algorithm?
   A) Start high-dose prednisone
   B) Start naproxen and schedule physical therapy
   C) Start methotrexate
   D) Start adalimumab (a TNF-inhibitor)
2. A 68-year-old male with OA of the knee and a history of GI bleeding is seeking pain relief. He has already failed weight loss and physical therapy. What is the most appropriate next step?
   A) Oral naproxen
   B) Topical diclofenac gel
   C) Total knee arthroplasty
   D) Oral hydrocodone
3. A 70-year-old female has a DXA scan showing a T-score of -2.9 at the femoral neck. Her labs show a Vitamin D level of 15 ng/mL. What is the correct treatment algorithm?
   A) Start alendronate 70 mg weekly immediately
   B) Start teriparatide immediately
   C) Aggressively replete Vitamin D, then initiate alendronate
   D) Start denosumab 60 mg subcutaneously
4. A 55-year-old male with a history of gout presents with an acute, severe flare in his ankle. He has CKD Stage 4. Which of the following is the safest and most appropriate treatment for the acute flare?
   A) Indomethacin 50 mg TID
   B) Oral prednisone 40 mg daily
   C) Allopurinol 300 mg daily
   D) High-dose colchicine
5. A patient with RA fails to reach low disease activity after 6 months of maximal-dose methotrexate.

What is the most appropriate "escalation" step in the algorithm?
A) Stop methotrexate and start sulfasalazine
B) Add a TNF-inhibitor (e.g., etanercept) to the methotrexate
C) Continue methotrexate and add high-dose prednisone D) Switch to long-term opioid management

6. Which of the following is the foundational, first-line algorithm for all patients with osteoarthritis of the knee? A) Acetaminophen 1000 mg TID
B) Intra-articular corticosteroid injection
C) Weight loss and physical therapy
D) Topical capsaicin cream
7. A 62-year-old male is being started on allopurinol for chronic tophaceous gout. What is the target serum uric acid (sUA) for this patient?
A) < 8.0 mg/dL
B) < 7.0 mg/dL
C) < 6.0 mg/dL
D) < 5.0 mg/dL
8. What is the primary purpose of co-prescribing colchicine 0.6 mg daily when initiating allopurinol?
A) To rapidly lower the serum uric acid
B) To prevent a "mobilization flare"
C) To treat the patient's acute flare
D) To prevent allopurinol hypersensitivity
9. A 75-year-old female sustains a hip fracture from a simple fall. Her T-score on a previous DXA was -2.0 (osteopenia). What is the correct diagnostic and therapeutic algorithm? A) She has osteopenia; start calcium and vitamin D only. B) The fracture is diagnostic of osteoporosis; start a bisphosphonate. C) The fall was the problem; no bone therapy is needed. D) She needs an anabolic agent like teriparatide.

10. A critical pitfall in managing RA is:
    A) Using methotrexate as a first-line agent.
    B) Delaying the initiation of a DMARD, relying only on NSAIDs.
    C) Titrating therapy to a "Treat-to-Target" goal.
    D) Screening for tuberculosis before starting a biologic.

Self-Assessment Questions

1. Describe the "Treat-to-Target" (T2T) algorithm for Rheumatoid Arthritis, including the first-line agent and the escalation steps.
2. What is the role of corticosteroids and NSAIDs in the RA treatment algorithm, and why are they not appropriate as monotherapy?
3. Outline the 5-step treatment algorithm for Osteoarthritis, starting from foundational non-pharmacological therapy.
4. A patient is diagnosed with osteoporosis (T-score -2.8). What is the first-line pharmacological algorithm, and what must be checked before initiating this therapy?
5. How does the treatment algorithm differ for a "high-risk" versus a "very high-risk" osteoporosis patient?
6. A patient presents with a classic acute gouty attack (podagra). What are the three first-line pharmacological options for this acute flare?
7. Why is urate-lowering therapy (e.g., allopurinol) not initiated during an acute gout flare?
8. Describe the "start low, go slow" algorithm for initiating allopurinol, including the sUA target and the mandatory concurrent prophylactic therapy.
9. What is the most critical, "cannot-miss" differential diagnosis for an acute, hot, swollen monoarticular joint, and why is it an emergency?
10. Identify two major pitfalls in the management of Osteoarthritis and two in the management of Osteoporosis.

Bibliography

1. Smolen JS, Aletaha D, Barton A, Burmester GR, Emery P, Firestein GS, et al. Rheumatoid arthritis. Nat Rev Dis Primers. 2018 Feb 8;4:18001.
2. Smolen JS, Landewé RBM, Bijlsma JWJ, Burmester GR, Combe B, Kerschbaumer A, et al. EULAR recommendations for the management of rheumatoid arthritis with synthetic and biological disease-modifying antirheumatic drugs: 2019 update. Ann Rheum Dis. 2020 Jun;79(6):685–99.
3. Singh JA, Saag KG, Bridges SL Jr, Akl EA, Bannuru RR, Sullivan MC, et al. 2015 American College of Rheumatology Guideline for the Treatment of Rheumatoid Arthritis. Arthritis Rheumatol. 2016 Jan;68(1):1–26.
4. Katz JN, Arant KR, Loeser RF. Diagnosis and Treatment of Hip and Knee Osteoarthritis: A Review. JAMA. 2021 Feb 9;325(6):568–78.
5. Kolasinski SL, Neogi T, Hochberg MC, Oatis C, Guyatt G, Block J, et al. 2019 American College of Rheumatology/Arthritis Foundation Guideline for the Management of Osteoarthritis of the Hand, Hip, and Knee. Arthritis Rheumatol. 2020 Feb;72(2):220–33.
6. Hunter DJ, Bierma-Zeinstra S. Osteoarthritis. Lancet. 2019 Apr 27;393(10182):1745–59.
7. Kanis JA, Cooper C, Rizzoli R, Reginster JY. European guidance for the diagnosis and management of osteoporosis in postmenopausal women. Osteoporos Int. 2019 Jan;30(1):3–44.
8. Shoback D, Rosen CJ, Black DM, Cheung AM, Murad MH, Eastell R. Pharmacological Management of Osteoporosis in Postmenopausal Women: An Endocrine Society Clinical Practice Guideline. J Clin Endocrinol Metab. 2020 Mar 1;105(3):dgaa048.
9. Eastell R, Rosen CJ, Black DM, Cheung AM, Murad MH, Shoback D. Pharmacological Management of Osteoporosis in Postmenopausal Women: An Endocrine Society Clinical Practice Guideline. J Clin Endocrinol Metab. 2019 May 1;104(5):1595–622.
10. FitzGerald JD, Dalbeth N, Mikuls T, Brignardello-Petersen R, Guyatt G, Abeles AM, et al. 2020 American College of Rheumatology Guideline for the Management of Gout. Arthritis Care Res (Hoboken). 2020 Jun;72(6):744–60.
11. Dalbeth N, Gosling AL, Gaffo A, Abhishek A. Gout. Lancet. 2021 May 15;397(10287):1843–55.
12. Qaseem A, Harris RP, Forciea MA. Management of Acute and Recurrent Gout: A Clinical Practice Guideline From the American College of Physicians. Ann Intern Med. 2017 Jan 3;166(1):58–68.
13. Neogi T. Gout. N Engl J Med. 2011 Aug 4;364(5):443–52.
14. Aringer M, Costenbader K, Daikh D, Brinks R, Mosca M, Ramsey-Goldman R, et al. 2019 European League Against Rheumatism/American College of Rheumatology Classification Criteria for Systemic Lupus Erythematosus. Arthritis Rheumatol. 2019 Sep;71(9):1400–12.
15. Martel-Pelletier J, Barr AJ, Cicuttini FM, Conaghan PG, Cooper C, Goldring MB, et al. Osteoarthritis. Nat Rev Dis Primers. 2016 Oct 27;2:16072.

CHAPTER 8

TREATMENT ALGORITHMS FOR INFECTIOUS DISEASES

Author

Mrs. Santhi Priya Adepu, Assistant Professor, Department of Pharmacology, Sir C.R. Reddy College of Pharmaceutical Sciences, Andhra Pradesh, India

Abstract

Infectious disease management is predicated on algorithms that integrate pathogen identification with host-specific factors. The algorithm for bacterial infections is stratified by the site of infection; community-acquired pneumonia (CAP) management is guided by CURB-65/PSI scores, dictating outpatient (e.g., macrolide, doxycycline) versus inpatient (e.g., ceftriaxone plus macrolide) therapy. Uncomplicated UTIs are treated with short-course antibiotics (e.g., nitrofurantoin), while skin infections are bifurcated into non-purulent (cellulitis) and purulent (abscess) algorithms. Viral infection algorithms are often time-sensitive. Influenza treatment with neuraminidase inhibitors is most effective within 48 hours of onset. Human Immunodeficiency Virus (HIV) follows a "treat-all" algorithm, initiating antiretroviral therapy (ART) with a 2- or 3-drug regimen immediately upon diagnosis. Fungal infection algorithms differentiate between prophylaxis, empiric, and definitive therapy, with echinocandins being first-line for suspected invasive candidiasis in critically ill patients. Parasitic disease algorithms, such as for malaria, are strictly species- and region-dependent, utilizing artemisinin-based combination therapies (ACTs) for uncomplicated *P. falciparum*. Antimicrobial stewardship principles, including de-escalation based on culture data, are integral to all algorithms.

Keywords: *Infectious Disease Algorithms, Antimicrobial Stewardship, Community-Acquired Pneumonia, HIV/ART, Sepsis, Empiric Therapy*

Learning Objectives

After completion of the chapter, the learners should be able to:

- Identify first-line antibiotic choices for common bacterial infections like acute otitis media and uncomplicated cystitis.
- Explain the algorithm for empiric antibiotic selection and the importance of de-escalation based on culture and sensitivity results.
- Formulate a treatment algorithm for a patient with influenza, including antiviral indications and supportive care.
- Differentiate the treatment algorithms for superficial fungal infections (e.g., tinea pedis) versus invasive systemic fungal infections (e.g., candidemia).
- Justify the choice of a specific antimalarial prophylactic regimen based on travel destination and drug resistance.

COMMON BACTERIAL INFECTIONS

Bacterial infections are managed via algorithms that balance the need for rapid, empiric therapy against the risk of antimicrobial resistance. The algorithm is typically stratified by the site of infection and host risk factors.

Community-Acquired Pneumonia (CAP)

CAP is an acute infection of the pulmonary parenchyma acquired outside of a hospital setting.

Pathophysiology

The pathophysiology of Community-Acquired Pneumonia (CAP) begins with the failure of host respiratory defenses (e.g., mucociliary escalator, cough reflex, alveolar macrophages) to clear an invading pathogen, most commonly *Streptococcus pneumoniae*. Following microaspiration or inhalation, the bacteria proliferate in the alveoli. This triggers a potent host inflammatory response, leading to the recruitment of neutrophils and the release of pro-inflammatory cytokines. The alveoli fill with an inflammatory exudate, red blood cells, and fibrin, a process known as consolidation. This consolidation of lung parenchyma, visible on chest X-ray, creates a physiologic shunt (perfusion without ventilation), which impairs gas exchange and leads to hypoxemia. Systemic symptoms (fever, chills, malaise) are driven by the systemic cytokine release.

Diagnosis

The diagnostic algorithm requires the presence of a new pulmonary infiltrate on chest radiograph combined with clinical signs of infection (e.g., fever, cough, purulent sputum, leukocytosis). Microbiological workup (sputum, blood cultures) is generally reserved for patients with severe disease.

Differential Diagnosis

The differential includes acute bronchitis (no infiltrate), heart failure (which can present with congestion and dyspnea), pulmonary embolism (can be pleuritic), and non-infectious pneumonitis.

Treatment Algorithm

The primary algorithm branch point is **site-of-care determination**, guided by a clinical risk score like **CURB-65** (Confusion, Urea > 7, Respiratory rate ≥ 30, Blood pressure < 90/60, age ≥ 65) or the Pneumonia Severity Index (PSI).

- **Algorithm 1: Outpatient (CURB-65 score 0-1)**
    - **No Comorbidities/Risk Factors:** Monotherapy with amoxicillin, doxycycline, or a macrolide (if local resistance is low).
    - **With Comorbidities (e.g., Heart/Lung/Liver/Renal disease, Diabetes, Asplenia):** Combination therapy with amoxicillin/clavulanate OR a cephalosporin *plus* a macrolide OR doxycycline; OR monotherapy with a respiratory fluoroquinolone (e.g., levofloxacin).
- **Algorithm 2: Inpatient - Non-Severe (CURB-65 score 2)**
    - **Standard:** IV beta-lactam (e.g., ceftriaxone) *plus* a macrolide (e.g., azithromycin).
    - **Alternative:** Respiratory fluoroquinolone monotherapy.
- **Algorithm 3: Inpatient - Severe (CURB-65 score 3-5; ICU admission)**

- **Standard:** IV beta-lactam *plus* a macrolide.
- **Risk for *Pseudomonas*:** Antipseudomonal beta-lactam (e.g., piperacillin-tazobactam) *plus* an anti-pseudomonal fluoroquinolone.
- **Risk for MRSA:** Add vancomycin or linezolid. The algorithm dictates de-escalation once sensitivities are known and a total duration of 5-7 days for most cases.

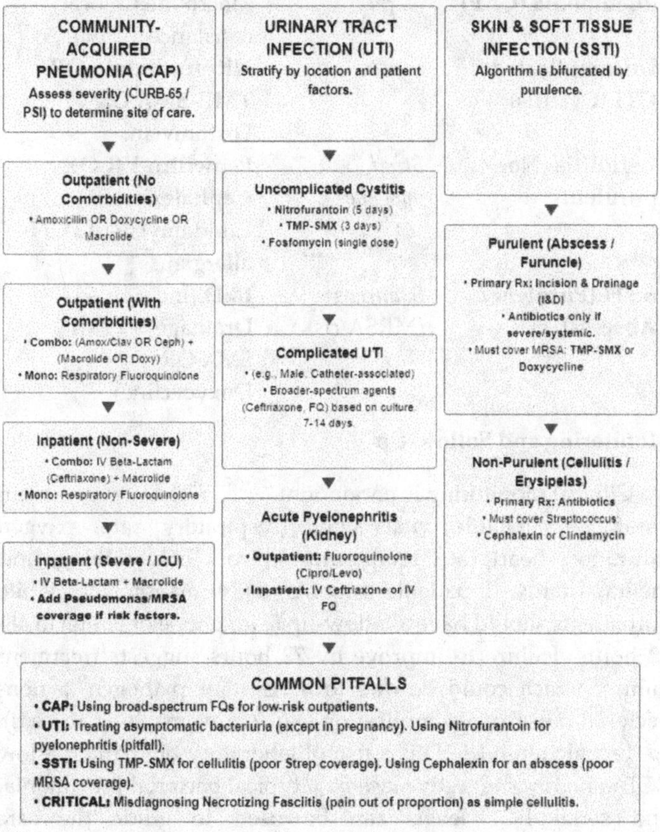

Figure 8.1: Common Bacterial Infections

Table 8.1: First-Line Outpatient Algorithms for Common Bacterial Infections

Infection	Likely Pathogen(s)	First-Line Algorithm (Healthy Adult)
Community-Acquired Pneumonia (CAP)	*S. pneumoniae, H. flu*	**Amoxicillin** OR **Doxycycline** OR Macrolide (if local resistance < 25%).
Uncomplicated UTI (Cystitis)	*E. coli*	**Nitrofurantoin** OR **TMP-SMX** OR Fosfomycin.
Cellulitis (Non-purulent)	*Strep. pyogenes*	**Penicillin VK** OR **Cephalexin** OR Clindamycin (if PCN-allergic).
SSTI (Purulent / Abscess)	*S. aureus* (MRSA risk)	**I&D** (Incision & Drainage) + (TMP-SMX OR Doxycycline).

Monitoring and Follow-Up

Clinical monitoring is paramount. The main parameters include vital signs (respiratory rate, oxygen saturation, heart rate, temperature), work of breathing, and mental status. Inpatients require daily assessment, while outpatients should have a follow-up (e.g., phone or clinic) in 48-72 hours. Failure to improve by 72 hours suggests treatment failure, which could be due to a resistant pathogen, a non-bacterial cause, or a complication (e.g., empyema, lung abscess).

Procalcitonin (PCT) is a useful laboratory biomarker; a low PCT is highly suggestive *against* a typical bacterial pneumonia, and serial PCT levels can be used to guide the safe discontinuation of antibiotics. A follow-up chest X-ray is *not* necessary for most patients who are clinically improving, as radiographic findings can lag behind clinical recovery by 4-6 weeks.

Long-Term Management / Secondary Prevention

The most effective secondary prevention strategies are vaccination and risk factor modification. Patients should be counseled on and receive both the **annual influenza vaccine** (as influenza is a major predisposing factor for bacterial pneumonia) and the **pneumococcal vaccine** (e.g., PCV20 or PCV15/PPSV23, based on age and comorbidities). **Smoking cessation** is critical, as smoking paralyzes the mucociliary escalator and is the strongest modifiable risk factor for CAP.

Patient Counseling Points

1. **Adherence:** "You must take the *entire* course of your antibiotics, even if you start to feel better after a few days. Stopping early can allow the infection to return or lead to antibiotic resistance."
2. **Expected Course:** "It is normal to cough for several weeks, even after the infection is gone. Your energy will also take time to return. The X-ray will take 4-6 weeks to clear."
3. **Warning Signs:** "You should start to feel slowly better in 48-72 hours. If you suddenly feel worse, or if you have new shortness of breath, chest pain, or high fever, you must seek care immediately."
4. **Prevention:** "The two best ways to prevent this from happening again are to get your flu shot every year, your pneumonia shot, and, if you smoke, to quit."

Common Pitfalls

A critical pitfall is miscalculating severity and under-treating a high-risk patient in the outpatient setting. Another is the overuse of broad-spectrum agents (fluoroquinolones, MRSA/Pseudomonas coverage) in low-risk patients, which drives resistance. Finally, failing to switch from IV to PO (oral) therapy when a patient is clinically stable is a common error.

Urinary Tract Infections (UTI)

UTIs are stratified into uncomplicated (cystitis), complicated (e.g., male, pregnant, catheter-associated), and pyelonephritis (kidney infection).

Pathophysiology

The pathophysiology of UTIs is typically an ascending infection. The process begins with colonization of the periurethral area by uropathogens (most commonly uropathogenic *E. coli*, or UPEC) from the gut. These bacteria possess "virulence factors," such as P-fimbriae (pili), which allow them to adhere to and ascend the urothelium of the urethra into the bladder, causing **cystitis**. The host responds with an inflammatory cascade, causing the typical symptoms of dysuria, frequency, and urgency. If the bacteria continue to ascend the ureters to the kidneys, **pyelonephritis** develops. This is a severe, invasive infection of the renal parenchyma, causing inflammation, tissue damage, and a systemic response (fever, chills, CVA tenderness).

Diagnosis

Diagnosis is based on symptoms (dysuria, frequency, urgency) and confirmed by urinalysis (pyuria, bacteriuria) and urine culture.

Differential Diagnosis

Differentials include vaginitis (yeast, BV), urethritis (e.g., STI like *Chlamydia* or *Gonorrhea*), and non-infectious interstitial cystitis.

Treatment Algorithm

- **Algorithm 1: Uncomplicated Cystitis (Non-pregnant female)**
  - **First-Line:** Nitrofurantoin 100 mg BID for 5 days OR Trimethoprim-sulfamethoxazole (TMP-SMX) DS BID for 3 days (if local resistance < 20%).
  - **Second-Line:** Fosfomycin 3g single dose. Fluoroquinolones are to be avoided.
- **Algorithm 2: Complicated UTI (e.g., Male, Obstruction, Catheter)**
  - Requires broader-spectrum agents based on

urine culture (e.g., ceftriaxone, fluoroquinolone) and a longer duration (7-14 days).

- **Algorithm 3: Acute Pyelonephritis**
    - **Outpatient (Mild, able to tolerate PO):** Ciprofloxacin or levofloxacin for 5-7 days.
    - **Inpatient (Severe, septic, unable to tolerate PO):** IV ceftriaxone or an IV fluoroquinolone. Therapy is tailored to culture results.

Monitoring and Follow-Up

For uncomplicated cystitis, monitoring is clinical. Symptoms should resolve within 24-48 hours of starting antibiotics. For pyelonephritis, monitoring involves tracking symptom resolution (fever, CVA tenderness) and laboratory markers (WBC, serum creatinine). Inpatients should improve within 48-72 hours; failure to do so warrants a renal CT scan to look for complications like a perinephric abscess or an obstructing kidney stone. A "test of cure" (follow-up urine culture) is *not* needed for uncomplicated cystitis but is recommended for pyelonephritis and in all pregnant patients.

Long-Term Management / Secondary Prevention

For patients with recurrent cystitis, prevention is crucial. Non-pharmacological strategies include counseling on post-coital voiding and adequate hydration. Pharmacological options for recurrent, well-documented infections include patient-initiated self-treatment, post-coital antibiotic prophylaxis, or, in severe cases, continuous low-dose antibiotic prophylaxis. Topical vaginal estrogen is a highly effective preventive measure for post-menopausal women with recurrent UTIs.

Patient Counseling Points

1. **Adherence:** "Finish the full antibiotic course. Even for a simple bladder infection, stopping early can lead to a more serious kidney infection (pyelonephritis)."
2. **Hydration:** "Drink plenty of water to help flush the bacteria from your system."
3. **Hygiene (for women):** "Always wipe from front to

back after using the toilet to prevent moving bacteria from the rectal area to the urethra."

4. **Pyelonephritis Warning Signs:** "A bladder infection (cystitis) is in your bladder. If you *ever* develop a fever, chills, or severe pain in your back or side, that means the infection may have moved to your kidneys, and you need to be seen by a doctor right away."

Common Pitfalls

The most common pitfall is treating "asymptomatic bacteriuria" (a positive urine culture with no symptoms) with antibiotics, which is a major driver of resistance and provides no benefit (exception: pregnancy). Another is using a 3-day course of TMP-SMX in an area with high resistance. Finally, using nitrofurantoin for pyelonephritis is a critical error, as it does not achieve adequate renal tissue concentrations.

Skin and Soft Tissue Infections (SSTI)

The SSTI algorithm is fundamentally bifurcated into purulent (abscess, furuncle) and non-purulent (cellulitis, erysipelas).

Treatment Algorithm

- **Algorithm 1: Purulent SSTI (High suspicion for *S. aureus* / MRSA)**
  - **Step 1:** The primary treatment is **incision and drainage (I&D).**
  - **Step 2 (Antibiotics):** Antibiotics are *only* indicated if the abscess is severe, associated with systemic signs (fever), or the patient is immunocompromised.
  - **Step 3 (Drug Choice):** Empiric coverage for MRSA is required (e.g., TMP-SMX, doxycycline).
- **Algorithm 2: Non-Purulent SSTI (Cellulitis - High suspicion for *Streptococcus*)**
  - **Step 1:** The primary treatment is **antibiotics.**
  - **Step 2 (Drug Choice):** Therapy must target *Streptococcus* (e.g., cephalexin, clindamycin).

- **Step 3 (Severe):** IV therapy (e.g., cefazolin) is used for severe, rapidly progressing, or systemically ill patients.

Common Pitfalls

The most common pitfall is treating cellulitis with TMP-SMX, which has poor streptococcal coverage. The inverse error is treating a purulent abscess with cephalexin, which has poor MRSA coverage. A critical, "cannot-miss" pitfall is misdiagnosing necrotizing fasciitis as simple cellulitis; clinical signs (pain out of proportion, crepitus, hemorrhagic bullae) demand immediate surgical exploration.

Case Study

A 30-year-old male presents to urgent care with a 3-day history of a "spider bite" on his forearm. On exam, you see a 4 cm, tender, red, fluctuant (tense, fluid-filled) nodule with a small purulent center. He has a 100.5°F fever.

Discussion

This is a classic **Purulent Skin & Soft Tissue Infection (SSTI)**, or abscess. The algorithm for SSTIs is critically bifurcated: purulent vs. non-purulent.

- **Non-purulent (Cellulitis):** Assumed *Strep* species. Treat with antibiotics (e.g., Cephalexin).
- **Purulent (Abscess):** Assumed *Staph. aureus* (with high risk of MRSA). Primary treatment is drainage.

Treatment Algorithm:

1. **Diagnosis:** Purulent SSTI (Abscess) with systemic signs (fever).
2. **Algorithm Step 1 (Primary):** The algorithm mandates **Incision and Drainage (I&D)** as the definitive treatment.
3. **Algorithm Step 2 (Antibiotics):** Because the patient has systemic signs (fever) and a surrounding ring of cellulitis, antibiotics are indicated (I&D alone is often sufficient for small, simple abscesses).
4. **Therapy:** The antibiotic algorithm must cover community-acquired **MRSA**.

- Start **Trimethoprim-Sulfamethoxazole (TMP-SMX) DS** one tablet BID for 7 days. (Doxycycline would also be a correct choice).
- A wound culture is sent from the drainage.

Outcome

The patient's abscess is drained in the clinic, providing immediate pain relief. He is started on TMP-SMX pending culture results and instructed on wound care.

VIRAL INFECTIONS

Viral treatment algorithms are often time-sensitive (influenza), require long-term adherence (HIV), or are rapidly evolving (COVID-19).

Influenza

Pathophysiology

Influenza is an acute respiratory illness caused by an orthomyxovirus (Type A or B). The virus's surface proteins, **hemagglutinin (HA)** and **neuraminidase (NA)**, are central to its pathophysiology. HA binds to sialic acid residues on the surface of respiratory epithelial cells, allowing viral entry. The virus replicates within the cell, and new virions are released by NA, which cleaves the sialic acid receptor. This viral replication leads to widespread destruction and desquamation of the ciliated respiratory epithelium, impairing the mucociliary defense mechanism. The abrupt onset of systemic symptoms (fever, myalgia, headache, malaise) is not due to viremia, but rather the massive and rapid induction of pro-inflammatory cytokines (e.g., interferons, TNF-α, IL-6).

Diagnosis

Diagnosis is clinical (acute onset fever, myalgia, cough) during peak season. Rapid antigen or molecular (PCR) tests confirm the diagnosis.

Treatment Algorithm

The algorithm is based on time-from-onset and host risk.

- **Step 1 (Symptom Onset < 48 Hours):**
    - **Algorithm:** Initiate a neuraminidase inhibitor (e.g., oseltamivir 75 mg BID for 5 days). This is recommended for all patients to shorten symptom duration.
- **Step 2 (Symptom Onset > 48 Hours):**
    - **Low-Risk Patient:** Treatment is symptomatic (antipyretics, hydration). Oseltamivir provides no benefit.
    - **High-Risk Patient (e.g., < 2 or > 65, pregnant, chronic disease, immunocompromised) OR Hospitalized:** Initiate oseltamivir *regardless* of symptom duration.

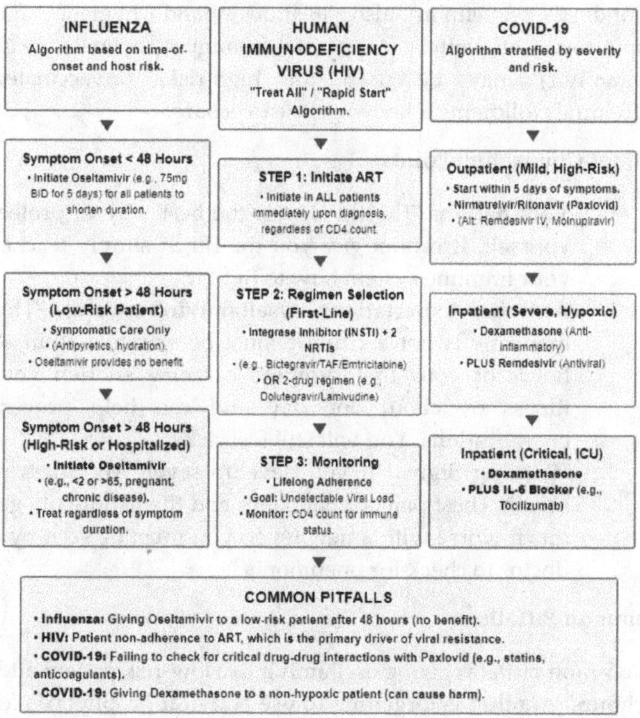
INFLUENZA
Algorithm based on time-of-onset and host risk.
Symptom Onset < 48 Hours
• Initiate Oseltamivir (e.g., 75mg BID for 5 days) for all patients to shorten duration.
Symptom Onset > 48 Hours (Low-Risk Patient)
• Symptomatic Care Only
• (Antipyretics, hydration).
• Oseltamivir provides no benefit.
Symptom Onset > 48 Hours (High-Risk or Hospitalized)
• Initiate Oseltamivir
• (e.g., <2 or >65, pregnant, chronic disease).
• Treat regardless of symptom duration.
HUMAN IMMUNODEFICIENCY VIRUS (HIV)
"Treat All" / "Rapid Start" Algorithm.
STEP 1: Initiate ART
• Initiate in ALL patients immediately upon diagnosis, regardless of CD4 count.
STEP 2: Regimen Selection (First-Line)
• Integrase Inhibitor (INSTI) + 2 NRTIs
• (e.g., Bictegravir/TAF/Emtricitabine)
• OR 2-drug regimen (e.g., Dolutegravir/Lamivudine)
STEP 3: Monitoring
• Lifelong Adherence
• Goal: Undetectable Viral Load
• Monitor: CD4 count for immune status.
COVID-19
Algorithm stratified by severity and risk.
Outpatient (Mild, High-Risk)
• Start within 5 days of symptoms.
• Nirmatrelvir/Ritonavir (Paxlovid)
• (Alt: Remdesivir IV, Molnupiravir)
Inpatient (Severe, Hypoxic)
• Dexamethasone (Anti-inflammatory)
• PLUS Remdesivir (Antiviral)
Inpatient (Critical, ICU)
• Dexamethasone
• PLUS IL-6 Blocker (e.g., Tocilizumab)
COMMON PITFALLS
• Influenza: Giving Oseltamivir to a low-risk patient after 48 hours (no benefit).
• HIV: Patient non-adherence to ART, which is the primary driver of viral resistance.
• COVID-19: Failing to check for critical drug-drug interactions with Paxlovid (e.g., statins, anticoagulants).
• COVID-19: Giving Dexamethasone to a non-hypoxic patient (can cause harm).

Figure 8.2: Viral Infections - Stratified Algorithms

Monitoring and Follow-Up

Monitoring is clinical, focused on symptom resolution and identifying complications. Symptoms typically peak at 48-72 hours and resolve over 5-7 days. The most feared complication is a secondary **bacterial pneumonia** (often *S. pneumoniae* or *S. aureus*), which should be suspected if a patient has "double-worsening" (i.e., starts to improve, then develops a high fever and productive cough). High-risk patients (e.g., elderly, pregnant, chronic lung disease) should be monitored closely for respiratory distress.

Long-Term Management / Secondary Prevention

The single most effective preventive strategy is **annual influenza vaccination**. Vaccination induces neutralizing antibodies against the HA protein, preventing viral entry. Secondary prevention also includes hand hygiene and respiratory etiquette. Antiviral chemoprophylaxis (e.g., oseltamivir) may be used for high-risk, unvaccinated individuals following a known, close exposure.

Patient Counseling Points

1. **Vaccination:** "The flu shot is the best way to protect yourself. It cannot *give* you the flu; it simply teaches your immune system how to fight it."
2. **Antiviral Expectations (Oseltamivir/Tamiflu):** "This medicine is not a cure. It must be started within 48 hours of your first symptom. It may shorten your illness by about one day and can help prevent complications. You will still feel sick."
3. **Warning Signs:** "If you develop severe shortness of breath, chest pain, or get better and then suddenly get much worse with a new fever, you must be seen by a doctor to check for pneumonia."

Common Pitfalls

A common pitfall is giving oseltamivir to a low-risk patient after 48 hours. Another is forgetting to use antiviral prophylaxis for high-risk household contacts.

Human Immunodeficiency Virus (HIV)

Pathophysiology

HIV is a retrovirus that attacks the human immune system. Its pathophysiology centers on the CD4+ T-helper lymphocyte. The virus's gp120 protein binds to the CD4 receptor and a co-receptor (CCR5 or CXCR4) on the T-cell surface, allowing viral entry. Once inside, the virus uses its reverse transcriptase enzyme to convert its viral RNA into double-stranded DNA. This "proviral DNA" is then permanently integrated into the host cell's own genome by the integrase enzyme. The T-cell is now a permanent "factory" for HIV, producing new virions that bud off (a process involving the protease enzyme) and infect other cells. This leads to a progressive destruction of CD4+ T-cells, which are the "conductors" of the entire immune response. Acquired Immunodeficiency Syndrome (AIDS) is diagnosed when the CD4 count drops below 200 cells/mm^3 or the patient develops an AIDS-defining opportunistic illness.

Diagnosis

Diagnosis is via 4th-generation antigen/antibody screening test, confirmed by an antibody differentiation assay or HIV-1/HIV-2 NAT.

Treatment Algorithm

The modern algorithm is "Treat All" or "Rapid Start."

- **Step 1: Initiate Antiretroviral Therapy (ART):** ART should be initiated in *all* individuals with HIV, regardless of CD4 count, to reduce morbidity and prevent transmission. Rapid Start (initiating on the same day of diagnosis) is preferred.
- **Step 2: Regimen Selection:**
    - **First-Line Algorithm:** A 2- or 3-drug regimen. The most common first-line regimen is an Integrase Strand Transfer Inhibitor (INSTI) *plus* two Nucleoside Reverse Transcriptase Inhibitors (NRTIs).
    - **Example:** Bictegravir/Tenofovir alafenamide/Emtricitabine (a single-pill

regimen).
    - **Alternative:** A 2-drug regimen such as Dolutegravir/Lamivudine is an option for many.
- **Step 3: Monitoring:** The algorithm requires lifelong adherence and monitoring of viral load (goal: undetectable) and CD4 count.

Table 8.2: Treatment Algorithms for Common Viral Infections

Virus	Primary Drug Class	Treatment Algorithm / Indication
Influenza	Neuraminidase Inhibitor	**Oseltamivir:** Start within 48h of symptoms, esp. in high-risk patients.
Herpes Simplex (HSV)	Nucleoside Analogs	**Acyclovir / Valacyclovir:** Episodic (start at prodrome) or Chronic Suppressive therapy.
COVID-19 (Mild-Mod)	Antiviral (e.g., Protease-I)	**Nirmatrelvir/Ritonavir (Paxlovid):** Start within 5 days of symptoms in high-risk patients.
Varicella-Zoster (Shingles)	Nucleoside Analogs	**Valacyclovir:** Start within 72h of rash onset to reduce post-herpetic neuralgia risk.

Monitoring and Follow-Up

HIV management requires lifelong, vigilant monitoring.

1. **Viral Load (HIV RNA):** This is the primary marker of treatment success. The goal of antiretroviral therapy (ART) is to achieve an "undetectable" viral load (e.g., <50 copies/mL) within 3-6 months. It is checked before starting ART, 2-8 weeks after, and then every 3-6 months once stable.
2. **CD4 Count:** This is the primary marker of immune *status* and risk for opportunistic infections (OIs). It is

checked at baseline and every 3-6 months.

3. **Genotypic Resistance Testing:** Performed at diagnosis and upon any virologic failure to guide ART selection.
4. **Safety Labs:** Routine monitoring of renal function, LFTs, and lipids is required, as many ART regimens can have long-term toxicities.

Long-Term Management / Secondary Prevention

The goal is to maintain an undetectable viral load, which allows for immune reconstitution (rising CD4 count) and a normal lifespan. This is achieved through **lifelong adherence to ART**. ART typically consists of three drugs from at least two classes (e.g., 2 NRTIs + 1 INSTI). Secondary prevention is focused on preventing OIs. Prophylactic antibiotics (e.g., trimethoprim-sulfamethoxazole for PJP) are initiated when the CD4 count drops below 200 and can be stopped once the count recovers above 200 on ART.

Patient Counseling Points

1. **U=U (Undetectable = Untransmittable):** "This is the most important concept in modern HIV care. If your medicine makes the virus 'undetectable' in your blood, you *cannot* transmit the virus to a sexual partner. Your medicine protects both you and them."
2. **Adherence is Lifelong:** "This medicine is not a cure; it is a permanent control. You must take your medicine every single day. Missing even a few doses can allow the virus to multiply and, worse, to develop resistance, which means your current pills will stop working."
3. **ART is Prevention:** "Starting and staying on your medication is the single most important thing you can do to live a long, healthy life and prevent progressing to AIDS."

Common Pitfalls

The primary pitfall is non-adherence, which leads to viral resistance. A diagnostic pitfall is failing to screen for HIV in patients presenting with opportunistic infections or "mono-like" syndromes (which can be acute retroviral syndrome).

COVID-19

Diagnosis

Diagnosis is via rapid antigen testing (home) or molecular testing (PCR).

Treatment Algorithm

The algorithm is stratified by severity.

- **Algorithm 1: Outpatient (Mild-Moderate Disease, High Risk for Progression):**
    - **Criteria:** Patient has risk factors (age > 65, obesity, chronic disease) but is not hypoxic.
    - **Treatment:** Initiate antiviral therapy *within 5 days of symptom onset*.
    - **First-Line:** Nirmatrelvir/Ritonavir (Paxlovid).
    - **Alternatives:** Remdesivir (IV), Molnupiravir.
- **Algorithm 2: Inpatient (Severe - Hypoxic, requiring O2):**
    - **Step 1 (Antiviral):** Remdesivir.
    - **Step 2 (Anti-inflammatory):** Dexamethasone (systemic corticosteroid).
- **Algorithm 3: Inpatient (Critical - Requiring ICU/Ventilation):**
    - **Step 1:** Dexamethasone.
    - **Step 2 (Immunomodulator):** Add an IL-6 receptor blocker (e.g., tocilizumab).
    - **Antiviral (Remdesivir) is often discontinued at this stage.**

Common Pitfalls

A common error is prescribing Paxlovid to a low-risk, vaccinated young person, where the benefit is minimal. A critical pitfall is failing to check for drug-drug interactions with Paxlovid (especially statins and anticoagulants). Inpatient, a pitfall is giving dexamethasone to a patient who is *not* hypoxic, which can cause harm.

Case Study

A 35-year-old high school teacher presents to his PCP in December with a **24-hour history** of *abrupt-onset* fever (102°F), severe muscle aches (myalgia), headache, and a dry cough. He "felt like he was hit by a truck." A rapid in-office test is positive for **Influenza A**.

Discussion

This is a classic, uncomplicated **Influenza** infection. The treatment algorithm is entirely **time-sensitive**. Antiviral therapy (Oseltamivir) is most effective when initiated within 48 hours of symptom onset.

Treatment Algorithm

1. **Diagnosis:** Influenza A.
2. **Algorithm (Time-Based):** The patient's symptom onset was 24 hours ago, placing him well **within the 48-hour window** for treatment.
3. **Therapy:** Start **Oseltamivir 75 mg BID for 5 days.**
4. **Counseling:** You must set expectations. This is *not* a "cure" like an antibiotic. It will, on average, shorten the duration of his illness by about 1 day and may reduce the risk of complications (like pneumonia).
5. **Supportive Care:** You also counsel him on the mainstays of treatment: rest, hydration, and antipyretics (e.g., acetaminophen or ibuprofen) for fever and myalgia.

Outcome

The patient is started on Oseltamivir and instructed on supportive care. He is told to return if he develops shortness of breath or "double-worsening" (gets better, then suddenly gets worse), which could signal a secondary bacterial pneumonia.

FUNGAL INFECTIONS

Fungal infection algorithms are critical in immunocompromised and critically ill patients, where delayed therapy is fatal.

Invasive Candidiasis (Candidemia)

Pathophysiology

Candida albicans is a dimorphic fungus that exists as a normal commensal (yeast form) in the oropharynx, GI tract, and vagina. Disease (candidiasis) occurs when a change in the host environment allows it to overgrow and transform into its pathogenic, invasive hyphal form. This is typically caused by local or systemic immunosuppression. **Oropharyngeal candidiasis (thrush)** is often seen with local immunosuppression (e.g., use of inhaled corticosteroids) or systemic (e.g., uncontrolled HIV/AIDS). **Esophageal candidiasis** is an AIDS-defining illness and implies severe immunodeficiency (CD4 < 100), as the fungus invades the esophageal mucosa, causing odynophagia (painful swallowing).

Diagnosis

Diagnosis is made via blood culture (e.g., *Candida albicans, glabrata*). Non-culture-based diagnostics (e.g., Beta-D-glucan) are supportive.

Treatment Algorithm

- **Algorithm 1: Empiric Therapy (Suspected, e.g., septic ICU patient with risk factors):**
    - **First-Line:** An echinocandin (e.g., caspofungin, micafungin). These are preferred due to efficacy and broad coverage (including azole-resistant *C. glabrata*).
- **Algorithm 2: Definitive Therapy (Confirmed Candidemia):**
    - **First-Line (Critically Ill):** Continue echinocandin.
    - **First-Line (Stable, *C. albicans*):** Step-down to

fluconazole (PO or IV) once sensitivities are known.

- **Step 3 (Duration):** Treat for 14 days *after* the first negative blood culture.
- **Step 4 (Mandatory Step):** All patients require a dilated ophthalmologic exam to rule out endophthalmitis.

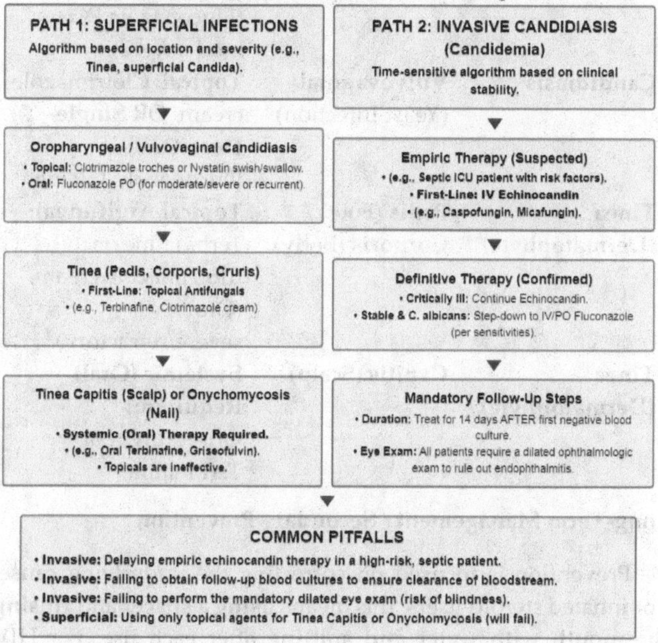

Figure 8.3: Fungal Infections - Stratified Algorithms

Table 8.3: Management Algorithms for Common Fungal Infections

Monitoring and Follow-Up

Monitoring is clinical. For thrush, the goal is the resolution of the white, "cheesy" plaques. For esophagitis, the goal is the resolution of odynophagia. If oral thrush is diagnosed in an adult with no obvious cause (e.g., inhaler use, recent antibiotics), the algorithm *must* include an HIV test. For recurrent thrush in an inhaler user, monitoring involves observing their inhaler technique

Infection	Type	First-Line Treatment Algorithm
Candidiasis	**Oropharyngeal** (Thrush)	**Topical:** Clotrimazole troches or Nystatin swish/swallow. (Fluconazole PO for mod-severe).
Candidiasis	**Vulvovaginal** (Yeast Infection)	**Topical:** Clotrimazole cream. OR **Single-Dose Oral:** Fluconazole 150 mg.
Tinea (Dermatophyte)	**Pedis** (Foot) / **Corporis** (Body)	**Topical Antifungal:** Terbinafine or Clotrimazole cream. (Oral if severe/refractory).
Tinea (Dermatophyte)	**Capitis** (Scalp)	**Systemic (Oral) Required:** Griseofulvin or Terbinafine.

Long-Term Management / Secondary Prevention

Prevention is focused on correcting the underlying cause. For inhaled steroid users, this means **using a spacer** and **rinsing the mouth with water and spitting** after each use. For HIV patients, the long-term prevention is successful ART. For patients with recurrent vulvovaginal candidiasis, a prophylactic (e.g., weekly) dose of oral fluconazole may be considered.

Patient Counseling Points

1. **Inhaler Technique (for Thrush):** "The white plaques in your mouth are a yeast infection caused by your steroid inhaler. This is very common. To prevent it, you must rinse your mouth with water and spit it out every single time you use your steroid inhaler. Using a 'spacer' device also helps."
2. **Topical vs. Systemic:** "For thrush, we can use a medicine that you 'swish and swallow' (Nystatin) or a

'troche' (Clotrimazole) that dissolves in your mouth. Because *your* infection has gone into your esophagus, causing pain when you swallow, we must use a *systemic* pill (Fluconazole) to treat it from the inside out."

Common Pitfalls

The most critical pitfall is delaying empiric therapy in a high-risk, septic patient. Another is failing to perform follow-up blood cultures to ensure clearance. Finally, failing to get the eye exam is a common omission that can lead to blindness.

Case Study

A 45-year-old male with poorly controlled Type 2 Diabetes presents with an itchy, red rash under his inguinal folds (groin). On exam, you see a "beefy red," moist plaque with small "satellite" papules and pustules extending beyond the main border.

Discussion

This presentation, especially the "beefy red" appearance and the "satellite lesions," is the hallmark of **Cutaneous Candidiasis (Intertrigo)**. It is *not* Tinea cruris ("jock itch"), which typically has an annular, scaling border. The algorithm is to treat the *Candida* and, critically, control the underlying risk factor (moisture + hyperglycemia).

Treatment Algorithm

1. **Diagnosis:** Cutaneous Candidiasis (Intertrigo).
2. **Algorithm (Topical):** First-line therapy is a topical antifungal that covers *Candida*.
    - **Therapy:** Start **Topical Clotrimazole cream** BID. (A topical azole is preferred over terbinafine, which is less effective against *Candida*). A mild topical steroid (e.g., hydrocortisone) can be added for 3-5 days to help with the inflammation.
3. **Risk Factor Control (Critical Step):** The primary goal is to modify the environment.

- **Counseling:** Instruct the patient to keep the area as **dry as possible** (e.g., using absorbent powders, drying thoroughly after bathing) and to work with his PCP to **improve his glycemic control**, as the high sugar "feeds" the yeast.

Outcome

The patient is started on topical clotrimazole. You spend most of the visit counseling him that the rash will only stay away if he keeps the area dry and manages his blood sugar.

PARASITIC DISEASES

Management algorithms are highly specific to the organism, its life cycle, and geographic resistance patterns.

Malaria

Pathophysiology

Malaria is a life-threatening protozoan disease caused by *Plasmodium* species, transmitted by the *Anopheles* mosquito. The pathophysiology begins when sporozoites are injected, travel to the liver, and undergo asexual reproduction (exo-erythrocytic stage). They then release merozoites, which invade red blood cells (RBCs). Inside the RBC, the parasite consumes hemoglobin and replicates, progressing from a "ring" form to a schizont. The **clinical illness is caused by the synchronous rupture of these schizonts**, which releases new merozoites (to infect more RBCs) and parasitic toxins/debris. This event triggers a massive cytokine cascade, causing the classic paroxysms of high fever, chills, and rigors. **Severe malaria**, caused by *P. falciparum*, is a medical emergency. Its unique pathophysiology involves the parasite expressing a protein (PfEMP1) that causes infected RBCs to *cytoadhere* (stick) to the endothelium of capillaries, leading to microvascular obstruction (sequestration) in the brain (cerebral malaria), kidneys (renal failure), and lungs (ARDS).

Diagnosis

The gold standard is peripheral blood smear (thick and thin) to identify the species and quantify parasitemia. Rapid diagnostic tests (RDTs) are used for screening.

Treatment Algorithm

The algorithm is a critical branch point: Uncomplicated vs. Severe.

- **Algorithm 1: Uncomplicated *P. falciparum* (from resistant area):**
  - **First-Line:** An artemisinin-based combination therapy (ACT).
  - **Example:** Artemether-lumefantrine.
- **Algorithm 2: Uncomplicated (Non-*falciparum*, e.g., *P. vivax, P. ovale*):**
  - **Step 1:** Chloroquine (if from a sensitive region).
  - **Step 2 (Radical Cure):** Add Primaquine or Tafenoquine to eradicate dormant liver hypnozoites (must check G6PD status first).
- **Algorithm 3: Severe Malaria (Any species, with end-organ damage, e.g., cerebral malaria):**
  - **First-Line:** Intravenous (IV) Artesunate.
  - **Step 2:** Follow with a full course of oral ACT once clinically stable.

Monitoring and Follow-Up

Monitoring for severe malaria is an ICU-level task. It involves:

1. **Parasitemia:** Serial blood smears (e.g., every 12-24 hours) to calculate the percentage of RBCs infected and to ensure it is decreasing with treatment.
2. **Neurologic Status:** Frequent GCS monitoring for cerebral malaria.

End-Organ Function: Monitoring urine output (for renal failure), Hgb (for severe anemia from hemolysis), and glucose (as quinine can cause hypoglycemia).

Table 8.4: Treatment Algorithms for Common Parasitic Diseases

Disease	Causative Parasite	First-Line Pharmacotherapy
Giardiasis	*Giardia lamblia* (Protozoa)	**Metronidazole** (Alt: Tinidazole).
Enterobiasis (Pinworm)	*Enterobius vermicularis* (Helminth)	**Albendazole** or Mebendazole or Pyrantel Pamoate. (Treat household).
Scabies	*Sarcoptes scabiei* (Ectoparasite)	**Topical Permethrin 5% cream.** (Oral Ivermectin as alternative).
Pediculosis (Lice)	*Pediculus humanus* (Ectoparasite)	**Topical Permethrin 1% lotion** or Pyrethrins.

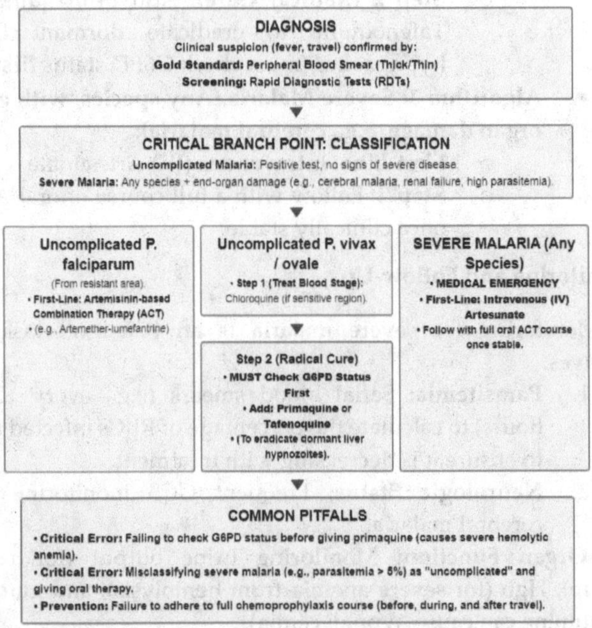

Figure 8.4: Parasitic Diseases - Malaria Algorithm

Long-Term Management / Secondary Prevention

The primary management is **prevention (prophylaxis).** For travelers to endemic areas, this is **chemoprophylaxis** (e.g., atovaquone-proguanil, doxycycline, or mefloquine) which must be taken before, during, and after travel. Other main preventive measures include DEET-containing insect repellent and permethrin-treated insecticide-treated bed nets (ITNs).

Patient Counseling Points

1. **Prophylaxis Adherence:** "This is one of the most important counseling points. You *must* take your 'malaria pill' exactly as prescribed, which includes *before* you go and *after* you return. No pill is 100%, so you must also prevent mosquito bites."
2. **Bite Prevention:** "Use DEET repellent on exposed skin and sleep under a treated bed net. The mosquitos that carry malaria bite most often from dusk until dawn."
3. **Fever Post-Travel:** "If you develop a fever *anytime,* even up to a year, after returning from a malaria-endemic area, you must go to an emergency room *immediately* and tell them, 'I traveled to a malaria zone.' This is a medical emergency."

Common Pitfalls

A critical pitfall is failing to check G6PD status before giving primaquine, which can induce severe hemolytic anemia. Another is misclassifying a patient with severe malaria (e.g., high parasitemia > 5%) as "uncomplicated" and giving oral therapy, which leads to treatment failure and death.

Case Study

A 28-year-old female presents for evaluation after returning from a 3-week backpacking trip through Southeast Asia. She complains of a fever (103.5°F) that seems to come and go, drenching chills, and a severe headache. She was prescribed Mefloquine for prophylaxis but admits she "missed a few doses."

Discussion

This is the classic presentation of **Malaria** in a returned traveler from an endemic area. This is a medical emergency until proven otherwise. The algorithm is to first diagnose, then identify the *species* and *severity*, as this dictates all treatment.

Treatment Algorithm

1. **Diagnosis (Algorithm Step 1):**
   - **Test:** Order an **emergent peripheral blood smear (thick and thin)** and a rapid diagnostic test (RDT).
   - **Result:** The thin smear identifies ***P. vivax***. The patient is awake, alert, and her parasitemia is 0.8%. She has **Uncomplicated *P. vivax* Malaria.**
2. **Treatment (Algorithm Step 2: Acute):** The algorithm for non-falciparum malaria in a chloroquine-sensitive area is:
   - **Therapy:** Start **Chloroquine** (oral, 3-day course).
3. **Treatment (Algorithm Step 3: Radical Cure):** This is the critical pitfall. *P. vivax* (and *P. ovale*) has dormant liver forms (hypnozoites) that will cause a relapse months later if not treated.
   - **Test:** First, you must check a **G6PD level.**
   - **Therapy:** Once the G6PD is confirmed normal, you start **Primaquine** daily for 14 days to kill the liver forms and achieve a "radical cure."

Outcome

The patient is started on Chloroquine to treat her acute infection. Her G6PD level is normal, so she is also prescribed a 14-day course of Primaquine to prevent relapse

Summary

Bacterial Infections: CAP management is stratified by CURB-65 score, guiding outpatient vs. inpatient (IV beta-lactam + macrolide) therapy. UTIs are stratified by complexity (uncomplicated vs. complicated). SSTIs are bifurcated into purulent (I&D ± MRSA coverage) and non-purulent (cellulitis, requiring Strep coverage).

Viral Infections: Influenza treatment (oseltamivir) is algorithmically guided by time-of-onset (< 48h) and host risk. HIV follows a "Treat All" algorithm with a 2- or 3-drug ART regimen. COVID-19 is stratified by severity (outpatient antivirals vs. inpatient steroids/antivirals).

Fungal Infections: Invasive candidiasis in septic patients requires empiric, first-line echinocandin therapy. Definitive therapy is guided by speciation and includes a mandatory eye exam.

Parasitic Diseases: Malaria algorithms are species-dependent. Uncomplicated P. falciparum requires an ACT. Severe malaria requires IV artesunate. P. vivax/ovale require a radical cure with primaquine (after G6PD testing).

Multiple Choice Questions

1. A 50-year-old healthy male with no comorbidities is diagnosed with CAP (CURB-65 = 0). Which is an appropriate first-line outpatient algorithm?
   A) Amoxicillin 1g TID
   B) Ceftriaxone 1g IV daily
   C) Piperacillin-tazobactam IV
   D) Ceftriaxone + Azithromycin
2. A 30-year-old female has a 3cm fluctuant, purulent abscess on her thigh with minimal surrounding erythema and no fever. What is the most appropriate management algorithm?
   A) Incision & Drainage + TMP-SMX
   B) Incision & Drainage alone
   C) Cephalexin
   D) Clindamycin
3. A 35-year-old male presents with a rapidly spreading, erythematous, hot, non-purulent rash on his lower leg. What is the most appropriate oral antibiotic choice?
   A) TMP-SMX
   B) Cephalexin
   C) Ciprofloxacin
   D) Doxycycline
4. A 22-year-old college student presents with 24 hours of fever, myalgia, and a positive influenza rapid test. What is the algorithm?
   A) Oseltamivir
   B) Amoxicillin
   C) Symptomatic care only
   D) Dexamethasone
5. A 65-year-old obese male with diabetes presents with COVID-19 (O2 sat 91% on room air). What is the first-line treatment algorithm?

A) Paxlovid
B) Dexamethasone + Remdesivir
C) Dexamethasone only
D) Symptomatic care only

6. An ICU patient develops septic shock. Blood cultures are drawn. Empiric therapy with piperacillin-tazobactam and vancomycin is started. He has risk factors for fungal infection. What is the next step?
A) Add empiric fluconazole
B) Add empiric echinocandin (e.g., caspofungin)
C) Wait for blood cultures to turn positive
D) Add empiric amphotericin B

7. A traveler returns from Africa with fever. A blood smear confirms P. falciparum malaria (2% parasitemia) with no signs of severe disease. What is the first-line algorithm?
A) IV Artesunate
B) Artemether-lumefantrine (oral)
C) Chloroquine (oral)
D) Primaquine (oral)

8. A patient with P. vivax malaria is treated with chloroquine. What is the mandatory next step in the algorithm to prevent relapse?
A) A 7-day course of IV artesunate
B) A 14-day course of primaquine after G6PD testing C) A single dose of tafenoquine
D) No further treatment is needed

9. A critical pitfall in managing a new diagnosis of pyelonephritis is:
A) Treating with oral ciprofloxacin
B) Treating with oral nitrofurantoin
C) Treating with IV ceftriaxone
D) Extending therapy to 7 days

10. A 40-year-old is diagnosed with HIV (CD4 500, viral load 50,000). What is the algorithm for ART?

    A) Defer ART until CD4 < 350

    B) Defer ART until symptomatic

    C) Initiate ART as soon as possible

    D) Initiate a 2-drug regimen of NRTIs only

Self-Assessment Questions

1. A 70-year-old male with CHF and diabetes presents with CAP. His CURB-65 score is 2. What is the first-line inpatient treatment algorithm?
2. A 25-year-old healthy female presents with a 2-day history of dysuria. Urinalysis is positive. What are the two appropriate first-line treatment algorithms, and what agent is contraindicated for this condition?
3. Differentiate the treatment algorithm for a 5cm purulent abscess versus a 5cm non-purulent, erythematous patch of cellulitis.
4. A 68-year-old nursing home resident presents with influenza symptoms for 72 hours. What is the correct algorithm for antiviral therapy?
5. A 30-year-old is newly diagnosed with HIV. What is the current algorithm for initiating ART, and what is a standard first-line regimen?
6. A 70-year-old with obesity and hypertension is diagnosed with COVID-19. He is not hypoxic. What is the treatment algorithm, and what is the time window for initiation?
7. An ICU patient develops sepsis and has a new positive blood culture for Candida. What is the first-line empiric agent, and what mandatory consultation is required?
8. What is the critical, "cannot-miss" differential for an acute, hot, swollen monoarticular joint that mimics gout?
9. A patient is diagnosed with P. vivax malaria. What is the 2-step treatment algorithm, and what test is mandatory before starting the second step?
10. What is the most common pitfall in the antibiotic management of asymptomatic bacteriuria?

Bibliography

1. Mandell LA, Wunderink RG, Anzueto A, Bartlett JG, Campbell GD, Dean NC, et al. Infectious Diseases Society of America/American Thoracic Society consensus guidelines on the management of community-acquired pneumonia in adults. Clin Infect Dis. 2007 Mar 1;44 Suppl 2:S27–72.
2. Metlay JP, Waterer GW, Long AC, Anzueto A, Brozek J, Crothers K, et al. Diagnosis and Treatment of Adults with Community-acquired Pneumonia. An Official Clinical Practice Guideline of the American Thoracic Society and Infectious Diseases Society of America. Am J Respir Crit Care Med. 2019 Oct 1;200(7):e45–e67.
3. Gupta K, Hooton TM, Naber KG, Wullt B, Colgan R, Miller LG, et al. International clinical practice guidelines for the treatment of acute uncomplicated cystitis and pyelonephritis in women: A 2010 update by the Infectious Diseases Society of America and the European Society for Microbiology and Infectious Diseases. Clin Infect Dis. 2011 Mar 1;52(5):e103–20.
4. Stevens DL, Bisno AL, Chambers HF, Dellinger EP, Goldstein EJC, Gorbach SL, et al. Practice guidelines for the diagnosis and management of skin and soft tissue infections: 2014 update by the Infectious Diseases Society of America. Clin Infect Dis. 2014 Jul 15;59(2):e10–52.
5. Fiore AE, Fry A, Bresee J, Uyeki TM. Antiviral agents for the treatment and chemoprophylaxis of influenza --- recommendations of the Advisory Committee on Immunization Practices (ACIP). MMWR Recomm Rep. 2011 Jan 21;60(1):1–24.
6. US Department of Health and Human Services. Guidelines for the Use of Antiretroviral Agents in Adults and Adolescents with HIV. [Accessed 2024 Oct 25]. Available from: https://www.google.com/search?q=https://clinicalinfo.hiv.gov/en/guidelines/hiv-clinical-guidelines-adult-and-adolescent-arv
7. Saag MS, Gandhi RT, Hoy JF, Landovitz RJ, Thompson MA, Sax PE, et al. Antiretroviral Drugs for Treatment and Prevention of HIV Infection in Adults: 2022 Recommendations of the International Antiviral Society-USA Panel. JAMA. 2022 Oct 18;328(15):1535–49.
8. World Health Organization. Guidelines for the treatment of malaria. 3rd ed. Geneva: World Health Organization; 2015.
9. Rossiter J, Al-Araji A, D'Ancona F, Johnson A, Wilson-Jones M, Johnson M. Treatment for uncomplicated Plasmodium vivax malaria: a systematic review and network meta-analysis. PLoS Negl Trop Dis. 2022 Jul 1;16(7):e0010536.
10. Pappas PG, Kauffman CA, Andes DR, Clancy CJ, Marr KA, Ostrosky-Zeichner L, et al. Clinical Practice Guideline for the Management of Candidiasis: 2016 Update by the Infectious Diseases Society of America. Clin Infect Dis. 2016 Feb 15;62(4):e1–50.
11. Cornely OA, Bassetti M, Calandra T, Garbino J, Kullberg BJ, Lortholary O, et al. ESCMID* guideline for the diagnosis and management of Candida diseases 2012: non-neutropenic adult patients. Clin Microbiol Infect. 2012 Dec;18 Suppl 7:19–37.

12. COVID-19 Treatment Guidelines Panel. Coronavirus Disease 2019 (COVID-19) Treatment Guidelines. National Institutes of Health. [Accessed 2024 Oct 25]. Available from: https://www.google.com/search?q=https://www.covid19treatmentguidelines.nih.gov/
13. Bhimraj A, Morgan RL, Shumaker AH, Lavergne V, Baden L, Cheng VC, et al. Infectious Diseases Society of America Guidelines on the Treatment and Management of Patients with COVID-19. Clin Infect Dis. 2020 Nov 23;ciaa1045.
14. Nicolle LE, Gupta K, Bradley SF, Colgan R, DeMuri GP, Drekonja D, et al. Clinical Practice Guideline for the Management of Asymptomatic Bacteriuria: 2019 Update by the Infectious Diseases Society of America. Clin Infect Dis. 2019 May 2;68(10):e83–e110.
15. Hooton TM, Bradley SF, Cardenas DD, Colgan R, Geerlings SE, Rice JC, et al. Diagnosis, prevention, and treatment of catheter-associated urinary tract infection in adults: 2009 International Clinical Practice Guidelines from the Infectious Diseases Society of America. Clin Infect Dis. 2010 Mar 1;50(5):625–63.

CHAPTER 9

TREATMENT ALGORITHMS FOR HEMATOLOGIC DISORDERS

Author

Miss Veera Naga Lalitha Nakkina, Pharm D Scholar, Koringa College of Pharmacy, Korangi, Tallarevu, Andhra Pradesh, India

Abstract

Hematologic treatment algorithms are fundamentally dictated by cell lineage, cell maturity, and functional defects. The algorithm for anemias begins with a morphological classification (microcytic, normocytic, macrocytic) based on Mean Corpuscular Volume (MCV). This pathway then uses specific tests (e.g., iron studies, B12/folate levels, reticulocyte count) to differentiate etiologies such as iron deficiency, B12/folate deficiency, or anemia of chronic disease, with treatment aimed at targeted repletion. In contrast, algorithms for leukemias are bifurcated by acuity (acute vs. chronic) and lineage (myeloid vs. lymphoid). Acute leukemias (AML, ALL) are medical emergencies requiring immediate induction chemotherapy. Chronic myeloid leukemia (CML) is managed with a first-line algorithm of oral tyrosine kinase inhibitors. Chronic lymphocytic leukemia (CLL) often follows a "watch and wait" algorithm until symptoms or cytopenias develop. Lymphoma algorithms diverge into Hodgkin (HL) and Non-Hodgkin (NHL) pathways. HL is treated with stage-adapted chemotherapy (e.g., ABVD). NHL algorithms are highly heterogeneous based on subtype, ranging from "watch and wait" for follicular lymphoma to aggressive R-CHOP for diffuse large B-cell lymphoma. Bleeding disorder algorithms differentiate between platelet and factor deficiencies. Immune thrombocytopenia is managed with first-line corticosteroids, while hemophilias require factor replacement algorithms (prophylactic or on-demand).

Keywords: *Anemia, Leukemia, Lymphoma, Bleeding Disorders, Chemotherapy, Targeted Therapy*

Learning Objectives

After completion of the chapter, the learners should be able to:

- Classify anemias based on MCV (microcytic, normocytic, macrocytic) and identify key follow-up tests for each.
- Explain the general treatment algorithm for Acute Myeloid Leukemia (AML), including induction and consolidation phases.
- Formulate a diagnostic and treatment algorithm for a patient presenting with new-onset microcytic anemia.
- Differentiate the staging and treatment algorithms for Hodgkin Lymphoma versus non-Hodgkin Lymphoma.
- Prioritize the management steps in the algorithm for a patient with a bleeding disorder (e.g., von Willebrand disease) requiring emergency surgery.

ANEMIAS

Anemia is defined as a reduction in the concentration of hemoglobin or the number of red blood cells. The management algorithm is not a single pathway but a diagnostic algorithm based on cell morphology, which then leads to etiology-specific treatment.

Iron Deficiency Anemia (IDA)

Pathophysiology

Iron deficiency anemia is the most common anemia worldwide. The pathophysiology is a direct consequence of insufficient iron supply for hemoglobin (Hgb) synthesis. Iron is a critical component of the heme molecule, which is the oxygen-carrying moiety within Hgb. The body's iron stores (primarily as ferritin) must be depleted *before* a drop in Hgb occurs. The most common cause in pre-menopausal women is chronic blood loss (menorrhagia). In men and post-menopausal women, the most common and ominous cause is chronic gastrointestinal blood loss (e.g., from a peptic ulcer or colon cancer). In resource-poor settings, nutritional deficiency is also a primary driver. The resulting RBCs are microcytic (small) and hypochromic (pale) because there is not enough hemoglobin to fill the cell.

Anemia of Chronic Disease / Inflammation (ACD)

Pathophysiology

Anemia of Chronic Disease (ACD) is the second most common anemia and is seen in patients with chronic inflammatory states (e.g., rheumatoid arthritis, IBD, chronic infection, malignancy). The pathophysiology is *not* a deficiency of iron, but a **functional iron deficiency** driven by inflammation. The main inflammatory cytokine is **hepcidin**, which is released by the liver. Hepcidin acts as the master iron regulator. It "locks" iron away: 1) it blocks iron absorption from the gut, and 2) it prevents the release of recycled iron from macrophages. Even though the patient has abundant iron stored in their ferritin, hepcidin prevents it from being released to the bone marrow for use in new RBCs. The result is an anemia that looks similar to IDA (often microcytic/normocytic) but occurs in the setting of a high ferritin (because the iron is trapped in storage).

Diagnosis and Classification

The diagnostic algorithm for anemia begins with a complete blood count (CBC) with differential. The first branch point is the Mean Corpuscular Volume (MCV), which classifies the anemia morphologically:

1. **Microcytic (MCV < 80 fL):** Small red blood cells.
2. **Normocytic (MCV 80-100 fL):** Normal-sized red blood cells.
3. **Macrocytic (MCV > 100 fL):** Large red blood cells.

Differential Diagnosis (Etiology)

The differential diagnosis is stratified by MCV:

- **Microcytic:** The differential includes iron deficiency anemia (IDA), thalassemia, anemia of chronic disease (ACD; can also be normocytic), and sideroblastic anemia.
- **Normocytic:** This is the broadest category. The algorithm is further stratified by the reticulocyte count. A high reticulocyte count implies hemolysis or acute blood loss (a correct bone marrow response). A low

reticulocyte count implies a production problem (e.g., ACD, aplastic anemia, renal failure).

- **Macrocytic:** The algorithm bifurcates into megaloblastic (impaired DNA synthesis) and non-megaloblastic causes. Megaloblastic anemia includes Vitamin B12 deficiency and folate deficiency. Non-megaloblastic causes include liver disease, alcoholism, and myelodysplastic syndrome (MDS).

Treatment Algorithm

The treatment algorithm is entirely dependent on the diagnosed etiology.

- **Iron Deficiency Anemia (IDA):** The algorithm begins with oral iron supplementation (e.g., ferrous sulfate) given with vitamin C to enhance absorption. For patients intolerant to oral iron or with severe malabsorption (e.g., IBD, post-bariatric surgery), the algorithm shifts to intravenous (IV) iron. It is also critical to investigate and treat the underlying cause of iron deficiency (e.g., occult GI bleeding).
- **Vitamin B12 Deficiency:** The algorithm is replacement, typically with intramuscular (IM) or subcutaneous (SC) cyanocobalamin, starting with loading doses followed by monthly maintenance. High-dose oral B12 can be used if absorption is intact.
- **Folate Deficiency:** The algorithm is simple replacement with oral folic acid.
- **Anemia of Chronic Disease (ACD):** The primary algorithm is to treat the underlying inflammatory condition (e.g., rheumatoid arthritis, IBD). If anemia is severe, particularly in the setting of CKD, the algorithm may involve erythropoiesis-stimulating agents (ESAs) after ensuring iron stores are replete.
- **Hemolytic Anemia:** The algorithm depends on the cause (e.g., corticosteroids for autoimmune hemolytic anemia, splenectomy for hereditary spherocytosis).

Table 9.1: Diagnostic Algorithm for Anemia Based on MCV

MCV Category	Initial Labs	Common Etiologies
Microcytic (< 80 fL)	**Iron Studies** (Ferritin, TIBC), Hgb Electrophoresis	Iron Deficiency, Thalassemia, Anemia of Chronic Disease (late).
Normocytic (80-100 fL)	**Reticulocyte Count,** LDH, Haptoglobin, Coombs'	**Low Retic:** Anemia of Chronic Disease, CKD, Aplastic Anemia. **High Retic:** Hemolysis, Acute Blood Loss.
Macrocytic (> 100 fL)	**B12 / Folate levels,** TSH, LFTs, Retic. Count	**Megaloblastic:** B12/Folate Deficiency. **Non-Megaloblastic:** Liver Disease, Alcoholism.

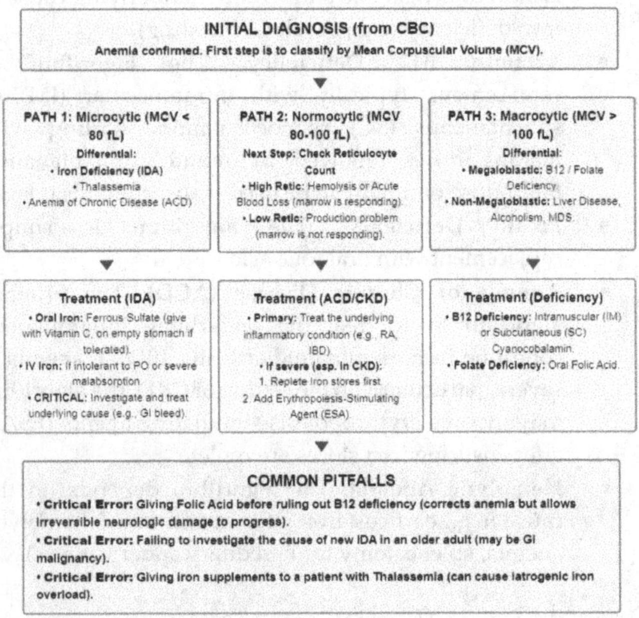
INITIAL DIAGNOSIS (from CBC)
Anemia confirmed. First step is to classify by Mean Corpuscular Volume (MCV).
PATH 1: Microcytic (MCV < 80 fL)
Differential:
• Iron Deficiency (IDA)
• Thalassemia
• Anemia of Chronic Disease (ACD)
PATH 2: Normocytic (MCV 80-100 fL)
Next Step: Check Reticulocyte Count
• High Retic: Hemolysis or Acute Blood Loss (marrow is responding).
• Low Retic: Production problem (marrow is not responding).
PATH 3: Macrocytic (MCV > 100 fL)
Differential:
• Megaloblastic: B12 / Folate Deficiency.
• Non-Megaloblastic: Liver Disease, Alcoholism, MDS.
Treatment (IDA)
• Oral Iron: Ferrous Sulfate (give with Vitamin C, on empty stomach if tolerated).
• IV Iron: If intolerant to PO or severe malabsorption.
• CRITICAL: Investigate and treat underlying cause (e.g., GI bleed).
Treatment (ACD/CKD)
• Primary: Treat the underlying inflammatory condition (e.g., RA, IBD).
• If severe (esp. in CKD):
1. Replete iron stores first.
2. Add Erythropoiesis-Stimulating Agent (ESA).
Treatment (Deficiency)
• B12 Deficiency: Intramuscular (IM) or Subcutaneous (SC) Cyanocobalamin.
• Folate Deficiency: Oral Folic Acid.
COMMON PITFALLS
• Critical Error: Giving Folic Acid before ruling out B12 deficiency (corrects anemia but allows irreversible neurologic damage to progress).
• Critical Error: Failing to investigate the cause of new IDA in an older adult (may be GI malignancy).
• Critical Error: Giving iron supplements to a patient with Thalassemia (can cause iatrogenic iron overload).

Figure 9.1: Anemia Diagnostic and Treatment Algorithm

Monitoring and Follow-Up

The primary monitoring parameter is the **hemoglobin** level, which should begin to rise within 2-3 weeks of starting iron supplementation. A complete blood count (CBC) and reticulocyte count should be checked at 4 weeks to confirm a response (a rise in reticulocytes, or new RBCs, should be seen within 7-10 days). A failure to respond suggests non-adherence, malabsorption, or incorrect diagnosis. More importantly, **ferritin** must be monitored. The goal is not just to normalize the Hgb, but to *replete the iron stores*. Oral iron should be continued for 3-6 *months* after the Hgb has normalized to fully replenish the ferritin stores.

Long-Term Management / Secondary Prevention

Long-term management is focused on identifying and **treating the underlying cause of iron loss**. In a man or post-menopausal woman with new IDA, the diagnostic algorithm *must* include an upper endoscopy and colonoscopy to rule out a GI malignancy. For a pre-menopausal woman, management of menorrhagia is crucial. Secondary prevention in high-risk groups (e.g., pregnant women, bariatric surgery patients) involves prophylactic low-dose iron supplementation.

Patient Counseling Points

1. **Iron Dosing and Side Effects:** "This is a critical counseling point. You should take your iron pill on an *empty stomach* to absorb it best, often with a glass of orange juice, as Vitamin C helps absorption. However, iron is very hard on the stomach and commonly causes constipation, nausea, and dark stools. If you can't tolerate it on an empty stomach, it is better to take it *with food* than to not take it at all."
2. **Constipation Management:** "You will almost certainly become constipated. You should start a stool softener (like docusate) or a gentle laxative (like Miralax) at the same time you start your iron."
3. **Duration of Therapy:** "This is not a quick fix. We are checking your blood count in a few weeks, but you will

need to take this pill for *many months*. Our goal is first to fix your blood count, and then to re-fill your body's 'iron savings account' (ferritin), which takes time."

Common Pitfalls in Management

A very common pitfall is prescribing iron supplementation to a patient with thalassemia; these patients are microcytic but often iron-overloaded, and iron can cause organ damage. Another error is initiating folic acid supplementation in a patient with severe macrocytic anemia *before* ruling out B12 deficiency; this can correct the anemia hematologically but allow irreversible neurologic damage from B12 deficiency to progress. Finally, failing to investigate the *cause* of iron deficiency in an older adult is a critical omission that can miss a GI malignancy.

Case Study

A 35-year-old pre-menopausal female (Ms. Yang) presents with a 6-month history of progressive fatigue, pallor, and "brain fog." She notes her menstrual periods have been very heavy. On exam, she has pale conjunctivae. Her CBC shows: Hgb **9.2 g/dL** (low), Hct 28% (low), and **MCV 74 fL** (low).

Discussion

The patient's CBC reveals a **microcytic anemia** (MCV < 80). The diagnostic algorithm for microcytic anemia is to first differentiate Iron Deficiency Anemia (IDA) from thalassemia or anemia of chronic disease. Given her history of heavy menses (chronic blood loss), IDA is the leading cause.

Treatment Algorithm

1. **Diagnosis (MCV-based):** Microcytic Anemia.
2. **Algorithm Step 1 (Diagnostic Labs):** You order **iron studies.**
    - **Ferritin: 5 ng/mL** (very low, < 15-30)
    - **Serum Iron:** Low
    - **TIBC:** High
    - This lab profile confirms the diagnosis of **Iron Deficiency Anemia**.

3. **Algorithm Step 2 (Treatment):**
   - **Repletion:** Start **oral Ferrous Sulfate 325 mg daily.**
   - **Counseling:** You counsel her to take it on an empty stomach with a glass of orange juice (Vitamin C) to enhance absorption, and warn her about expected side effects (constipation, dark stools).
4. **Algorithm Step 3 (Address Cause):** The anemia will recur unless the cause is treated. You refer her to a GYN to manage her menorrhagia.
5. **Follow-up:** Re-check CBC in 4 weeks to see a rise in Hgb. The algorithm *requires* continuing iron for **3-6 months *after*** her Hgb normalizes to replete her ferritin stores.

Outcome

Ms. Yang is started on oral iron supplementation and referred to GYN to manage the underlying cause of her chronic blood loss.

LEUKEMIAS

Leukemias are malignant proliferative disorders of hematopoietic cells. The treatment algorithms are highly specific and are bifurcated by acuity (acute vs. chronic) and cell lineage (myeloid vs. lymphoid).

Pathophysiology

A. Acute Myeloid Leukemia (AML)

Acute Myeloid Leukemia (AML) is a cancer of the myeloid bloodline. The pathophysiology is a **maturation arrest**. A hematopoietic stem cell in the bone marrow acquires a genetic mutation (e.g., *FLT3, NPM1*) that causes it to proliferate uncontrollably and, critically, *fail to differentiate* into a mature cell (like a neutrophil). This results in the massive overproduction and accumulation of immature, non-functional "blasts." These blasts crowd out the entire bone marrow, leading to a failure of all other cell lines. This "bone marrow failure" is what causes the clinical presentation: **anemia** (from lack of RBCs, causing fatigue), **thrombocytopenia** (from lack of platelets, causing bleeding/bruising), and **neutropenia** (from lack of *functional* neutrophils, leading to severe infections, even though the total WBC count may be high).

Chronic Myeloid Leukemia (CML

Chronic Myeloid Leukemia (CML) is a myeloproliferative neoplasm. The pathophysiology is elegant and specific: it is driven by a single, hallmark genetic mutation known as the **Philadelphia chromosome**. This is a translocation between chromosomes 9 and 22, t(9;22), which creates a new, fused "fusion gene" called **BCR-ABL**. This new gene produces a new, constitutively "on" tyrosine kinase enzyme. This BCR-ABL kinase acts as a powerful, non-stop "gas pedal" for the myeloid cell line, causing the massive overproduction of *all* mature and maturing myeloid cells, especially neutrophils. This results in a spectacularly high WBC count (often > 100,000) and splenomegaly (as the spleen fills with these excess cells).

Diagnosis and Classification

Diagnosis is made by peripheral blood smear and confirmed by bone marrow aspiration and biopsy, which includes cytogenetics, flow cytometry, and molecular studies.

1. **Acute Leukemias (AML, ALL):** Characterized by > 20% blasts (immature cells) in the bone marrow and a rapid, fulminant course with cytopenias.
2. **Chronic Leukemias (CML, CLL):** Characterized by an overproduction of mature-appearing but dysfunctional cells and a more indolent course.

Differential Diagnosis

The differential for acute leukemia includes aplastic anemia or severe viral infections (e.g., EBV, HIV) which can also cause profound pancytopenia. The differential for CML (high WBC with mature neutrophils) includes a "leukemoid reaction" (a benign response to severe infection or inflammation). The differential for CLL (high lymphocyte count) includes other lymphoproliferative disorders.

Treatment Algorithm

- **Acute Myeloid Leukemia (AML):** AML (except Acute Promyelocytic Leukemia) is a medical emergency. The algorithm is emergent induction chemotherapy, most commonly the "7+3" regimen (7 days of cytarabine and 3 days of an anthracycline). The goal is to achieve remission. This is followed by a consolidation algorithm (e.g., high-dose cytarabine) or allogeneic stem cell transplant based on risk stratification (cytogenetics, molecular markers).
- **Acute Promyelocytic Leukemia (APL):** This AML subtype has a unique algorithm and is also an emergency due to high risk of DIC. The algorithm is immediate initiation of All-Trans-Retinoic Acid (ATRA) and arsenic trioxide (ATO), even on suspicion, which induces differentiation of the malignant promyelocytes.
- **Acute Lymphoblastic Leukemia (ALL):** The algorithm is also emergent induction chemotherapy, but with a different, multi-agent regimen (e.g., vincristine, prednisone, anthracycline, asparaginase). A critical component is CNS prophylaxis (intrathecal chemotherapy), as ALL commonly relapses in the CNS.
- **Chronic Myeloid Leukemia (CML):** The algorithm for CML was revolutionized by targeted therapy. The first-line treatment is an oral Tyrosine Kinase Inhibitor (TKI) that targets the *BCR-ABL* fusion protein, such as Imatinib. The algorithm then involves routine molecular monitoring (quantitative PCR for *BCR-ABL* transcripts) to ensure treatment milestones are met.
- **Chronic Lymphocytic Leukemia (CLL):** The algorithm for asymptomatic, early-stage CLL is "watch and wait," as treatment does not improve survival. Treatment is initiated only for "active disease" (e.g., significant B symptoms, progressive cytopenias, massive lymphadenopathy). The modern first-line algorithm involves oral targeted agents, such as a BTK inhibitor (e.g., ibrutinib, acalabrutinib) or a BCL-2 inhibitor (venetoclax).

Table 9.2: Differentiating Acute vs. Chronic Leukemias

Feature	Acute Leukemia (AML/ALL)	Chronic Leukemia (CML/CLL)
Onset	Sudden, Rapid	Insidious, Slow
Cell Type	**> 20% Blasts** (Immature) in bone marrow.	Predominantly **Mature-**appearing cells.
Symptoms	"B Symptoms" (fever, night sweats), Bleeding, Infections.	Often asymptomatic, found on routine CBC. (Fatigue, lymphadenopathy).
Marker	**Auer Rods** (AML), **t(9;22)** (Ph+ ALL)	**t(9;22) BCR-ABL** (CML), **Smudge Cells** (CLL).

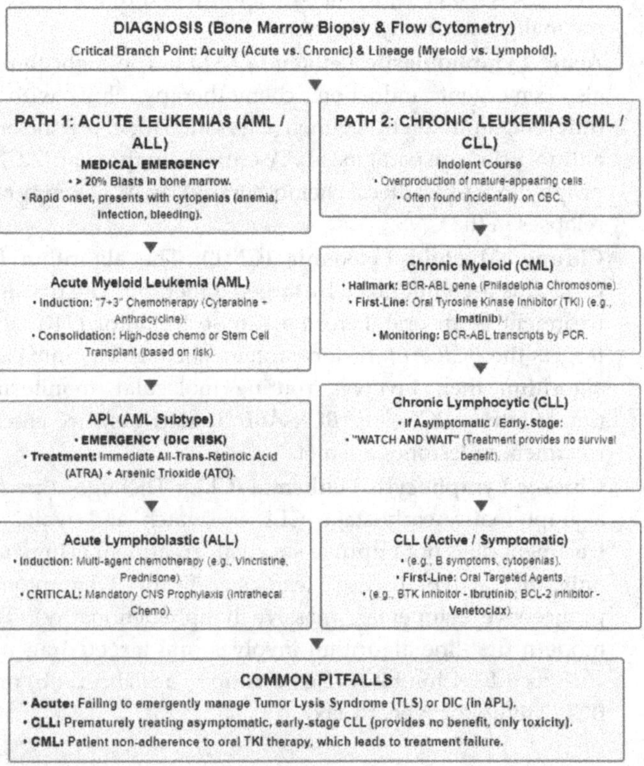
DIAGNOSIS (Bone Marrow Biopsy & Flow Cytometry)
Critical Branch Point: Acuity (Acute vs. Chronic) & Lineage (Myeloid vs. Lymphoid).
PATH 1: ACUTE LEUKEMIAS (AML / ALL)
MEDICAL EMERGENCY
• > 20% Blasts in bone marrow.
• Rapid onset, presents with cytopenias (anemia, infection, bleeding).
PATH 2: CHRONIC LEUKEMIAS (CML / CLL)
Indolent Course
• Overproduction of mature-appearing cells.
• Often found incidentally on CBC.
Acute Myeloid Leukemia (AML)
• Induction: "7+3" Chemotherapy (Cytarabine + Anthracycline).
• Consolidation: High-dose chemo or Stem Cell Transplant (based on risk).
Chronic Myeloid (CML)
• Hallmark: BCR-ABL gene (Philadelphia Chromosome).
• First-Line: Oral Tyrosine Kinase Inhibitor (TKI) (e.g., Imatinib).
• Monitoring: BCR-ABL transcripts by PCR.
APL (AML Subtype)
• EMERGENCY (DIC RISK)
• Treatment: Immediate All-Trans-Retinoic Acid (ATRA) + Arsenic Trioxide (ATO).
Chronic Lymphocytic (CLL)
• If Asymptomatic / Early-Stage:
• "WATCH AND WAIT" (Treatment provides no survival benefit).
Acute Lymphoblastic (ALL)
• Induction: Multi-agent chemotherapy (e.g., Vincristine, Prednisone).
• CRITICAL: Mandatory CNS Prophylaxis (Intrathecal Chemo).
CLL (Active / Symptomatic)
• (e.g., B symptoms, cytopenias).
• First-Line: Oral Targeted Agents.
• (e.g., BTK inhibitor - Ibrutinib; BCL-2 inhibitor - Venetoclax).
COMMON PITFALLS
• Acute: Failing to emergently manage Tumor Lysis Syndrome (TLS) or DIC (in APL).
• CLL: Prematurely treating asymptomatic, early-stage CLL (provides no benefit, only toxicity).
• CML: Patient non-adherence to oral TKI therapy, which leads to treatment failure.

Figure 9.2: Leukemias - Treatment Algorithms

Monitoring and Follow-Up

Monitoring during induction chemotherapy is an intensive inpatient process. It involves daily CBCs to monitor for profound pancytopenia and daily monitoring for **Tumor Lysis Syndrome** (TLS) with labs for uric acid, potassium, phosphorus, and creatinine. The patient is monitored for "neutropenic fever," which is a medical emergency. After the patient's counts recover, a **bone marrow biopsy** is performed (e.g., around day 14 and day 28) to confirm "remission" (defined as <5% blasts in the marrow). Long-term monitoring involves frequent CBCs and surveillance for "minimal residual disease" (MRD) using highly sensitive molecular or flow cytometry tests.

Long-Term Management / Secondary Prevention

The management is emergent. The first phase is **induction chemotherapy** (e.g., "7+3" regimen) to achieve remission. The second phase is **consolidation therapy** to prevent relapse. The algorithm for consolidation is based on the patient's cytogenetic and molecular risk profile. "Favorable" risk patients may receive high-dose chemotherapy. "Unfavorable" risk patients are managed with the only curative option: an **allogeneic stem cell transplant**.

Patient Counseling Points

1. **"This is an Emergency"**: "This is an 'acute' leukemia, which means it develops very quickly and is life-threatening. We must start chemotherapy in the hospital within the next day or two. The goal is a cure, but the treatment is very aggressive."
2. **Infection Risk (Neutropenia):** "The chemotherapy will wipe out your bone marrow and your immune system, leaving you with zero white blood cells to fight infection. A *fever* (100.4°F) is a life-threatening emergency, and you must tell us immediately. You will be in a protective room and must be strict about hand hygiene."
3. **Blood Product Support:** "You will require multiple blood and platelet transfusions over the next few weeks

to keep you alive while your bone marrow is recovering."

Common Pitfalls in Management

The most critical pitfall in acute leukemia is failing to recognize and emergently manage oncologic emergencies, such as tumor lysis syndrome (TLS), hyperleukocytosis, and DIC (especially in APL). In CML, non-adherence to oral TKI therapy is a major pitfall leading to treatment failure. In CLL, the most common error is prematurely treating an asymptomatic patient, which exposes them to therapy side effects with no survival benefit.

Case Study

A 55-year-old male (Mr. Barnes) presents for an annual physical. He feels well, though he mentions "feeling full" after small meals. His exam is notable for an enlarged spleen (splenomegaly). His routine CBC is abnormal: **WBC 122,000/µL** (high), Hgb 11.5 (low), Platelets 480,000 (high). The differential shows a "left-shift" with a predominance of mature neutrophils.

Discussion

This presentation (massive leukocytosis with mature cells, splenomegaly) is the hallmark of a **chronic leukemia**, specifically **Chronic Myeloid Leukemia (CML)**

This is *not* an acute leukemia, which would present with >20% immature blasts and rapid onset of symptoms. The CML algorithm requires specific genetic confirmation.

Treatment Algorithm

1. **Diagnosis (Suspected):** Chronic Myeloid Leukemia (CML).
2. **Algorithm Step 1 (Confirm):** Order a peripheral blood FISH or PCR test to look for the **BCR-ABL fusion gene (Philadelphia chromosome)**. The test comes back **positive**.
3. **Algorithm Step 2 (Treatment):** The first-line algorithm for CML is a targeted oral Tyrosine Kinase Inhibitor (TKI).

    - **Therapy:** Start **Imatinib 400 mg once daily**.
4. **Algorithm Step 3 (Monitoring):** The goal is not just a normal CBC, but a deep molecular remission.
    - **Follow-up:** You schedule regular follow-ups to monitor his *BCR-ABL* transcript levels via quantitative PCR, with the goal of achieving a major molecular response by 12 months.

Outcome

Mr. Barnes is diagnosed with CML and started on Imatinib, a highly effective, lifelong oral therapy.

LYMPHOMAS

Lymphomas are malignancies of mature lymphocytes that form solid tumors in lymph nodes and other tissues. The diagnostic and treatment algorithm is fundamentally split into two major families: Hodgkin Lymphoma and Non-Hodgkin Lymphoma.

Pathophysiology

Hodgkin Lymphoma is a B-cell lymphoma defined by a unique pathologic finding: the presence of large, malignant **Reed-Sternberg (RS) cells**. The paradox of HL is that these RS cells make up only ~1% of the tumor mass. The other 99% of the tumor is a massive, non-malignant inflammatory infiltrate (lymphocytes, eosinophils, plasma cells) that is *recruited* by the RS cells. The RS cells release cytokines that create this inflammatory environment, which in turn supports their survival. The disease typically arises in a single lymph node (often cervical) and spreads in a *contiguous, predictable, stepwise* pattern to adjacent lymph nodes, which is important to its staging and treatment

DLBCL is the most common non-Hodgkin lymphoma (NHL). Unlike Hodgkin's, it is an aggressive, rapidly growing tumor *composed entirely* of malignant, large B-lymphocytes. It does not spread predictably; it is often disseminated at diagnosis and can arise in "extranodal" sites (e.g., GI tract, brain). The pathophysiology is heterogeneous, driven by various genetic mutations that lead to uncontrolled B-cell proliferation.

Diagnosis and Classification

The definitive diagnostic algorithm is an excisional lymph node biopsy. Fine-needle aspiration is insufficient.

1. **Hodgkin Lymphoma (HL):** Characterized by the presence of pathognomonic Reed-Sternberg cells in the biopsy. It typically spreads in an orderly, contiguous fashion.
2. **Non-Hodgkin Lymphoma (NHL):** A large, heterogeneous group of over 60 subtypes, classified by cell of origin (B-cell vs. T-cell) and behavior (indolent vs. aggressive).

Differential Diagnosis

The primary differential for lymphadenopathy is infection (e.g., infectious mononucleosis/EBV, HIV, cat-scratch disease) or autoimmune disease (e.g., lupus, sarcoidosis). The presence of "B symptoms" (fever, night sweats, unintentional weight loss > 10%) strongly suggests lymphoma.

Treatment Algorithm

The staging algorithm for both HL and NHL is the Ann Arbor staging system (Stage I-IV), which is determined by PET/CT scan and bone marrow biopsy.

- **Hodgkin Lymphoma (HL):** The algorithm is stage-dependent.
    - **Early-Stage (I/II):** The algorithm is combined-modality therapy: a shorter course of chemotherapy (e.g., ABVD regimen) followed by involved-site radiation therapy (ISRT).
    - **Advanced-Stage (III/IV):** The algorithm is a full course of combination chemotherapy (e.g., ABVD or BEACOPP).
- **Non-Hodgkin Lymphoma (NHL):** The algorithm is entirely dependent on the specific subtype.
    - **Aggressive NHL (e.g., Diffuse Large B-Cell Lymphoma, DLBCL):** The algorithm is curative-intent, first-line

immunochemotherapy, most commonly R-CHOP (Rituximab, Cyclophosphamide, Doxorubicin, Vincristine, Prednisone).

- **Indolent NHL (e.g., Follicular Lymphoma):** The algorithm is similar to CLL. If asymptomatic, the algorithm is "watch and wait." If symptomatic, the algorithm is typically rituximab-based, with or without chemotherapy (e.g., R-CVP or bendamustine-rituximab).

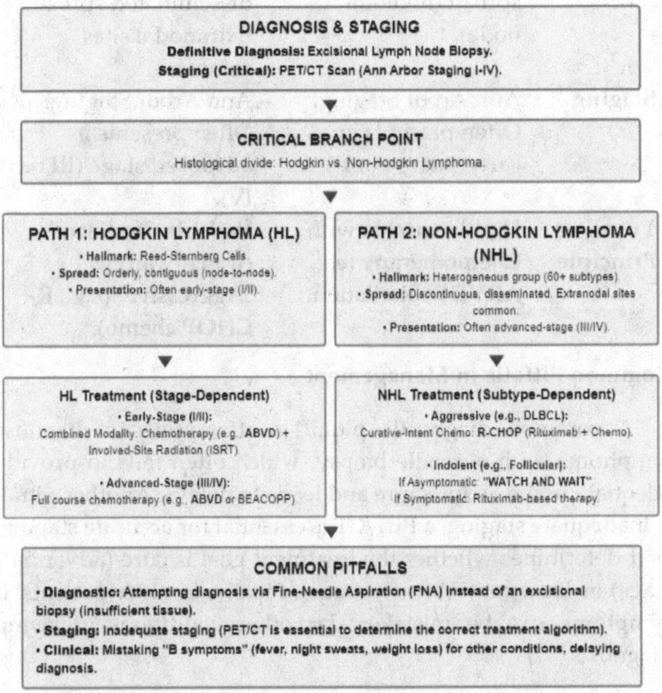

Figure 9.3: Lymphomas - Treatment Algorithms

Table 9.3: Differentiating Hodgkin vs. Non-Hodgkin Lymphoma

Feature	Hodgkin Lymphoma (HL)	Non-Hodgkin Lymphoma (NHL)
Cell	**Reed-Sternberg (RS) Cell** (minority of cells in tumor).	Malignant B-cells or T-cells.
Spread	**Contiguous,** orderly spread (node-to-node).	**Non-contiguous,** disseminated spread. Extranodal sites common.
Staging	Ann Arbor Staging. Often presents in early stage (I or II).	Ann Arbor Staging. Often presents in advanced stage (III or IV).
Tx Principle	Highly curable with Chemotherapy (e.g., **ABVD**) ± Radiation.	Variable. "Indolent" (watch/wait) vs. "Aggressive" (e.g., **R-CHOP** chemo).

Common Pitfalls in Management

A common diagnostic pitfall is attempting to diagnose lymphoma with a needle biopsy, which often fails to provide adequate tissue architecture and leads to delays. Another pitfall is inadequate staging; a PET/CT is essential for accurate staging, as it determines whether the treatment goal is cure (advanced-stage) or local control (early-stage). Finally, in older patients, B symptoms can be mistaken for other conditions, delaying diagnosis.

Monitoring and Follow-Up

The primary monitoring tool is the **PET-CT scan**. An "interim" PET scan is often performed after 2 cycles of chemotherapy (e.g., ABVD). The response on this scan (using the "Deauville score") is highly prognostic and can be used to de-escalate therapy (e.g., drop a drug) if the response is excellent. After completion of therapy, a final PET-CT is done to confirm remission. Long-term monitoring involves clinical follow-up for relapse and, crucially, for the **late-term toxicities** of treatment, especially cardiovascular disease (from chest radiation) and secondary malignancies (from chemotherapy and radiation).

Long-Term Management / Secondary Prevention

Hodgkin Lymphoma is considered one of the most curable cancers. The algorithm is based on stage. Early-stage (I/II) "favorable" disease is treated with a "combined modality" approach: a short course of chemotherapy (e.g., 2-4 cycles of ABVD) followed by low-dose "involved-site" radiation therapy (ISRT). Advanced-stage (III/IV) disease is treated with chemotherapy alone (e.g., 6 cycles of ABVD or escalated BEACOPP).

Patient Counseling Points

1. **"This is a Highly Curable Cancer":** "This is the 'good' lymphoma, if there is one. With modern treatment, the cure rate, even for advanced-stage disease, is extremely high (80-90%)."
2. **Chemo Side Effects:** "The main side effects of your chemo (ABVD) are nausea, hair loss, and low blood counts. One drug, Bleomycin, can rarely cause lung damage, so we will monitor your breathing."
3. **Long-Term Follow-Up is Lifelong:** "Our job is to cure you, and then to keep you healthy for the next 50 years. The radiation and chemo can have 'late effects' that appear 10-20 years later, like heart or thyroid problems. You will need to be monitored for these for the rest of your life."

Case Study

A 24-year-old female (Ms. Smith) presents with a single, painless, "rubbery" lymph node in the left side of her neck, which she first noticed 2 months ago. She also reports a 15-lb unintentional weight loss and drenching night sweats.

Discussion

This is the classic presentation for **Hodgkin Lymphoma (HL)**: a young adult with "B symptoms" (fever, night sweats, weight loss) and localized, non-tender lymphadenopathy. The algorithm requires a tissue biopsy for diagnosis, followed by PET scanning for staging.

Treatment Algorithm

1. **Diagnosis (Step 1):** The algorithm mandates an **excisional lymph node biopsy** (a needle biopsy is often insufficient).
2. **Pathology:** The biopsy reveals **Reed-Sternberg cells** amidst a mixed inflammatory background, confirming **Hodgkin Lymphoma**.
3. **Staging (Step 2):** A full-body **PET/CT scan** is performed. It shows avid uptake in her left cervical nodes and in a cluster of mediastinal nodes, all on the same side of the diaphragm. This is **Stage IIB** ("B" for her B symptoms).
4. **Treatment (Step 3):** The algorithm is stage-dependent. For Stage IIB (early-stage, but unfavorable due to B symptoms), she requires combination chemotherapy. **Therapy:** Start the **ABVD chemotherapy regimen**.

Outcome

Ms. Smith is diagnosed with Stage IIB Hodgkin Lymphoma and is started on a curative-intent ABVD chemotherapy regimen. She is counseled that her prognosis is excellent

BLEEDING DISORDERS

Bleeding disorder algorithms focus on identifying the defective component of hemostasis: platelets (primary hemostasis) or coagulation factors (secondary hemostasis).

Pathophysiology

von Willebrand Disease is the most common *inherited* bleeding disorder. The pathophysiology is a deficiency or dysfunction of **von Willebrand Factor (vWF)**. vWF has two primary jobs in clotting: 1) it acts as the "glue" that allows platelets to adhere to a site of blood vessel injury (primary hemostasis), and 2) it acts as the "chaperone" protein that carries and protects Factor VIII from degradation (secondary hemostasis). In vWD, a lack of vWF means platelets can't stick properly, and Factor VIII levels are low. This creates a "double-hit" defect, causing the characteristic **mucocutaneous bleeding** (easy bruising, heavy menses, nosebleeds) from the platelet defect, and, in severe cases, joint bleeding (like hemophilia) from the Factor VIII defect.

ITP is an *acquired* autoimmune disorder. The pathophysiology is the production of **autoantibodies (IgG) that target the patient's own platelets**. These antibody-coated platelets are recognized as "foreign" by the spleen and are destroyed by splenic macrophages. This leads to an isolated, often severe, thrombocytopenia (low platelet count), while all other cell lines (WBC, Hgb) are normal. The bone marrow is working overtime to produce new platelets (megakaryocytes are high), but they are destroyed in the circulation as soon as they are released.

Diagnosis and Classification

The initial algorithm involves a CBC (for platelet count) and coagulation studies (PT/INR and PTT).

- **Thrombocytopenia or Platelet Dysfunction:** Suspected if platelet count is low or bleeding time is prolonged with normal coags.
- **Coagulation Factor Deficiency:** Suspected if PT or PTT is prolonged with a normal platelet count.

Differential Diagnosis (Etiology)

- **Isolated Thrombocytopenia:** Differential includes Immune Thrombocytopenia (ITP), drug-induced, or viral.
- **Thrombocytopenia + Microangiopathic Hemolysis:** This is a medical emergency. The differential is Thrombotic Thrombocytopenic Purpura (TTP) vs. Hemolytic Uremic Syndrome (HUS) vs. Disseminated

Intravascular Coagulation (DIC).

- **Prolonged PTT:** Differential includes Hemophilia A (Factor VIII), Hemophilia B (Factor IX), or von Willebrand Disease (vWD, as vWF stabilizes FVIII).
- **Prolonged PT/INR:** Differential includes liver disease or warfarin use.
- **Prolonged PT and PTT + Thrombocytopenia:** This pattern strongly suggests DIC.

Treatment Algorithm

- **Immune Thrombocytopenia (ITP):** The algorithm is triggered by platelet count (e.g., < 30,000/μL) or active bleeding.
    - **First-Line:** High-dose corticosteroids (e.g., prednisone or dexamethasone) or IV Immunoglobulin (IVIG) for rapid platelet increase.
    - **Second-Line (for refractory/chronic):** TPO-receptor agonists (e.g., romiplostim, eltrombopag) or rituximab.
- **Thrombotic Thrombocytopenic Purpura (TTP):** This is a medical emergency. The algorithm is immediate, emergent plasmapheresis (PEX) to remove anti-ADAMTS13 autoantibodies and replenish functional ADAMTS13.
- **von Willebrand Disease (vWD):** The algorithm is based on type.
    - **Type 1 (Mild):** Desmopressin (DDAVP) to stimulate vWF release from endothelial cells.
    - **Type 2/3 (Severe):** vWF-containing factor concentrates.
- **Hemophilia A/B:** The algorithm involves factor replacement (recombinant FVIII or FIX). This can be prophylactic (to prevent bleeds) or on-demand (to treat active bleeds).
- **Disseminated Intravascular Coagulation (DIC):** The primary and most critical algorithm is to **treat the underlying cause** (e.g., antibiotics for sepsis, surgical control of trauma). The hematologic algorithm is

supportive: replace components only if actively bleeding (e.g., platelets for thrombocytopenia, cryoprecipitate for low fibrinogen).

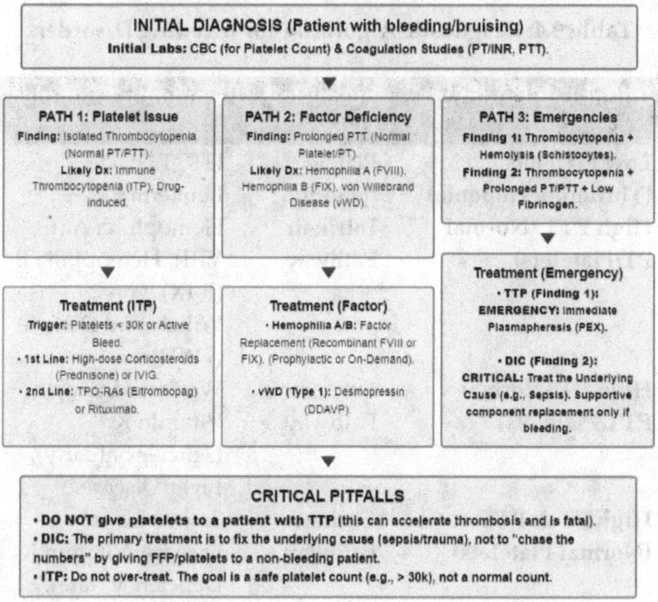

Figure 9.4: Bleeding Disorders

Monitoring and Follow-Up

Monitoring is largely clinical, asking about bleeding symptoms (e.g., duration of menses, frequency of epistaxis). Laboratory monitoring involves checking a "vWD panel," which includes vWF antigen (the amount of protein), vWF activity (how well it works), and the Factor VIII level.

Long-Term Management / Secondary Prevention

Management is based on bleeding severity.

- **Mild-Moderate Bleeding (e.g., for dental work, heavy menses):** The first-line treatment is **Desmopressin (DDAVP).** This is *not* a blood product; it is a hormone that forces the body to release its own stored vWF and Factor VIII from the blood vessel walls.

Severe Bleeding / Major Surgery: For severe (Type 3) vWD or in situations where DDAVP is ineffective, the algorithm is **vWF/Factor VIII concentrate infusion**

Table 9.4: Diagnostic Algorithm for Bleeding Disorders

Initial Lab Finding	Suspected Defect	Common Examples
Low Platelets (Thrombocytopenia)	Platelet quantity.	ITP, TTP, DIC, Leukemia.
High PTT (Normal PT/Platelets)	**Intrinsic** Pathway.	Hemophilia A (F-VIII), Hemophilia B (F-IX), von Willebrand Disease (vWD).
High PT (Normal PTT/Platelets)	**Extrinsic** Pathway.	**Warfarin** therapy, Vitamin K Deficiency (early), Liver Disease.
High PT & PTT (Normal Platelets)	**Common** Pathway.	Severe Liver Disease, Vitamin K Deficiency (late), DIC.

Patient Counseling Points

1. **"It's a 'Sticky' Problem":** "This is a common, usually mild, inherited bleeding disorder. You are not a 'free-bleeder.' The problem is that your platelets, which are the first-line responders to a cut, are not 'sticky' enough to form a strong plug."
2. **DDAVP (Desmopressin):** "For a dental procedure or a bad nosebleed, we can give you a nasal spray (DDAVP) that is a hormone. It 'squeezes' your blood vessels and forces them to release your own clotting factors, which temporarily fixes the problem."
3. **Avoid Aspirin/NSAIDs:** "You must *never* take Aspirin, Ibuprofen, or Naproxen. These drugs *also* make your platelets less sticky, and for you, this is like pouring gasoline on a fire. You must use Tylenol (acetaminophen) for pain."

B. Immune Thrombocytopenia (ITP)

Monitoring and Follow-Up

The primary monitoring tool is the **CBC**, specifically the platelet count. In the acute phase, this is checked daily or weekly to assess response to therapy. The goal is not a *normal* platelet count, but a *safe* one (e.g., > 30-50k/μL) to prevent major bleeding.

Long-Term Management / Secondary Prevention

The treatment algorithm is risk-stratified. Patients with a platelet count > 30k and no bleeding may be observed.

- **First-line:** For patients with significant bleeding or a count < 30k, the first-line therapy is **corticosteroids** (e.g., prednisone or high-dose dexamethasone) to suppress the immune system. **IVIG** may also be given in emergencies to rapidly, but temporarily, "distract" the spleen.
- **Second-line (for relapse):** For patients who relapse after steroids, the algorithm moves to second-line agents, which include **splenectomy** (to remove the site of destruction) or **TPO-receptor agonists** (e.g., romiplostim, eltrombopag) which are drugs that "stimulate" the bone marrow to produce more platelets.

Patient Counseling Points

1. **"Your Immune System is Eating Your Platelets":** "This is an autoimmune disease. Your immune system is mistaking your own platelets for an infection and is creating antibodies to destroy them. The 'factory' in your bone marrow is working fine, but the 'product' is being destroyed as soon as it's made."
2. **"Goal is 'Safe,' Not 'Normal'":** "We are starting you on steroids to calm your immune system down. Our goal is not to get your platelet count back to 300,000. Our goal is to get it to a *safe* level (e.g., above 30,000-50,000) so you are not at risk for a serious bleed."
3. **Bleeding Precautions:** "Until your count is safe, you must be on 'bleeding precautions.' This means no

contact sports, be careful with sharp objects, and use a soft-bristle toothbrush. If you hit your head, you must go to an ER, even if you feel fine. For a cut that won't stop bleeding, you must seek care."

Common Pitfalls in Management

The most lethal pitfall in hematology is **giving platelets to a patient with TTP**. This can accelerate thrombosis and is contraindicated; the correct treatment is PEX. In DIC, a common error is "chasing the numbers" and giving blood products (like FFP) to a non-bleeding patient, which can "fuel the fire" and worsen the thrombotic component of DIC. In ITP, a common pitfall is over-treating an asymptomatic patient with a stable platelet count (e.g., 40,000/μL), as the goal is to prevent bleeding, not to normalize the platelet count.

Case Study

A 28-year-old female (Ms. Kent) presents to the ED with a 2-day history of a new, widespread petechial rash on her legs and "blood blisters" in her mouth (wet purpura). She feels well. Her CBC is: Hgb 13.5 (normal), WBC 7.0 (normal), and **Platelets 4,000/μL** (critically low). PT and PTT are normal.

Discussion

This is **isolated thrombocytopenia**. The normal Hgb, WBC, and coagulation studies rule out DIC, TTP, and leukemia. The diagnosis is **Immune Thrombocytopenia (ITP)**. Her platelet count of 4,000 and the presence of wet purpura put her at very high risk for a spontaneous intracranial hemorrhage. This is a medical emergency.

Treatment Algorithm

1. **Diagnosis:** Severe, symptomatic Immune Thrombocytopenia (ITP).
2. **Algorithm (First-Line):** The algorithm is triggered by bleeding or a platelet count < 30k. She requires immediate therapy to raise her platelet count.
3. **Therapy (Step 1 - Suppress):** Start **High-Dose Corticosteroids.**

  - o **Regimen: Dexamethasone 40 mg daily for 4 days.**

4. **Therapy (Step 2 - Rapid Blockade):** Due to her high-risk features (wet purpura, Plt < 10k), you also give **IV Immunoglobulin (IVIG) 1 g/kg (one dose)**. This will rapidly "distract" the spleen from destroying platelets.
5. **Monitoring:** She is admitted to the hospital, placed on bleeding precautions, and her platelet count is monitored daily.

Outcome

Ms. Kent is admitted and started on Dexamethasone and IVIG. Her platelet count rises to 55,000 within 48 hours. She is monitored for a durable response to the steroids.

Summary

Anemias: The algorithm begins with morphological classification (MCV). Treatment is targeted to the specific deficiency identified (e.g., oral iron for IDA, IM B12 for B12 deficiency).

Leukemias: Acute leukemias (AML/ALL) are emergencies requiring induction chemotherapy. Chronic leukemias (CML, CLL) have distinct algorithms: CML is treated with first-line TKIs (e.g., Imatinib), while asymptomatic CLL is managed with "watch and wait."

Lymphomas: The algorithm requires an excisional biopsy and PET/CT staging. Hodgkin Lymphoma is treated with stage-adapted chemotherapy (e.g., ABVD). Non-Hodgkin Lymphoma algorithms are subtype-specific (e.g., R-CHOP for aggressive DLBCL, "watch and wait" for indolent follicular).

Bleeding Disorders: The algorithm differentiates platelet vs. factor issues. ITP is managed with first-line corticosteroids/IVIG. TTP is a medical emergency requiring plasmapheresis. Hemophilia is managed with factor replacement. DIC management requires treating the underlying cause.

Multiple Choice Questions

1. A 68-year-old male presents with fatigue. Labs show Hgb 9.1 g/dL, MCV 72 fL, and high ferritin. What is the most likely diagnosis?
   A) Iron Deficiency Anemia
   B) Vitamin B12 Deficiency
   C) Anemia of Chronic Disease
   D) Folate Deficiency
2. A patient with known macrocytic anemia (B12 deficiency) is treated with folic acid alone. Which of the following is the most likely adverse outcome?
   A) Worsening of the anemia
   B) Progression of irreversible neurologic symptoms
   C) Development of iron overload
   D) Acute kidney injury
3. A 45-year-old male presents with a WBC count of 150,000/μL, mostly mature neutrophils. The BCR-ABL fusion gene is positive. What is the first-line treatment algorithm?
   A) "7+3" Induction Chemotherapy
   B) R-CHOP Chemotherapy
   C) Imatinib
   D) "Watch and wait"
4. A 70-year-old female is diagnosed with asymptomatic, early-stage Chronic Lymphocytic Leukemia (CLL). What is the appropriate management?
   A) "Watch and wait"
   B) Ibrutinib
   C) Venetoclax
   D) FCR Chemotherapy
5. A 30-year-old female presents with fever, night sweats, and a new, painless cervical lymph node. Biopsy reveals Reed-Sternberg cells. What is the most likely diagnosis? A) Non-Hodgkin Lymphoma

B) Hodgkin Lymphoma
C) Infectious Mononucleosis
D) Acute Lymphoblastic Leukemia

6. What is the standard, first-line, curative-intent algorithm for Diffuse Large B-Cell Lymphoma (DLBCL)?
A) ABVD
B) R-CHOP
C) "Watch and wait"
D) Imatinib

7. A 25-year-old female presents with petechiae. Platelet count is 8,000/μL. PT and PTT are normal. What is the first-line treatment for presumed ITP?
A) Platelet transfusion
B) High-dose corticosteroids
C) Eltrombopag
D) Splenectomy

8. A 30-year-old patient presents with fever, confusion, thrombocytopenia, and schistocytes. ADAMTS13 activity is <10%. What is the emergent, life-saving algorithm?
A) Immediate platelet transfusion
B) Emergent plasmapheresis (PEX)
C) High-dose IVIG
D) Hemodialysis

9. A patient with sepsis develops oozing from IV sites. Labs show thrombocytopenia, prolonged PT/INR, prolonged PTT, and low fibrinogen. What is the most important step in the algorithm?
A) Administer fresh frozen plasma (FFP) immediately.
B) Administer platelets immediately.
C) Treat the underlying sepsis with antibiotics.
D) Administer heparin.

10. A 10-year-old boy with known Hemophilia A has a severe bleed. What is the treatment?

A) Desmopressin (DDAVP)
B) Recombinant Factor VIII
C) Recombinant Factor IX
D) IVIG

Self-Assessment Questions

1. Describe the diagnostic algorithm for anemia, starting from the CBC. What are the three main MCV categories and a primary differential for each?
2. What is a major pitfall of using folic acid to treat macrocytic anemia?
3. Compare and contrast the typical presentation and first-line treatment algorithm for Acute Myeloid Leukemia (AML) vs. Chronic Myeloid Leukemia (CML).
4. What is the "watch and wait" algorithm, and for which two chronic hematologic malignancies is it a standard approach?
5. What is the unique, emergent treatment algorithm for Acute Promyelocytic Leukemia (APL), and why is it so urgent?
6. Differentiate the treatment algorithm for early-stage Hodgkin Lymphoma vs. aggressive, advanced-stage Non-Hodgkin Lymphoma (like DLBCL).
7. A patient presents with isolated thrombocytopenia (platelet count 15,000/μL) and new petechiae. What is the likely diagnosis and the first-line treatment algorithm?
8. A patient presents with thrombocytopenia, schistocytes on peripheral smear, and renal failure. What are the top differentials, and what is the single most critical pitfall to avoid in treatment?
9. Explain the treatment algorithm for Type 1 von Willebrand Disease (vWD) versus Hemophilia A.
10. What is the *primary* treatment algorithm for Disseminated Intravascular Coagulation (DIC)?

Bibliography

1. National Heart, Lung, and Blood Institute. Evidence-Based Management of Sickle Cell Disease: Expert Panel Report, 2014. Rockville, MD: National Institutes of Health; 2014.
2. Camaschella C. Iron-deficiency anemia. N Engl J Med. 2015 May 7;372(19):1832–43.
3. Lachner C, St L, Schrier SL. Approach to the adult patient with anemia. In: UpToDate, Post TW (Ed), UpToDate, Waltham, MA. (Accessed on October 25, 2025).
4. Döhner H, Estey EH, Amadori S, Appelbaum FR, Büchner T, Burnett AK, et al. Diagnosis and management of acute myeloid leukemia in adults: recommendations from an international expert panel, on behalf of the European LeukemiaNet. Blood. 2010 Jan 21;115(3):453–74.
5. Sanz MA, Fenaux P, Tallman MS, Estey EH, Löwenberg B, Naoe T, et al. Management of acute promyelocytic leukemia: updated recommendations from an expert panel of the European LeukemiaNet. Blood. 2019 Apr 11;133(15):1630–43.
6. Jabbour E, O'Brien S, Konopleva M, Kantarjian H. New insights into the mechanisms of action of tyrosine kinase inhibitors. Nat Rev Clin Oncol. 2015 Apr;12(4):203–18.
7. Hallek M. Chronic lymphocytic leukemia: 2020 update on diagnosis, risk stratification, and treatment. Am J Hematol. 2019 Nov;94(11):1266–87.
8. Eich H, Diehl V, Görgen H, Pabst T, Markova J, Debus J, et al. Intensified chemotherapy and dose-reduced involved-field radiotherapy in patients with early-stage unfavorable Hodgkin's lymphoma: final analysis of the German Hodgkin Study Group HD14 trial. J Clin Oncol. 2010 Sep 20;28(27):4199–206.
9. Coiffier B, Thieblemont C, Van Den Neste E, Le B, M, E. et al. Long-term outcome of patients in the LNH-98.5 trial, the first randomized study comparing R-CHOP to CHOP chemotherapy in DLBCL patients: a study by the Groupe d'Etudes des Lymphomes de l'Adulte. Blood. 2010 Oct 21;116(16):2917–24.
10. Rummel MJ, Niederle N, Maschmeyer G, Banat GA, von Grünhagen U, Losem C, et al. Bendamustine plus rituximab versus CHOP plus rituximab as first-line treatment for patients with indolent and mantle-cell lymphomas: an open-label, multicentre, randomised,

phase 3 non-inferiority trial. Lancet. 2013 Apr 6;381(9873):1203–10.
11. Neunert C, Lim W, Crowther M, Cohen A, Solberg L Jr, Crowther MA. The American Society of Hematology 2011 evidence-based practice guideline for immune thrombocytopenia. Blood. 2011 Apr 21;117(16):4190–207.
12. George JN. Clinical practice. Thrombotic thrombocytopenic purpura. N Engl J Med. 2006 May 18;354(20):2142–51.
13. Leebeek FWG, Eikenboom J. Von Willebrand disease. N Engl J Med. 2016 Nov 17;375(20):1961–72.
14. Srivastava A, Santagostino E, Dougall A, Kitchen S, Sutherland M, Pipe SW, et al. WFH Guidelines for the Management of Hemophilia, 3rd edition. Haemophilia. 2020 Aug;26 Suppl 6:1–158.
15. Levi M, Toh CH, Thachil J, Watson HG. Guidelines for the diagnosis and management of disseminated intravascular coagulation. British Committee for Standards in Haematology. Br J Haematol. 2009 Apr;145(1):24–33.

CHAPTER 10

TREATMENT ALGORITHMS FOR RENAL DISORDERS

Author

Dr. Shannumukha Sainath A, Assistant Professor,
Department of Pharmacy Practice, Nirmala College of Pharmacy (Autonomous), Kadapa, Andhra Pradesh, India

Abstract

Treatment algorithms for renal disorders are stratified by acuity, etiology, and the pattern of glomerular injury. The management of Chronic Kidney Disease (CKD) is a staged algorithm based on GFR and albuminuria (KDIGO criteria). This pathway focuses on slowing progression via foundational therapies, including aggressive blood pressure control (primarily with RAS blockade), glycemic control (notably with SGLT2 inhibitors), and lifestyle modifications. The algorithm extends to the systematic management of secondary complications, including anemia with iron and erythropoiesis-stimulating agents, and mineral-bone disorder with phosphate binders and vitamin D sterols. In contrast, the Acute Kidney Injury (AKI) algorithm is a diagnostic pathway to rapidly determine and reverse the etiology. It bifurcates into pre-renal (requiring volume resuscitation), intrinsic (supportive care, nephrotoxin removal), and post-renal (urinary decompression). The algorithm for glomerulonephritis (GN) is driven by serology and renal biopsy. Crescentic, rapidly progressive GN (RPGN) necessitates an emergent algorithm of high-dose corticosteroids combined with either cyclophosphamide or rituximab, and plasmapheresis for anti-GBM disease. Nephrotic syndrome management is also etiology-specific based on biopsy, with the algorithm for adult minimal change disease centered on high-dose corticosteroids, while algorithms for focal segmental glomerulosclerosis or membranous nephropathy involve more complex immunosuppressive regimens.

Keywords: *Chronic Kidney Disease, Acute Kidney Injury, Glomerulonephritis, Nephrotic Syndrome, KDIGO, RAS Blockade*

Learning Objectives

After completion of the chapter, the learners should be able to:

- Define the stages of Chronic Kidney Disease (CKD) based on GFR and albuminuria.
- Explain the management algorithm for life-threatening hyperkalemia in a patient with Acute Kidney Injury (AKI).
- Apply the KDIGO guideline algorithm for managing blood pressure and proteinuria in a patient with diabetic nephropathy.
- Differentiate the diagnostic and therapeutic algorithms for pre-renal, intra-renal, and post-renal AKI.
- Justify the use of immunosuppressive therapy in the algorithm for a patient with biopsy-proven, new-onset nephrotic syndrome

CHRONIC KIDNEY DISEASE

Chronic Kidney Disease (CKD) is defined as abnormalities of kidney structure or function, present for more than 3 months, with implications for health. The management algorithm is a long-term strategy focused on staging, slowing progression, and managing systemic complications.

Pathophysiology

The pathophysiology is a final common pathway resulting from numerous primary insults, such as diabetes mellitus and hypertension. The initial insult (e.g., hyperglycemic damage to the glomerulus) leads to the loss of functional nephrons. In response, the remaining, viable nephrons undergo **adaptive hyperfiltration** to maintain the overall glomerular filtration rate (GFR). This compensatory hyperfiltration, while beneficial in the short term, is the central mechanism of progressive disease. The increased intra-glomerular pressure and flow (hyperfiltration) leads to mechanical stress, podocyte injury, and glomerulosclerosis. This, in turn, causes the loss of more nephrons, creating a vicious, self-perpetuating cycle of nephron loss, adaptive hyperfiltration, and further nephron loss, leading to end-stage renal disease (ESRD).

Diagnosis and Staging

The diagnostic and staging algorithm for CKD is based on the Kidney Disease: Improving Global Outcomes (KDIGO) guidelines. This framework classifies CKD using two main parameters: the cause, the Glomerular Filtration Rate (GFR) category (G1-G5, based on eGFR), and the albuminuria category (A1-A3, based on urine albumin-to-creatinine ratio, ACR). GFR categories range from G1 (GFR ≥ 90 ml/min/1.73m^2) to G5 (GFR < 15, or End-Stage Renal Disease, ESRD). Albuminuria categories range from A1 (< 30 mg/g) to A3 (> 300 mg/g). This GFR/ACR grid forms a "heat map" that stratifies the risk for progression and mortality, thereby guiding the algorithm for monitoring frequency and therapeutic intensity.

Differential Diagnosis (Etiology)

The differential diagnosis for CKD is an investigation into its underlying cause, which is a critical part of the initial algorithm. The most common causes in Western populations are diabetic nephropathy and hypertensive nephrosclerosis. Other important etiologies include glomerulonephritis (e.g., IgA nephropathy), genetic disorders (e.g., autosomal dominant polycystic kidney disease), chronic tubulointerstitial nephritis (e.g., from drugs or autoimmune disease), and chronic obstructive uropathy.

Treatment Algorithm

The treatment algorithm for CKD is multifactorial, with the primary goal of slowing GFR decline and managing complications. The foundational algorithm for slowing progression involves:

1. **Blood Pressure Control:** Aggressive BP targets are important. Angiotensin-Converting Enzyme (ACE) inhibitors or Angiotensin II Receptor Blockers (ARBs) are first-line agents, especially in the presence of albuminuria (A2 or A3), due to their specific renal-protective, anti-proteinuric effects.
2. **Glycemic Control:** In patients with diabetes, strict glycemic control is essential. SGLT2 inhibitors (e.g.,

dapagliflozin, empagliflozin) are now a pillar of therapy for both diabetic and non-diabetic proteinuric CKD, as they have been shown to significantly slow GFR decline.

3. **Lifestyle Modification:** This includes sodium restriction (to enhance diuretic and RAS blockade efficacy), dietary protein moderation, and smoking cessation.

Table 10.1: CKD Staging and Core Management Algorithm (KDIGO)

GFR Stage	GFR (mL/min/1.73 m²)	Albuminuria (AER)	Management Goals
G1 / G2	≥ 60 (with damage)	A1 (<30) / A2 (30-300) / A3 (>300)	Diagnose/Treat underlying cause. **BP Control.** Risk reduction.
G3a / G3b	45-59 / 30-44	(as above)	All above + **SGLT2i** (if T2DM/HF/proteinuria). Monitor anemia, bone health.
G4	15-29	(as above)	All above + Prepare for Renal Replacement Therapy (RRT). Manage hyper-K, acidosis.
G5	< 15	(as above)	**Initiate RRT** (Dialysis or Transplant). Manage uremia, fluid overload.

AER = Albumin Excretion Rate (mg/day or mg/g creatinine)

A parallel algorithm involves the systematic management of CKD complications:

- **Anemia:** The algorithm is triggered when hemoglobin

levels fall. It involves first repleting iron stores (oral or IV iron) and then, if Hb remains low, initiating an erythropoiesis-stimulating agent (ESA).

- **Mineral and Bone Disorder (CKD-MBD):** This algorithm involves monitoring phosphorus, calcium, and parathyroid hormone (PTH). Treatment is stepwise, beginning with dietary phosphate restriction, followed by oral phosphate binders, and finally, the use of active vitamin D sterols (e.g., calcitriol) or calcimimetics to control secondary hyperparathyroidism.
- **Metabolic Acidosis:** If serum bicarbonate falls, the algorithm dictates initiation of oral sodium bicarbonate or sodium citrate to maintain levels within the normal range, which may slow CKD progression.
- **Renal Replacement Therapy (RRT):** For G5 CKD, the algorithm involves timely patient education on RRT modalities (hemodialysis, peritoneal dialysis, transplantation) and surgical referral for dialysis access (e.g., AV fistula) creation.

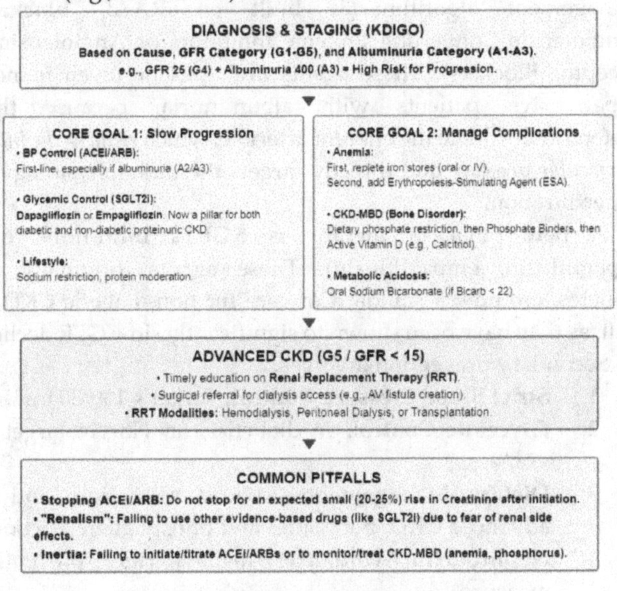

Figure 10.1: Chronic Kidney Disease

Monitoring and Follow-Up

CKD management requires lifelong, vigilant monitoring of two main parameters: GFR (estimated by serum creatinine and eGFR) and albuminuria (measured by a urine albumin-to-creatinine ratio, UACR). Patients are monitored at 3- to 6-month intervals. The goal is to slow the *rate of eGFR decline* and *reduce albuminuria*. Monitoring also includes:

1. **Blood Pressure:** This is the most critical parameter to monitor. Strict BP control is paramount.
2. **Electrolytes:** Monitoring for hyperkalemia, hyperphosphatemia, and hypocalcemia.
3. **Anemia:** A CBC is monitored to screen for anemia of CKD (due to decreased erythropoietin production by the failing kidney).
4. **Bone Health:** Monitoring PTH and phosphate levels to manage secondary hyperparathyroidism.

Long-Term Management / Secondary Prevention

The goal is to slow the progression to ESRD. The entire management algorithm is built on **RAAS blockade** (Angiotensin-Converting Enzyme inhibitors or Angiotensin II Receptor Blockers). These agents are first-line, even in non-hypertensive patients with albuminuria, because they preferentially dilate the efferent arteriole, which *reduces the intra-glomerular pressure* and directly targets the pathophysiology of hyperfiltration.

A new pillar of therapy is **SGLT2 inhibitors** (e.g., dapagliflozin, empagliflozin). These agents, originally for diabetes, are now a standard of care for non-diabetic CKD as well, as they have been shown to significantly slow GFR decline.

Secondary prevention involves:

1. **Strict Blood Pressure Control:** Target < 130/80 mmHg.
2. **Glycemic Control:** In diabetics, an HbA1c target of ~7.0%.
3. **Dietary Management:** Sodium restriction, and in advanced CKD, potassium and phosphate restriction.
4. **Nephrotoxin Avoidance:** This is a critical preventive measure.

Patient Counseling Points

1. **"This is a 'Silent' Disease":** "This is the most important thing to know. Kidney disease is silent; you will not *feel* sick until your kidney function is less than 10-15%. Our goal is to treat this disease now, while you feel well, to *prevent* you from ever feeling sick or needing dialysis."
2. **"Your Kidneys are 'Leaking' Protein":** "The main sign of kidney damage is a 'leaky filter,' which lets protein spill into your urine. Our primary goal is to stop this leak. The most important medicine for this is an 'ACE inhibitor' or 'ARB' (e.g., Lisinopril). This pill is *more* than a blood pressure pill; it is a 'kidney-protection' pill, and you must take it even if your blood pressure is normal."
3. **The "No-Fly List" for Your Kidneys:** "There are medicines that are now dangerous for you. You must *never* take NSAIDs, which are pills like Ibuprofen (Advil, Motrin) or Naproxen (Aleve). These can permanently damage your kidneys. You must use Tylenol (acetaminophen) for pain. You must also be very careful with CT scan contrast dye."
4. **Blood Pressure is Everything:** "Controlling your blood pressure is the single most important thing you can do, besides your kidney-protection pill, to slow this disease down."

Common Pitfalls in Management

A common pitfall is therapeutic inertia, particularly the failure to initiate or titrate ACE inhibitors/ARBs in patients with albuminuria. A critical error is stopping an ACE inhibitor due to a small, expected "bump" (e.g., 20-25%) in serum creatinine upon initiation; this rise reflects a beneficial change in glomerular hemodynamics and the drug should be continued. Another pitfall is "renalism," where other evidence-based therapies (e.g., for heart failure) are withheld due to fear of renal side effects. Finally, failing to monitor and treat CKD-MBD can lead to severe bone disease and cardiovascular calcification.

Case Study

A 62-year-old male (Mr. Singh) with a 10-year history of Type 2 Diabetes and Hypertension presents for a routine check-up. His BP is 145/88 mmHg. His labs show: Serum Creatinine 1.8 mg/dL (eGFR **40 mL/min/1.73m²**) and a Urine Albumin-to-Creatinine Ratio (UACR) of **350 mg/g.**

Discussion

This patient meets the criteria for **Chronic Kidney Disease (CKD).** The algorithm requires staging based on GFR and Albuminuria (KDIGO criteria).

- **G-Stage:** GFR is 40, placing him in **Stage G3b** (30-44).
- **A-Stage:** UACR is 350, placing him in **Stage A3** (>300).
- This is **CKD Stage G3bA3**, placing him at very high risk for progression. The algorithm mandates aggressive treatment to slow this progression, especially BP control and SGLT2 inhibition.

Treatment Algorithm

1. **Diagnosis:** CKD Stage G3bA3, secondary to Diabetic Nephropathy.
2. **Algorithm (BP Control):** His BP is 145/88, which is above the goal of <130/80. He is already on Lisinopril (an ACEi).
    - **Action:** Increase **Lisinopril** dose and add a diuretic.
3. **Algorithm (Progression Slowing):** He has T2DM, a GFR > 20, and a UACR > 200. The algorithm **mandates** a new pillar of therapy:
    - **Action:** Start an **SGLT2 inhibitor**, such as **Dapagliflozin 10 mg daily**, for its proven renal and cardiovascular benefits.
4. **Follow-up:** Re-check labs (K+, Creatinine) in 2 weeks. A small, expected bump in creatinine after starting an SGLT2i is acceptable.

Outcome

Mr. Singh is started on Dapagliflozin 10 mg daily and his BP regimen is intensified. The goal is to reduce his UACR and slow his GFR decline.

ACUTE KIDNEY INJURY

Acute Kidney Injury (AKI) is an abrupt decline in kidney function. Unlike the chronic management algorithm of CKD, the AKI algorithm is a rapid diagnostic pathway to identify and reverse the underlying cause.

Pathophysiology

The pathophysiology is classified by location.

- **Pre-renal AKI:** This is the most common cause and is a purely hemodynamic problem. The kidney structure is *normal*, but it is being under-perfused. This is due to true volume depletion (e.g., dehydration, hemorrhage) or a decrease in effective arterial blood volume (e.g., in heart failure or sepsis). The kidney responds appropriately by avidly conserving sodium and water (producing concentrated, low-sodium urine).
- **Post-renal AKI:** This is an obstructive problem. Kidney function is normal, but urine is blocked from being excreted, causing back-pressure that stops filtration. This is commonly due to benign prostatic hyperplasia (BPH) or a kidney stone.
- **Intrinsic AKI:** This is true kidney *damage*. The most common cause is **Acute Tubular Necrosis (ATN)**. ATN pathophysiology is ischemic or toxic damage to the renal tubular cells. In a "pre-renal" state (hypoperfusion), if the low blood flow is severe and prolonged, it converts to an "intrinsic" injury (ATN), and the tubular cells die. This "muddy brown cast" in the urine is the sloughed, dead tubular cells.

Diagnosis and Staging

AKI is diagnosed based on a rise in serum creatinine (sCr) or a fall in urine output (UOP), as defined by KDIGO. Staging (Stage 1-3) is based on the magnitude of sCr rise (e.g., Stage 1: 1.5-1.9x baseline; Stage 3: > 3.0x baseline or initiation of RRT).

Differential Diagnosis (Etiology)

The AKI treatment algorithm is fundamentally an algorithm to differentiate its three main etiological categories:

1. **Pre-renal:** Caused by renal hypoperfusion. This is the most common cause and includes hypovolemia (e.g., dehydration, hemorrhage), low cardiac output (e.g., cardiorenal syndrome), and systemic vasodilation (e.g., sepsis).
2. **Intrinsic:** Caused by direct damage to the kidney parenchyma. This is most commonly Acute Tubular Necrosis (ATN) from ischemia (e.g., prolonged pre-renal state) or nephrotoxins (e.g., contrast dye, NSAIDs, antibiotics). Other intrinsic causes include Acute Interstitial Nephritis (AIN), glomerulonephritis, and vascular causes.
3. **Post-renal:** Caused by downstream urinary tract obstruction (e.g., benign prostatic hyperplasia, kidney stones, pelvic malignancy).

Treatment Algorithm

The algorithm is a stepwise process of exclusion and intervention:

- **Step 1: Rule out Post-renal Obstruction.** The first step is a renal/bladder ultrasound. If obstruction is found (e.g., hydronephrosis), the algorithm is urinary decompression (e.g., Foley catheter, urology consultation for stents or nephrostomy tubes).
- **Step 2: Assess Volume Status.** If non-obstructive, the algorithm differentiates pre-renal from intrinsic. This involves a thorough physical exam (orthostatics, JVP, edema) and diagnostic aids (e.g., passive leg raise, ultrasound of IVC).
- **Step 3: Treat Pre-renal AKI.** If the patient is hypovolemic (pre-renal), the algorithm is immediate volume resuscitation with intravenous fluids.
- **Step 4: Treat Intrinsic AKI (ATN).** If the patient is euvolemic or hypervolemic, or does not respond to fluids, a diagnosis of intrinsic AKI (most commonly

ATN) is made. The algorithm for ATN is supportive:

- o Stop all nephrotoxic medications.
- o Dose-adjust all renally-cleared medications.
- o Manage complications: loop diuretics for volume overload, medical management for hyperkalemia (e.g., insulin/glucose, calcium gluconate), and bicarbonate for severe acidosis.

- **Step 5: Initiate RRT (Dialysis).** The algorithm dictates initiation of RRT for refractory complications, commonly remembered by the "AEIOU" mnemonic: Acidosis, Electrolyte abnormalities (especially hyperkalemia), Intoxication, Overload (volume), and Uremia (e.g., pericarditis, encephalopathy).

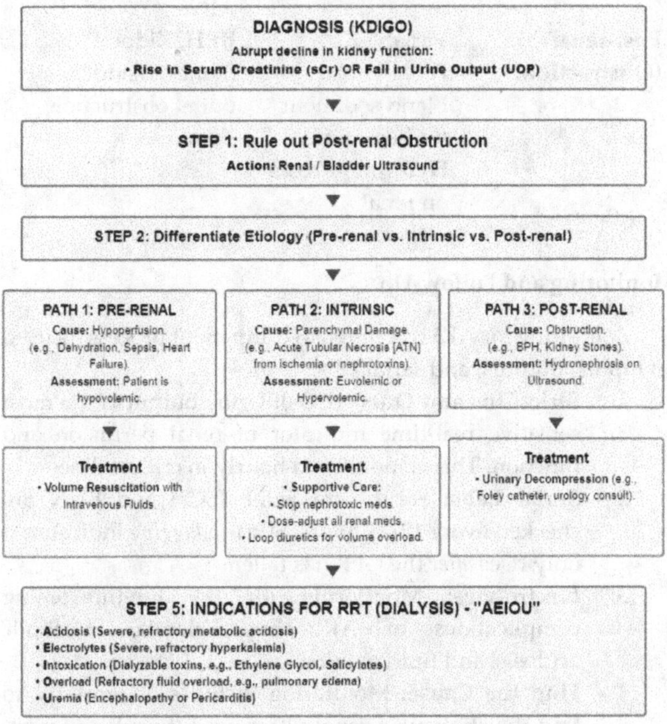

Figure 10.2: Acute Kidney Injury - Management Algorithm

Table 10.2: Diagnostic Algorithm for Acute Kidney Injury (AKI)

AKI Type	Findings (Urine)	Common Etiologies
Pre-renal (Hypoperfusion)	**FeNa < 1%, U-Na < 20.** Bland sediment. High BUN/Cr ratio (> 20:1).	**Volume Depletion** (e.g., Dehydration, Hemorrhage), Sepsis, NSAIDs, ACEi/ARBs.
Intrinsic (Renal)	**FeNa > 2%, U-Na > 40. Casts** (e.g., Muddy Brown Casts for ATN).	**Acute Tubular Necrosis (ATN)** (Ischemia or Nephrotoxin), Glomerulonephritis, AIN.
Post-renal (Obstruction)	Variable FeNa/U-Na. Bland sediment (or hematuria). **Hydronephrosis** on renal ultrasound.	**BPH,** Kidney Stones, Bladder outlet obstruction, Tumor.

Monitoring and Follow-Up

Monitoring for AKI is an intensive, inpatient process focused on inputs, outputs, and serial labs.

1. **Strict "Ins and Outs" (I/Os):** Urine output is the most sensitive real-time indicator of renal perfusion and function. This is monitored hourly in critical illness.
2. **Serial Labs:** Serum creatinine (SCr) and BUN are checked every 12-24 hours. SCr is a *lagging* indicator; it only rises *after* the GFR has fallen.
3. **Electrolytes:** Monitoring for the life-threatening complications of AKI: hyperkalemia, metabolic acidosis, and fluid overload.
4. **Find the Cause:** Monitoring includes a "workup" to find the etiology: a renal ultrasound (to rule out post-renal obstruction) and a "Fractional Excretion of Sodium" (FENa) to distinguish pre-renal (<1%) from

intrinsic-ATN (>2%).

Long-Term Management / Secondary Prevention

The long-term management of a patient who has recovered from an AKI episode is now recognized as critical. A single episode of AKI is a massive risk factor for the future development of **Chronic Kidney Disease**. Follow-up involves a nephrology clinic visit 1-3 months post-discharge to:

1. Confirm that serum creatinine has returned to its true baseline.
2. Screen for new-onset CKD (e.g., persistent albuminuria or eGFR < 60).
3. Institute secondary prevention measures, which are identical to those for CKD: aggressive BP control, RAAS blockade if albuminuric, and, most importantly, strict avoidance of nephrotoxins (NSAIDs, IV contrast).

Patient Counseling Points

1. **"Your Kidneys Took a 'Hit'"**: "Your kidneys were injured during your illness (e.g., from the infection/low blood pressure). The good news is they are recovering, but they are not as strong as they were before."
2. **"You are Now at High Risk"**: "Having an episode of acute kidney injury is like having a 'heart attack of the kidney.' It means you are now at a very high risk of developing *chronic* kidney disease in the future. We must be very aggressive in protecting them from now on."
3. **The "No-Fly List" is Now Permanent:** "You must *never* take Ibuprofen or Naproxen (NSAIDs) again. Your kidneys are too sensitive now. You must also *always* tell any doctor or nurse that you have 'had a kidney injury' *before* you get any CT scan with IV contrast dye."
4. **Stay Hydrated:** "Your kidneys are most vulnerable when you are dehydrated. You must be very careful to drink plenty of fluids, especially when you are sick with a fever, vomiting, or diarrhea."

Common Pitfalls in Management

The most common pitfall is failing to get a timely renal ultrasound to rule out a reversible post-renal cause. Another critical error is administering a large fluid bolus to a patient who is already volume-overloaded (e.g., cardiorenal syndrome), thereby worsening pulmonary edema. In ATN, a common omission is failing to review the medication list and stop all nephrotoxic agents. Finally, mistaking Acute Interstitial Nephritis (AIN)—often allergic, presenting with rash, fever, and eosinophils—for simple ATN can be a pitfall, as AIN may respond to corticosteroids.

Case Study

A 78-year-old male (Mr. Johnson) from a nursing home is brought to the ED for acute confusion and agitation. The staff notes he has not produced any urine in his catheter bag for the past 12 hours. His baseline creatinine is 1.2 mg/dL. His current creatinine is **4.9 mg/dL**.

Discussion

This is a clear case of **Acute Kidney Injury (AKI)**. The algorithm for AKI is a rapid diagnostic pathway to determine the cause: Pre-renal, Intrinsic, or Post-renal. The history of anuria (no urine) and his known history of BPH (benign prostatic hyperplasia) places **Post-renal obstruction** at the top of the differential.

Treatment Algorithm

1. **Diagnosis:** AKI (Stage 3)
2. **Algorithm Step 1 (Rule out Post-renal):** A **bedside bladder ultrasound** is performed. It shows a massively distended bladder (700 mL).
    - *Alternative:* If no bladder scanner, the algorithm would be to first **flush the Foley catheter**. It is found to be clogged with sediment.
3. **Algorithm Step 2 (Treat):** The algorithm for post-renal AKI is immediate decompression.

- **Action:** The clogged Foley catheter is removed and a new one is placed. It immediately drains **800 mL of urine**.

4. **Monitoring:** His creatinine is re-checked 6 hours later and has already dropped to 3.5 mg/dL. He is monitored for "post-obstructive diuresis."

Outcome

The patient had an **obstructive, Post-renal AKI** caused by a blocked Foley catheter. His kidney function is expected to return to baseline simply by relieving the obstruction.

GLOMERULONEPHRITIS

Glomerulonephritis (GN) is a group of diseases that cause inflammation in the glomeruli. The treatment algorithm is dictated by the clinical presentation (acuity) and the underlying etiology, which must be confirmed by serology and renal biopsy.

Pathophysiology

The pathophysiology is almost always **immune-mediated.** This can be due to:

1. **Immune Complex Deposition:** Antibodies and antigens form complexes that get "stuck" in the glomerulus, triggering an intense inflammatory response. This is the mechanism in **IgA Nephropathy** (the most common GN, where IgA complexes deposit) and **Post-Streptococcal GN** (where Strep antigens and antibodies deposit).
2. **Anti-GBM Disease:** Autoantibodies directly attack the glomerular basement membrane (GBM) itself (e.g., Goodpasture's syndrome).
3. **Pauci-Immune GN:** Inflammation is caused by ANCA (Anti-Neutrophil Cytoplasmic Antibodies) which directly activate neutrophils in the glomerular capillaries, with few or no immune deposits.

This inflammation causes a "nephritic" picture: the glomerular filter is damaged and "broken," leading to **hematuria** (red blood cell casts, "coca-cola" urine), moderate proteinuria, and acute kidney injury with hypertension.

Diagnosis and Classification

GN typically presents as a "nephritic" syndrome, characterized by hematuria (with dysmorphic red blood cells and RBC casts on urine microscopy), variable proteinuria (usually non-nephrotic), edema, hypertension, and oliguria. The most urgent classification is Rapidly Progressive Glomerulonephritis (RPGN), defined as a nephritic syndrome with a rapid decline in GFR (e.g., 50% loss in < 3 months).

Differential Diagnosis (Etiology)

The differential diagnosis is based on the "serologic footprint" and confirmed by biopsy findings (immunofluorescence and light microscopy).

1. **Anti-GBM Disease (Goodpasture's):** Positive anti-GBM antibodies. Biopsy shows linear IgG staining.
2. **Pauci-Immune GN (ANCA-associated vasculitis):** Positive ANCA (c-ANCA/PR3 or p-ANCA/MPO). Biopsy shows no or minimal immune deposits ("pauci-immune") and crescent formation.
3. **Immune-Complex GN:** Positive ANA/anti-dsDNA (Lupus Nephritis), low complement (Post-infectious GN, MPGN), or normal serology (IgA Nephropathy). Biopsy shows granular immune deposits.

Treatment Algorithm

The algorithm for RPGN is a medical emergency:

- **Step 1 (High Suspicion):** If a patient presents with AKI and a nephritic urine sediment (RBC casts), immediately send broad serologies (ANCA, anti-GBM, ANA, complement).
- **Step 2 (Emergent Immunosuppression):** Do not wait for serology results or biopsy if clinical suspicion for RPGN is high. The algorithm dictates immediate initiation of high-dose, pulse-dose intravenous steroids (e.g., methylprednisolone 500-1000mg for 3 days).
- **Step 3 (Induction Therapy):** Concurrently, initiate a

second agent. The choice is typically between Rituximab (now often preferred) or Cyclophosphamide (oral or IV).

- **Step 4 (Plasmapheresis):** If anti-GBM disease is confirmed or suspected, or in cases of severe ANCA vasculitis with pulmonary hemorrhage, the algorithm requires the immediate addition of plasmapheresis.
- **Step 5 (Biopsy):** A renal biopsy should be obtained emergently to confirm the diagnosis and guide long-term therapy, but treatment should not be delayed to obtain it.

For less aggressive GN (e.g., mild IgA nephropathy), the algorithm is non-emergent, focusing on supportive care with ACE inhibitors/ARBs to control proteinuria and blood pressure.

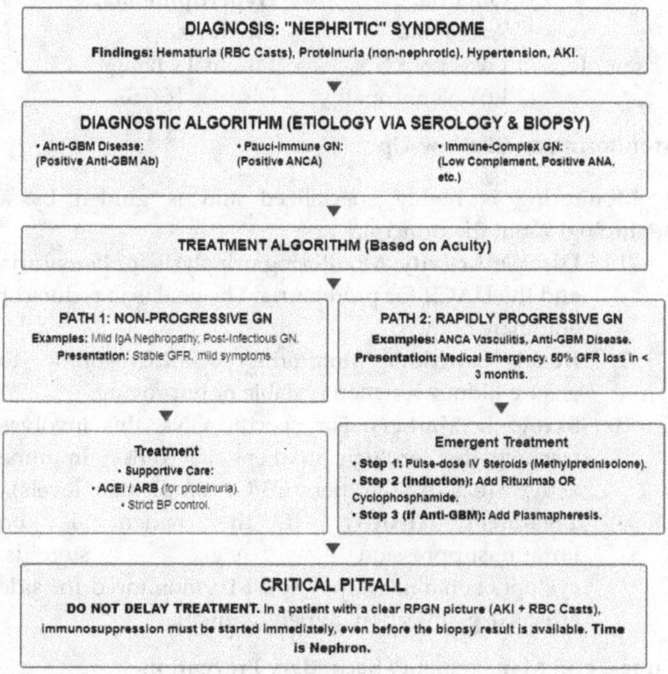

Figure 10.3: Glomerulonephritis - Management Algorithm

Table 10.3: Differentiating Nephritic vs. Nephrotic Syndromes

Feature	Nephritic Syndrome	Nephrotic Syndrome
Pathology	**Inflammatory** process (Glomerulitis).	**Damage** to podocytes / glomerular basement membrane.
Proteinuria	Mild-Moderate (< 3.5 g/day).	**Heavy** (> 3.5 g/day).
Hematuria	**Yes** (dysmorphic RBCs, RBC casts).	No (or microscopic).
Signs	**Hypertension,** Oliguria, Azotemia.	**Edema** (anasarca), **Hyperlipidemia,** Lipiduria.
Example	Post-Strep GN, IgA Nephropathy.	Minimal Change Disease, FSGS.

Monitoring and Follow-Up

Monitoring is highly specialized and is guided by a nephrologist, but the principles are:

1. **Disease Activity:** Monitoring urinalysis for hematuria and the UACR for proteinuria. The goal is to reduce or eliminate both.
2. **Renal Function:** Monitoring eGFR/Creatinine to ensure kidney function is stable or improving.
3. **Serologic Markers:** For specific GNs, this involves tracking the serologic markers that reflect immune activity (e.g., ANCA titers, C3/C4 complement levels).
4. **Treatment Toxicity:** If the patient is on immunosuppression (e.g., steroids, cyclophosphamide), they must be monitored for side effects (e.g., infection, hyperglycemia).

Long-Term Management / Secondary Prevention

Management is etiology-specific. For a self-limited process like Post-Streptococcal GN, management is purely supportive (BP control, diuretics). For chronic GNs like IgA Nephropathy, the algorithm is focused on **slowing progression**. This involves RAAS blockade (ACEi/ARB) to reduce proteinuria and strict BP control. For aggressive, rapidly-progressing GNs (like ANCA vasculitis), the algorithm is **aggressive immunosuppression** with high-dose corticosteroids and cyclophosphamide or rituximab to "shut down" the immune system.

Patient Counseling Points

1. **"Your Immune System is Attacking Your Kidney Filter":** "You have a condition where your own immune system is causing inflammation in your kidney's filters. This is why you are seeing blood in your urine and your blood pressure is high."
2. **"We Have Two Goals":** "Our first goal is to 'cool down' this inflammation, often with strong medicines that suppress your immune system, like prednisone. Our second goal, which is for the rest of your life, is to protect your kidneys from the long-term damage. We do this with a 'kidney-protection' (ACEi/ARB) pill."
3. **Sodium and Blood Pressure:** "Because your kidney filter is inflamed, it cannot handle salt. You must be on a strict low-salt diet. This, combined with your blood pressure medicine, is the most important thing you can do to protect your kidneys."
4. **Infection Risk (if on immunosuppression):** "This medicine (e.g., prednisone) weakens your immune system. You must be very careful to avoid sick people, wash your hands, and call us *immediately* if you develop a fever."

Common Pitfalls in Management

The single most critical pitfall is **delaying treatment**. Waiting for a definitive renal biopsy result before starting immunosuppression in a patient with a clear RPGN picture can lead to irreversible GFR loss and dialysis-dependence. Another pitfall is missing the "pulmonary-renal syndrome" (hemoptysis + hematuria) as a red-flag sign of anti-GBM disease or ANCA vasculitis. Finally, dismissing hematuria as being from a simple UTI without performing urine microscopy for dysmorphic RBCs or casts is a common diagnostic error.

Case Study

A 28-year-old male (Mr. Chen) presents to the ED with a 3-day history of "smoky, Coca-Cola-colored urine" (hematuria) and significant swelling around his eyes and in his legs. His BP is 170/100 mmHg. His urinalysis shows **3+ blood, 2+ protein, and RBC casts.**

Discussion

This is the classic **"Nephritic" Syndrome**. The presence of **RBC casts** is pathognomonic (confirmatory) for **Glomerulonephritis (GN)**. The acute onset, hypertension, and AKI (his creatinine is 2.5 mg/dL) suggest a **Rapidly Progressive Glomerulonephritis (RPGN)**, which is a medical emergency.

Treatment Algorithm

1. **Diagnosis:** Acute Nephritic Syndrome, highly concerning for RPGN.
2. **Algorithm Step 1 (Emergent Labs):** Immediately send serologies: **ANCA**, **anti-GBM**, C3/C4, ANA.
3. **Algorithm Step 2 (Emergent Treatment):** Do *not* wait for lab results. The algorithm for suspected RPGN is to start immediate, high-dose immunosuppression to save the kidneys.
   - **Therapy:** Start **IV Methylprednisolone (Solu-Medrol) 1000 mg daily** for 3 days.
4. **Algorithm Step 3 (Induction):** Plan to add a second agent.
   - **Therapy:** Prepare to start **Cyclophosphamide** or **Rituximab** (pending serology results).
5. **Algorithm Step 4 (Definitive Dx):** Schedule an **emergent renal biopsy** to confirm the exact etiology (e.g., ANCA vasculitis, Anti-GBM disease, or Lupus Nephritis).

Outcome

Mr. Chen is admitted and started on pulse-dose steroids. His ANCA serology comes back positive (p-ANCA/MPO), and the biopsy confirms pauci-immune crescentic GN. He is started on a Rituximab induction regimen.

NEPHROTIC SYNDROME

Nephrotic syndrome is a clinical syndrome defined by a specific tetrad of findings. The treatment algorithm is focused on managing the complications of the syndrome and treating the specific underlying glomerular disease.

Pathophysiology

Nephrotic Syndrome is characterized by a classic tetrad: **heavy proteinuria** (>3.5 g/day), **hypoalbuminemia** (low albumin in the blood), **edema** (anasarca), and **hyperlipidemia**. The pathophysiology is a profound derangement of the glomerular filtration barrier, specifically **injury to the podocytes** (the cells that wrap the filter). This injury causes the podocyte "foot processes" to be effaced (flattened), leading to a massive, non-inflammatory "leak" of protein (mostly albumin) into the urine. This is different from the "inflammatory" leak in nephritis.

The loss of albumin in the urine (hypoalbuminemia) lowers the plasma oncotic pressure, causing fluid to shift from the blood vessels into the tissues, leading to massive edema. The liver, in a non-specific attempt to compensate for the low albumin, ramps up production of *all* proteins, including lipoproteins, leading to hyperlipidemia.

Diagnosis and Classification

Diagnosis is clinical, based on the presence of the tetrad:

1. Heavy proteinuria (e.g., > 3.5 grams per day or urine protein:creatinine ratio > 3500 mg/g)
2. Hypoalbuminemia (serum albumin < 3.0 g/dL)
3. Peripheral edema
4. Hyperlipidemia

Differential Diagnosis (Etiology)

In adults, new-onset nephrotic syndrome mandates a renal biopsy to determine the etiology. The differential diagnosis includes:

- **Minimal Change Disease (MCD):** Most common cause in children, but accounts for ~15-20% of adult cases.
- **Focal Segmental Glomerulosclerosis (FSGS):** Can be primary (idiopathic) or secondary (e.g., from obesity, HIV, or prior kidney injury).
- **Membranous Nephropathy (MN):** Often primary (idiopathic, associated with anti-PLA2R antibodies) or secondary to malignancy, infections (HBV), or lupus.
- **Other Causes:** Diabetic nephropathy is the most common overall cause of proteinuria, but may not always present as a full nephrotic syndrome. Amyloidosis is a critical "cannot-miss" diagnosis.

Treatment Algorithm

The algorithm is two-pronged: general supportive care and disease-specific therapy.

General Supportive Algorithm (for all etiologies):

- **Edema:** Loop diuretics (often requiring high doses or combinations) and sodium restriction.
- **Hyperlipidemia:** High-intensity statin therapy.
- **Thrombosis Risk:** Prophylactic anticoagulation is initiated based on an algorithm considering serum albumin (e.g., strongly consider if albumin < 2.5 g/dL) and other risk factors, due to the high risk of renal vein thrombosis and other VTE.
- **Proteinuria:** ACE inhibitors or ARBs are used to reduce proteinuria.

Disease-Specific Algorithm (based on biopsy):

- **Minimal Change Disease (MCD):** The first-line algorithm is high-dose oral corticosteroids (e.g., prednisone 1mg/kg/day) for an extended period (e.g., 8-16 weeks) followed by a slow taper.
- **Focal Segmental Glomerulosclerosis (FSGS):** The algorithm also often starts with high-dose steroids, but resistance is common. Calcineurin inhibitors (e.g., tacrolimus) or rituximab may be required.
- **Primary Membranous Nephropathy (MN):** The

algorithm is risk-stratified based on GFR, anti-PLA2R antibody levels, and degree of proteinuria. Low-risk patients may be monitored with supportive care alone. High-risk patients are treated with immunosuppression, with Rituximab now considered a first-line agent.

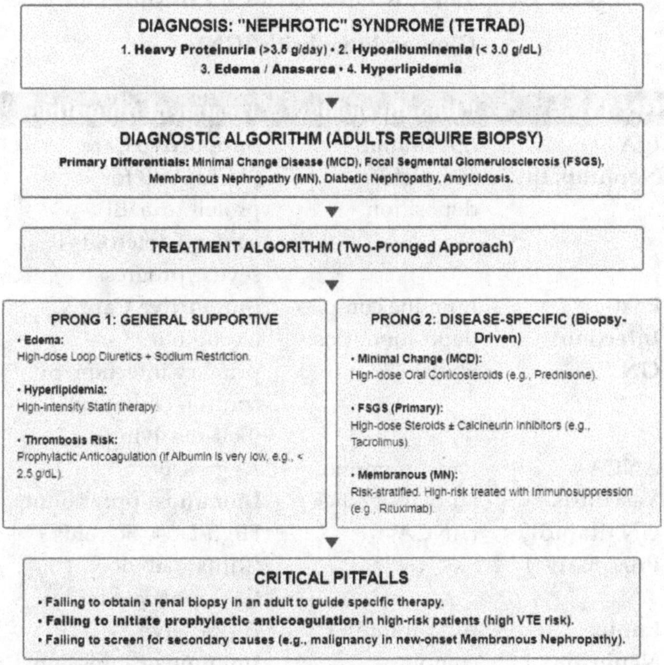

Figure 10.4: Nephrotic Syndrome - Management Algorithm

Monitoring and Follow-Up

Monitoring is focused on tracking the *amount of proteinuria* and the *complications* of the syndrome.

1. **Proteinuria:** This is the primary marker of disease activity and response to treatment. It is monitored with serial UACR or 24-hour urine protein collections. The goal is "remission" (proteinuria < 300 mg/day).
2. **Fluid Status:** Daily weights are the best way to monitor

fluid status. The patient is monitored for peripheral and pulmonary edema.

3. **Complications:** The patient is at high risk for **thrombosis (clots)** because they are also "leaking" their natural anticoagulant proteins (like Antithrombin III) into the urine. They must be monitored for DVT/PE.

Table 10.4: Simplified Management Principles for Glomerulonephritis (GN)

GN Type	Pathophysiology	Treatment Algorithm
IgA Nephropathy	IgA immune complex deposition.	**Supportive Care** (ACEi/ARB for proteinuria, BP control). (Steroids if severe/progressive).
Post-Infectious GN	Immune complex deposition (post-Strep).	**Supportive Care** (Antibiotics for primary infection, BP control, Diuretics). (Self-resolving).
ANCA-Vasculitis GN (Rapidly Progressive)	Pauci-immune, auto-antibodies (ANCA).	**Aggressive Immunosuppression:** High-Dose Steroids + (Rituximab or Cyclophosphamide).
Lupus Nephritis (SLE)	Auto-immune complex deposition.	**Aggressive Immunosuppression:** Steroids + (Mycophenolate Mofetil or Cyclophosphamide).

Long-Term Management / Secondary Prevention

The management algorithm is etiology-specific, based on the findings of a renal biopsy.

- **Minimal Change Disease (common in children):** The pathophysiology is podocyte damage from a presumed T-cell dysfunction. It is highly responsive to

corticosteroids, which are the first-line treatment.

- **Focal Segmental Glomerulosclerosis (FSGS):** This is a pattern of scarring. The algorithm is more complex, involving RAAS blockade and often prolonged immunosuppression (e.g., steroids, calcineurin inhibitors).
- **Diabetic Nephropathy:** This is the most common cause of nephrotic syndrome in adults. The algorithm is *not* immunosuppression, but the CKD algorithm: strict RAAS blockade, strict BP control, strict glucose control, and SGLT2 inhibitors.

Patient Counseling Points

1. **"Your Kidney Filter is 'Leaky,' Not 'Inflamed'":** "This is a different kind of kidney problem. Your filter isn't inflamed; it's just 'leaky,' allowing massive amounts of protein (albumin) to spill out of your blood and into your urine."
2. **"Salt and Water are Your Enemy":** "Because you have lost the protein that holds fluid in your blood, your body is like a 'water-logged' sponge. The most important thing you can do is to be on a *very strict* low-salt diet (< 2 grams/day) and take your 'water pills' (diuretics) to get rid of the dangerous extra fluid."
3. **"This is a 'Clotty' State":** "This is a critical risk. When you leak protein, you also leak out your body's *natural blood thinners*. This means your blood is 'sticky' and you are at a very high risk for developing a blood clot in your legs or lungs. You must tell us if you have any new leg swelling or sudden chest pain."
4. **"We Must Find the Cause":** "Our treatment depends on *why* your filter is leaky. For some causes, we use 'steroids' to fix it. For other causes (like diabetes), we use 'kidney-protection' pills."

Common Pitfalls in Management

A major pitfall is failing to obtain a renal biopsy in an adult with new-onset nephrotic syndrome, and incorrectly assuming the etiology. A critical safety pitfall is forgetting to initiate prophylactic anticoagulation in high-risk patients (e.g., severe hypoalbuminemia), leading to preventable VTE. Another common error is under-dosing diuretics; patients are often intravascularly volume-depleted but extravascularly overloaded, and diuretics must be used aggressively but cautiously. Finally, in MN, failing to screen for secondary causes (especially malignancy in older adults) is a significant omission.

Case Study

A 42-year-old female (Ms. Davis) presents with a 2-week history of profound, generalized swelling. Her legs are "like water balloons" (anasarca), her face is puffy, and her abdomen is distended. Her labs show: 24-hour urine protein **10.2 grams/day** (massive proteinuria), Serum Albumin **1.8 g/dL** (low), and high cholesterol.

Discussion

This is the classic, severe presentation of **Nephrotic Syndrome** (heavy proteinuria, hypoalbuminemia, edema, hyperlipidemia). The algorithm in an adult is two-pronged: 1) Manage the severe complications. 2) Biopsy to find the cause and provide specific treatment.

Treatment Algorithm

1. **Diagnosis:** Nephrotic Syndrome.
2. **Algorithm (Part 1: Manage Complications):**
    - **Edema:** Start aggressive **IV Furosemide (Lasix)** to remove fluid.
    - **Thrombosis Risk:** Her albumin is 1.8 g/dL (critically low, < 2.5). The algorithm *mandates* starting prophylactic **anticoagulation (e.g., Enoxaparin)**, as she is at extremely high risk for blood clots (e.g., DVT, PE).
    - **Lipids:** Start a **high-intensity statin (e.g., Atorvastatin 40 mg)**.
3. **Algorithm (Part 2: Find Cause):**
    - **Action:** A **renal biopsy** is performed.
    - **Result:** The biopsy shows **Minimal Change Disease (MCD)**.

4. **Algorithm (Part 3: Disease-Specific):** The first-line treatment for adult MCD is:
    - **Therapy:** Start **high-dose oral Prednisone 1 mg/kg/day**.

Outcome

Ms. Davis is admitted, diuresed with IV Lasix, started on Enoxaparin for clot prevention, and initiated on high-dose prednisone. She is expected to go into a full remission within several weeks.

Summary

Chronic Kidney Disease (CKD): The algorithm is a chronic, staged (by GFR/albuminuria) pathway. It focuses on slowing progression with RAS blockade and SGLT2 inhibitors, and systematically managing complications like anemia, acidosis, and MBD.

Acute Kidney Injury (AKI): The algorithm is a rapid diagnostic pathway to determine etiology. It follows a stepwise approach: 1. Rule out post-renal (ultrasound), 2. Assess volume (differentiate pre-renal from intrinsic), 3. Treat (fluids for pre-renal, supportive care for intrinsic).

Glomerulonephritis (GN): This algorithm is triggered by a "nephritic" picture (hematuria, RBC casts). Rapidly Progressive GN (RPGN) is a medical emergency requiring an algorithm of immediate pulse-dose steroids and cyclophosphamide/rituximab, often before a definitive biopsy.

Nephrotic Syndrome (NS): This algorithm is triggered by the "nephrotic" tetrad (heavy proteinuria, hypoalbuminemia, edema, hyperlipidemia). In adults, it requires a biopsy. The algorithm is two-pronged: 1. General management (diuretics, statins, anticoagulation), 2. Etiology-specific immunosuppression (e.g., steroids for MCD, rituximab for MN).

Multiple Choice Questions

1. According to the KDIGO staging algorithm, a patient with a GFR of 25 ml/min/1.73m^2 and an ACR of 400 mg/g is classified as:
   A) G3a A2
   B) G3b A3
   C) G4 A3
   D) G5 A1
2. A 58-year-old male with Type 2 Diabetes and CKD (G3a A3) has a BP of 145/90 mmHg. Which medication provides both antihypertensive and specific anti-proteinuric benefits?
   A) Losartan
   B) Amlodipine
   C) Hydrochlorothiazide
   D) Metoprolol
3. A 70-year-old male with BPH presents with anuria and a serum creatinine of 5.2 mg/dL. A bladder ultrasound shows 600 mL post-void residual. What is the immediate next step?
   A) Administer a 1L normal saline bolus.
   B) Insert a Foley catheter.
   C) Administer IV furosemide.
   D) Order an ANCA and anti-GBM serology.
4. A patient in the ICU develops AKI after a prolonged hypotensive episode. Urine microscopy shows muddy brown casts. What is the treatment algorithm?
   A) Fluid resuscitation and IV antibiotics
   B) Supportive care and avoidance of nephrotoxins
   C) High-dose oral corticosteroids
   D) Emergent plasmapheresis
5. Which of the following is not one of the "AEIOU" indications for emergent dialysis in AKI?
   A) Refractory hyperkalemia
   B) Uremic pericarditis
   C) Severe metabolic acidosis

D) Asymptomatic hypoalbuminemia

6. A patient presents with AKI, hematuria, and a positive p-ANCA test. Biopsy confirms pauci-immune crescentic GN. What is the first-line induction algorithm?
   A) High-dose oral prednisone alone
   B) Pulse-dose steroids plus rituximab or cyclophosphamide
   C) Plasmapheresis and IVIG
   D) Lisinopril and supportive care
7. A 40-year-old adult presents with new-onset nephrotic syndrome. A biopsy confirms Minimal Change Disease. What is the first-line treatment?
   A) High-dose oral corticosteroids
   B) Rituximab
   C) Cyclosporine
   D) Supportive care and observation
8. A patient with nephrotic syndrome and a serum albumin of 2.1 g/dL is at highest risk for which complication, which may require a prophylactic algorithm?
   A) Venous thromboembolism (VTE)
   B) Spontaneous bacterial peritonitis
   C) Severe hyperkalemia
   D) Hypoglycemia
9. A patient with known CKD (G4) is started on an ACE inhibitor. The creatinine rises from 2.5 to 3.0 mg/dL (a 20% increase) within one week. What is the most appropriate action?
   A) Stop the ACE inhibitor immediately due to AKI.
   B) Continue the ACE inhibitor and re-check labs in 1-2 weeks.
   C) Add an ARB for dual-RAS blockade.
   D) Send the patient for a renal ultrasound to rule out obstruction.

10. A 65-year-old male presents with nephrotic syndrome. Biopsy shows membranous nephropathy, and serology is positive for anti-PLA2R antibodies. What other screening is a mandatory part of the algorithm?
    A) Age-appropriate malignancy screening
    B) HIV and Hepatitis C testing
    C) Genetic testing for FSGS
    D) Echocardiogram for Fabry disease

Self-Assessment Questions

1. What are the two main parameters used for the KDIGO staging of CKD, and what are the GFR/ACR values for the highest-risk category?
2. Outline the pharmacological algorithm for slowing CKD progression in a patient with Type 2 Diabetes and albuminuria.
3. Describe the stepwise diagnostic algorithm for a patient presenting with new-onset AKI.
4. What are the "AEIOU" indications for initiating renal replacement therapy in severe AKI?
5. What clinical and laboratory findings differentiate a "nephritic" syndrome from a "nephrotic" syndrome?
6. A patient presents with AKI, hemoptysis, and RBC casts. What is the differential diagnosis, and what is the emergent treatment algorithm?
7. What is the rationale for using plasmapheresis in Anti-GBM disease but not typically in pauci-immune GN (unless severe)?
8. What are the three components of the general supportive treatment algorithm for all patients with nephrotic syndrome?
9. Compare the first-line disease-specific treatment algorithm for adult Minimal Change Disease vs. high-risk primary Membranous Nephropathy.
10. What is the most critical pitfall related to "timing" in the management of RPGN, and what is the most critical pitfall related to "medication omission" in high-risk nephrotic syndrome?

Bibliography

1. Kidney Disease: Improving Global Outcomes (KDIGO) CKD Work Group. KDIGO 2012 clinical practice guideline for the evaluation and management of chronic kidney disease. Kidney Int Suppl. 2013;3(1):1–150.
2. Kidney Disease: Improving Global Outcomes (KDIGO) AKI Work Group. KDIGO clinical practice guideline for acute kidney injury. Kidney Int Suppl. 2012;2(1):1–138.
3. Kidney Disease: Improving Global Outcomes (KDIGO) Glomerulonephritis (GN) Work Group. KDIGO clinical practice guideline for glomerulonephritis. Kidney Int Suppl. 2012;2(2):139–274.
4. Wanner C, Inzucchi SE, Lachin JM, Fitchett D, von Eynatten M, Mattheus M, et al. Empagliflozin and Progression of Kidney Disease in Type 2 Diabetes. N Engl J Med. 2016 Jul 28;375(4):323–34.
5. The EMPA-KIDNEY Collaborative Group. Empagliflozin in Patients with Chronic Kidney Disease. N Engl J Med. 2023 Jan 5;388(2):117–27.
6. Kidney Disease: Improving Global Outcomes (KDIGO) CKD-MBD Work Group. KDIGO 2017 clinical practice guideline update for the diagnosis, evaluation, prevention, and treatment of Chronic Kidney Disease–Mineral and Bone Disorder (CKD-MBD). Kidney Int Suppl. 2017;7(1):1–59.
7. Kidney Disease: Improving Global Outcomes (KDIGO) Anemia Work Group. KDIGO clinical practice guideline for anemia in chronic kidney disease. Kidney Int Suppl. 2012;2(4):279–335.
8. Lameire N, Bagga A, Cruz D, De Maeseneer J, Endre Z, Kellum JA, et al. Acute kidney injury: an increasing global concern. Lancet. 2013 Jul 13;382(9887):170–9.
9. Walsh M, Merkel PA, Peh CA, Szpirt W, Puéchal X, Fujimoto S, et al. Plasma Exchange and Glucocorticoids in Severe ANCA-Associated Vasculitis. N Engl J Med. 2020 Feb 13;382(7):622–31.
10. Hogan JJ, Mocanu M, Berns JS. The medical evaluation and management of the adult with minimal change disease. Clin J Am Soc Nephrol. 2016 Mar 7;11(3):525–35.
11. Fervenza FC, Appel GB, Barbour SJ, Rovin BH, Lafayette RA, Aslam N, et al. Rituximab or Cyclosporine in the Treatment of Membranous Nephropathy. N Engl J Med. 2019 Jul 4;381(1):36–46.
12. Ponticelli C, Glassock RJ. Glomerulonephritis: treatment of membranous nephropathy in the 21st century. J Nephrol. 2019 Oct;32(5):705–14.
13. Rovin BH, Caster DJ, Cattran DC, Gibson KL, Hogan JJ, Moeller MJ, et al. Management and treatment of glomerular diseases (part 1): conclusions from a Kidney Disease: Improving Global Outcomes (KDIGO) Controversies Conference. Kidney Int. 2019 Jan;95(1):37–47.
14. Llach F. Thromboembolic complications in nephrotic syndrome. Kidney Int. 1985 Dec;28(6):835–42.

CHAPTER 11

TREATMENT ALGORITHMS FOR DERMATOLOGIC CONDITIONS

Author

Mrs. Udaya Kumari Tula, Research Associate Scientist, DSK Biopharma Inc. Pharmaceutical Company, Morrisville, North Carolina, USA

Abstract

Dermatologic treatment algorithms are organized by etiology and clinical morphology. The algorithm for common skin infections is etiology-specific. Bacterial infections like cellulitis are treated with systemic antibiotics targeting Gram-positives, whereas superficial impetigo responds to topical mupirocin. Fungal infections (tineas) are managed with an algorithm progressing from topical azoles or terbinafine to oral terbinafine or fluconazole for extensive disease or onychomycosis. Viral infections like HSV require episodic or suppressive oral antivirals (e.g., valacyclovir). Autoimmune skin disorder algorithms aim for inflammation control. Plaque psoriasis follows a stepwise algorithm from high-potency topical corticosteroids and vitamin D analogs, to phototherapy, and finally to systemic agents or biologics for moderate-to-severe disease. Bullous pemphigoid management prioritizes high-potency topical or systemic corticosteroids. Dermatitis algorithms are centered on barrier repair and inflammation suppression. Atopic dermatitis is managed with a foundational algorithm of emollients, followed by topical corticosteroids or calcineurin inhibitors. Skin cancer algorithms are dictated by tumor type and risk. Basal cell and squamous cell carcinomas are treated with an algorithm based on location and risk, primarily surgical excision or Mohs micrographic surgery. Melanoma management is a stage-dependent algorithm involving wide local excision, sentinel node biopsy for staging, and systemic immunotherapy or targeted therapy for advanced, metastatic disease.

Keywords: *Dermatitis, Psoriasis, Skin Infections, Skin Cancer, Melanoma, Treatment Algorithm*

Learning Objectives

After completion of the chapter, the learners should be able to:

- Identify first-line topical treatments for psoriasis, atopic dermatitis, and acne vulgaris.
- Explain the stepwise treatment algorithm for plaque psoriasis, from topical agents to phototherapy and systemic biologics.
- Select the correct antibiotic algorithm for a patient with non-purulent cellulitis versus a purulent skin abscess.
- Differentiate the surgical and medical management algorithms for basal cell carcinoma (BCC) versus invasive cutaneous melanoma.
- Justify the choice of Mohs micrographic surgery over standard excision for a non-Dermatologic skin cancer in a high-risk area.

COMMON SKIN INFECTIONS

The management algorithms for common skin infections are stratified by the causative organism: bacterium, fungus, or virus. An accurate diagnosis based on clinical presentation and, if necessary, microscopy or culture, is the first step in the algorithm.

Pathophysiology

Cellulitis (Non-purulent)

Cellulitis is an acute, spreading infection of the dermis and subcutaneous tissues. The pathophysiology begins with a breach in the skin barrier (e.g., a fissure, insect bite, tinea pedis, or trauma). This breach allows bacteria, most commonly Group A *Streptococcus* (e.g., *S. pyogenes*) or *Staphylococcus aureus*, to bypass the epidermis and proliferate. The bacteria release toxins and enzymes (like hyaluronidase and streptokinase) that break down the extracellular matrix, allowing the infection to spread rapidly along fascial planes. The host's potent inflammatory response, characterized by vasodilation and neutrophil infiltration, is responsible for the clinical signs: intense, warm erythema, edema, and pain.

Tinea Corporis (Ringworm)

Tinea corporis is a superficial fungal infection of the glabrous (non-hairy) skin caused by dermatophytes (e.g., *Trichophyton rubrum*). The pathophysiology begins when fungal arthrospores adhere to the stratum corneum (the outermost dead layer of skin). The fungus then germinates, and its hyphae spread *radially* through the stratum corneum, digesting keratin as a food source. The fungus *only* lives in this dead keratin layer. The characteristic "ringworm" appearance (an annular plaque with central clearing and a scaling, active border) is a direct result of this growth pattern. The inflammation and scaling at the border represent the active, advancing front of the fungus, while the "central clearing" represents the area where the immune system has begun to clear the infection.

Diagnosis and Classification

- **Bacterial:** Infections like impetigo present with honey-crusted plaques. Cellulitis and erysipelas present as spreading, tender, erythematous, and edematous skin. A purulent focus (abscess or furuncle) suggests a staphylococcal, often MRSA, etiology.
- **Fungal (Dermatophytosis/Tinea):** These infections are classified by location (e.g., *tinea corporis* - body, *tinea pedis* - foot, *tinea cruris* - groin, *onychomycosis* - nail). The classic presentation is an annular (ring-shaped), scaling plaque with central clearing. Diagnosis is confirmed by KOH microscopy of skin scrapings, which reveals septate hyphae.
- **Viral:** Herpes Simplex (HSV) presents as grouped vesicles on an erythematous base, progressing to pustules and erosions. Varicella-Zoster Virus (VZV) reactivation (shingles) causes a dermatomal vesicular eruption. Human Papillomavirus (HPV) causes verrucae (warts).

Differential Diagnosis

The differential for bacterial cellulitis includes stasis dermatitis, which is often bilateral and lacks the acute, tender warmth of infection. Tinea corporis can mimic nummular eczema or psoriasis. Herpes simplex can be mistaken for bacterial impetigo or fungal infections, especially *tinea faciei*.

Treatment Algorithm

Bacterial Infections

- Impetigo: The algorithm for limited disease is topical mupirocin. For widespread infection, oral antibiotics (e.g., cephalexin) are required.
- Non-purulent Cellulitis/Erysipelas: The algorithm targets *Streptococcus*. Oral cephalexin, dicloxacillin, or clindamycin is first-line.
- Purulent Cellulitis/Abscess: This algorithm must cover MRSA. The primary treatment for an abscess is incision and drainage. Antibiotics (e.g., trimethoprim-sulfamethoxazole or doxycycline) are added based on severity.

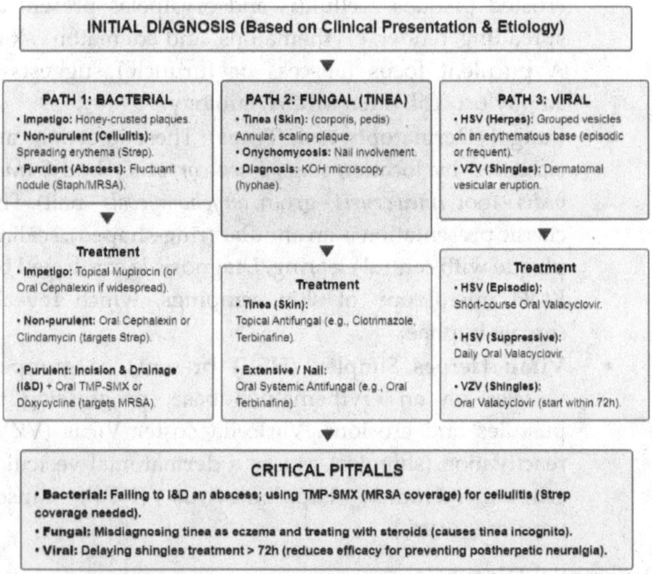

Figure 11.1: Common Skin Infections - Management Algorithm

Fungal Infections

- Tinea (Skin): The first-line algorithm for localized *tinea corporis, cruris,* or *pedis* is a topical antifungal cream (e.g., clotrimazole, ketoconazole, terbinafine) applied daily for 2-4 weeks.

- Extensive Tinea or Onychomycosis: If the infection is widespread, fails topical therapy, or involves the nails, the algorithm shifts to oral systemic therapy. Oral terbinafine is first-line for onychomycosis and most tineas.

Table 11.1: Treatment Algorithm for Common Skin Infections

Infection Type	Example(s)	Presentation	First-Line Treatment Algorithm
Bacterial	Impetigo	Honey-colored crusts.	**Topical:** Mupirocin. **Oral:** Cephalexin (if widespread).
Bacterial	Cellulitis	Spreading, warm, tender erythema.	**Oral:** Cephalexin (covers *Strep*). Add TMP-SMX (if MRSA suspected).
Fungal	Tinea Pedis / Corporis	Annular, scaling plaque, central clearing.	**Topical:** Terbinafine or Clotrimazole cream.
Viral	Herpes Zoster (Shingles)	Dermatomal, vesicular rash.	**Oral Antiviral:** Valacyclovir (start within 72h).

Viral Infections:

- HSV (Oro-labial/Genital): The algorithm is based on frequency and severity.
  - Episodic: For acute outbreaks, a short course of oral valacyclovir, acyclovir, or famciclovir is initiated

within 72 hours of onset.

- Suppressive: For patients with frequent recurrences, a lower-dose daily antiviral is used for long-term suppression.

Varicella-Zoster (Shingles)

The algorithm is oral valacyclovir or acyclovir initiated within 72 hours of rash onset to reduce the duration of rash and the risk of postherpetic neuralgia

Cellulitis

Monitoring and Follow-Up

Clinical monitoring is paramount. The aim is to **mark the borders of the erythema** with a skin marker at the time of diagnosis. This provides an objective measure of progression. The patient should show signs of clinical improvement (e.g., reduction in fever, pain, and, crucially, no further spread of the erythema) within 24-48 hours of starting effective antibiotics. Outpatients should have a follow-up check (in-person or phone) at 48 hours. Inpatients require daily monitoring of vital signs and the infection site. Failure to improve warrants investigation for a resistant organism (MRSA), a deeper infection (abscess, necrotizing fasciitis), or an incorrect diagnosis (e.g., stasis dermatitis).

Long-Term Management / Secondary Prevention

The primary long-term management is **risk factor reduction**. For patients with recurrent cellulitis, the algorithm focuses on identifying and managing the portal of entry. This includes:

1. **Treating Tinea Pedis:** This is a very common and often-overlooked entry point. All patients with cellulitis of the leg should have their feet inspected and treated for athlete's foot.
2. **Lymphedema Management:** Patients with chronic edema or lymphedema (e.g., post-surgery or due to venous insufficiency) require meticulous skin care, emollients, and often compression therapy to reduce the "culture medium" of static lymph fluid.
3. **Prophylactic Antibiotics:** For patients with 3-4

episodes per year despite other measures, low-dose daily oral penicillin or erythromycin may be considered.

Patient Counseling Points

1. **Elevation:** "The most important non-antibiotic treatment is to elevate your leg above the level of your heart. This uses gravity to help drain the swelling, which reduces pain and helps the antibiotic get to the infection."
2. **Warning Signs:** "We have marked the edge of the infection. If you see this redness spreading *past* the line, or if you develop a high fever, severe pain, or any blisters, you must come back to the emergency room immediately. This could be a sign of a more dangerous infection."
3. **Find the Cause:** "This infection got in through a small crack in your skin. We must find it. This often means treating any athlete's foot you might have between your toes, or using lotion daily to prevent dry, cracked skin."

Ring worm

Monitoring and Follow-Up

Monitoring is clinical. The goal is the resolution of erythema, scaling, and pruritus. Patients are instructed to apply topical antifungal cream (e.g., clotrimazole, terbinafine) not just to the ring, but to at least 2 cm of normal-looking skin *beyond* the active border. A common error is stopping treatment as soon as the rash looks better; treatment must be continued for 1-2 weeks *after* the rash has completely resolved to eradicate subclinical spores. Failure to improve on topical therapy warrants a re-evaluation of the diagnosis or consideration of oral antifungal therapy.

Long-Term Management / Secondary Prevention

Prevention is focused on hygiene and moisture control. This includes drying the skin thoroughly after bathing, especially in skin folds. Patients should be advised to avoid sharing towels or clothing. In athletes (e.g., wrestlers, *tinea corporis gladiatorum*), this involves showering immediately after practice and not sharing equipment. Any household pets, particularly new kittens, should be checked by a veterinarian as they can be asymptomatic carriers of dermatophytes (e.g., *Microsporum canis*).

Patient Counseling Points

1. **"This is Not a Worm":** "The name 'ringworm' is very misleading. This is not a worm; it is a common, superficial fungal infection of the skin, just like athlete's foot. It is very treatable."
2. **How to Apply Cream:** "You must apply the cream not just to the red ring, but to a border of normal skin around it. Keep applying the cream for at least one full week *after* the rash is completely gone to prevent it from coming back."
3. **Avoid Steroids:** "Do not put any steroid cream (like hydrocortisone) on this. A steroid will make the rash *look* less red, but it is 'food' for the fungus and will make the infection spread and drive deeper into the skin. This is a very common mistake."

Common Pitfalls in Management

A common pitfall is misdiagnosing tinea corporis as nummular eczema and prescribing topical steroids alone; this can worsen the infection (*tinea incognito*). In bacterial infections, a critical error is failing to cover MRSA in a purulent infection or not performing an incision and drainage on a fluctuant abscess. In shingles, delaying antiviral therapy beyond the 72-hour window significantly reduces its efficacy in preventing postherpetic neuralgia.

Case Study

A 48-year-old male with Type 2 Diabetes presents to urgent care with a 2-day history of a rapidly expanding, red, hot, and tender rash on his left lower leg. The exam shows a well-demarcated, erythematous plaque with no central purulence, fluctuance, or abscess. He has a fever of 101.1°F.

Discussion

This is the classic presentation of **non-purulent cellulitis**. The algorithm is bifurcated from purulent SSTIs (like an abscess). For non-purulent cellulitis, the primary pathogen is assumed to be *Streptococcus*, and the treatment algorithm must cover it.

Treatment Algorithm

1. **Diagnosis:** Non-purulent cellulitis (a bacterial infection).
2. **Algorithm (Non-Purulent):** The primary treatment is antibiotics. Drainage is not possible.
3. **Therapy:** The antibiotic choice must cover *Streptococcus*.
    - **Action:** Start **Cephalexin 500 mg QID for 7 days**. (Note: TMP-SMX or Doxycycline, which cover MRSA, would be *incorrect* first-line monotherapy here as they have poor *Strep* coverage).
4. **Counseling:** You draw a line around the border of the erythema and instruct the patient to elevate his leg. He is told to return immediately if the redness spreads past the line or his fever persists.

Outcome

The patient is started on Cephalexin and his symptoms begin to improve within 36 hours. You also treat his tinea pedis ("athlete's foot"), which was the likely portal of entry for the bacteria.

AUTOIMMUNE SKIN DISORDERS

Autoimmune skin disorders are chronic, inflammatory conditions where the immune system attacks components of the skin. Management algorithms are typically stepwise, aiming to control inflammation and induce remission.

Psoriasis

Pathophysiology

Psoriasis is a chronic, immune-mediated inflammatory disease with a strong genetic predisposition. The pathophysiology is a profound dysregulation of the skin's immune system, primarily driven by the **IL-23/Th17 axis**. In psoriasis, a trigger (e.g., infection, trauma) causes dendritic cells to release Interleukin-23 (IL-23). IL-23 activates T-helper 17 (Th17) cells, which in turn release a cascade of pro-inflammatory cytokines, especially **IL-17** and **TNF-α**. These cytokines signal to the keratinocytes (skin cells) to **hyperproliferate**. Normally, keratinocytes mature and shed over ~28 days. In psoriasis, this process is accelerated to ~3-5 days. This rapid turnover and incomplete maturation are what create the characteristic, thick, silvery-scaled plaque.

Diagnosis and Differential

Psoriasis, most commonly plaque psoriasis, is a chronic inflammatory disease presenting as well-demarcated, erythematous plaques with silvery scale, typically on extensor surfaces (elbows, knees), the scalp, and the lumbosacral area. Diagnosis is clinical. The differential includes seborrheic dermatitis (greasier scale, in scalp and face), nummular eczema (coin-shaped, very pruritic), and tinea corporis.

Treatment Algorithm

The psoriasis algorithm is stepwise, based on disease severity (Body Surface Area, BSA, and quality of life impact):

Mild-to-Moderate (e.g., < 10% BSA):

- **First-line:** High-potency topical corticosteroids (e.g., clobetasol) combined with topical vitamin D analogs (e.g., calcipotriene).

- o **Sensitive Areas (Face/Folds):** Lower-potency steroids or topical calcineurin inhibitors (e.g., tacrolimus).

Moderate-to-Severe (e.g., > 10% BSA or refractory):

- o **Second-line:** Phototherapy (narrowband UVB).
- o **Third-line (Systemic):** If phototherapy fails or is impractical, the algorithm moves to systemic agents. This includes oral agents (e.g., methotrexate, acitretin, apremilast) or, most effectively, biologic agents (e.g., TNF-α inhibitors, IL-17 inhibitors, IL-23 inhibitors).

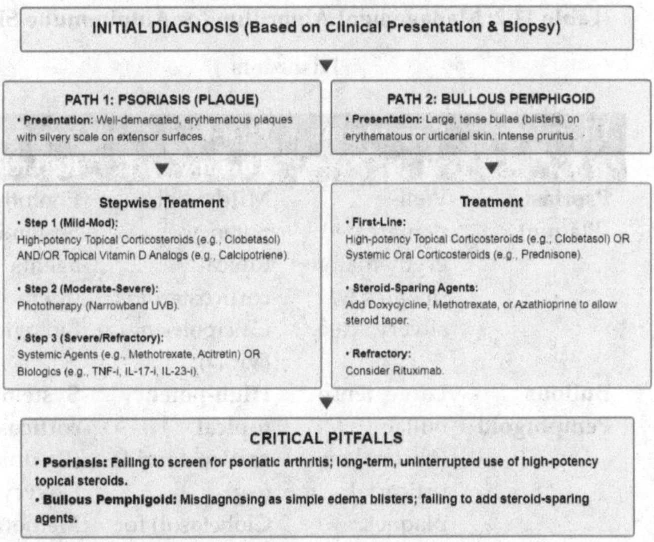

Figure 11.2: Autoimmune Skin Disorders - Management Algorithm

Monitoring and Follow-Up

Monitoring is based on disease severity and treatment type.

1. **Clinical Assessment:** The primary monitoring tool is a clinical exam to assess the Body Surface Area (BSA) involved, as well as plaque thickness, erythema, and

scale (e.g., PASI score).

2. **Comorbidity Screening:** Psoriasis is a systemic inflammatory disease. Monitoring *must* include annual screening for **psoriatic arthritis** (asking about joint pain/stiffness), **metabolic syndrome** (BP, lipids, glucose), and mental health (depression).
3. **Treatment-Specific Monitoring:** Patients on phototherapy require regular skin exams to monitor for skin cancer. Patients on systemic methotrexate require baseline and serial monitoring of LFTs and CBC. Patients on biologics require baseline and annual screening for tuberculosis.

Table 11.2: Management Algorithm for Autoimmune Skin Disorders

Disorder	Presentation	First-Line Therapy	Second-Line / Refractory
Psoriasis (Plaque)	Well-demarcated, erythematous plaques w/ silvery scale.	**Mild:** High-potency topical corticosteroids, Calcipotriene (Vit D).	Phototherapy, Systemic agents (Methotrexate, Biologics).
Bullous Pemphigoid	Large, tense bullae (blisters) on urticarial plaques. Pruritus.	**High-potency topical corticosteroids** (e.g., Clobetasol) for localized.	**Systemic corticosteroids** (Prednisone), Doxycycline, Methotrexate.

Long-Term Management / Secondary Prevention

Long-term management is focused on chronic disease control, not a cure. The goal is to minimize skin involvement and manage comorbidities. This involves a long-term, stepwise therapeutic plan, often involving rotation of therapies to minimize cumulative toxicity. Secondary prevention includes lifestyle modifications (smoking cessation, weight loss, stress reduction) which can all reduce disease severity. Patients must also be counseled to avoid known triggers, such as skin trauma (the Koebner phenomenon) and certain medications (e.g., beta-blockers, lithium) that can flare psoriasis.

Patient Counseling Points

1. **"This is an 'Inside-Out' Disease":** "Psoriasis is not just a 'skin-deep' problem. It is an autoimmune condition, meaning your immune system is overactive and is sending the wrong signals to your skin, telling it to grow too fast. Our treatments work by 'calming down' this overactive immune system."
2. **"This is a Marathon, Not a Sprint":** "This is a chronic, lifelong condition. We do not have a cure, but we have excellent, safe treatments to control it. The goal is to find a long-term plan that keeps your skin clear and is safe for you."
3. **"It's More Than Just Skin":** "Because this is a whole-body inflammatory disease, it puts you at a higher risk for other conditions like arthritis, high blood pressure, and diabetes. It is very important that you see your primary care doctor for regular check-ups to screen for these."

Common Pitfalls

A common pitfall is the long-term, uninterrupted use of high-potency topical steroids, leading to skin atrophy. Another is failing to screen psoriasis patients for comorbidities; psoriasis is a systemic disease associated with psoriatic arthritis, metabolic syndrome, and cardiovascular disease. Finally, abrupt cessation of systemic steroids can cause a severe "rebound" flare.

Bullous Pemphigoid

Pathophysiology

Bullous Pemphigoid is the most common autoimmune blistering disease. The pathophysiology is the production of **autoantibodies (IgG) against two 'hemidesmosomal' proteins**: BP180 and BP230. Hemidesmosomes are the "spot welds" that anchor the bottom layer of the epidermis (keratinocytes) to the top layer of the dermis (the basement membrane). When these autoantibodies bind, they trigger a massive inflammatory cascade, recruiting eosinophils and neutrophils. These cells release proteases that degrade the hemidesmosomes, causing the epidermis to "unzip" or separate from the dermis. This separation creates a "sub-epidermal" split, which then fills with fluid, forming the characteristic large, *tense* bullae (blisters). The bullae are tense because the "roof" of the blister is the entire, intact epidermis.

Diagnosis and Differential

Bullous Pemphigoid (BP) is an autoimmune blistering disease of the elderly. It presents as large, tense bullae (blisters) on erythematous or urticarial skin, and is intensely pruritic. Diagnosis is confirmed by skin biopsy for routine histology and direct immunofluorescence (DIF), which shows linear IgG and C3 deposits at the dermo-epidermal junction. The main differential is Pemphigus Vulgaris, which involves flaccid blisters and, crucially, oral mucosal erosions (less common in BP).

Treatment Algorithm

The algorithm aims to stop blistering and relieve pruritus.

- **First-line:** High-potency topical corticosteroids (e.g., clobetasol ointment) applied to the entire body surface is a first-line option, especially in Europe, as it has fewer systemic side effects.
- **Alternative First-line:** Systemic oral corticosteroids (e.g., prednisone 0.5-1.0 mg/kg/day) are also first-line and achieve rapid control.
- **Steroid-Sparing Agents:** To minimize long-term steroid toxicity, a steroid-sparing agent (e.g., doxycycline, methotrexate, or azathioprine) is often added to the algorithm. Refractory cases may require rituximab.

Monitoring and Follow-Up

Monitoring is focused on assessing disease activity and, just as importantly, monitoring for the severe side effects of therapy (typically high-dose steroids).

1. **Disease Activity:** The primary monitoring parameter is a **blister count**. The goal is to stop the formation of *new* blisters and relieve the intense pruritus.
2. **Steroid Side Effects:** In this elderly population, monitoring *must* include regular checks of blood glucose (for new-onset diabetes), blood pressure, and mental status. Bone protection (with calcium, Vitamin D, and often a bisphosphonate) and PJP prophylaxis (with trimethoprim-sulfamethoxazole) must be initiated with high-dose steroids.

Long-Term Management / Secondary Prevention

The goal is to induce remission (stop new blister formation) and then taper the patient off systemic steroids as quickly as possible. This is achieved by adding a **"steroid-sparing" agent** early in the treatment course. Common second-line agents include doxycycline (which has anti-inflammatory properties), methotrexate, or azathioprine. This allows for a slow taper of prednisone over many months, minimizing its long-term toxicity. The disease often "burns out" after 1-5 years, and therapies can sometimes be discontinued.

Patient Counseling Points

1. **"Your Immune System is Attacking Your Skin's 'Glue'":** "You have an autoimmune condition where your body is making antibodies that attack the 'glue' holding your top layer of skin onto the bottom layer. This is causing the layers to separate and form these large, deep blisters."
2. **"Our Goal: Stop New Blisters":** "Our first-line treatment is a strong steroid, like prednisone, to quickly 'shut down' your immune system and stop it from making these antibodies. Our first goal is to see *no new blisters* forming. This is how we know the medicine is working."
3. **"The Treatment Can Be a 'Double-Edged Sword'":** "The steroids are very effective, but they have strong side effects, especially at high doses. They can raise

your blood sugar and blood pressure, weaken your bones, and increase your risk of infection. We will be starting other medicines to protect you from these side effects, and we will add a 'steroid-sparing' medicine so we can lower the steroid dose as soon as possible."

Common Pitfalls

A pitfall is mistaking BP for simple "blisters from edema" in an elderly patient, delaying diagnosis. The most critical pitfall is managing long-term, high-dose systemic steroids without adequate prophylaxis for side effects (e.g., bone protection, PJP prophylaxis).

Case Study

A 38-year-old male (Mr. Smith) presents with a 6-month history of "stubborn, scaly patches" on his elbows, knees, and scalp. The exam reveals sharply demarcated, erythematous plaques with a thick, silvery scale. He has mild itching. His Body Surface Area (BSA) is estimated at 5%.

Discussion

This is the hallmark presentation of **Plaque Psoriasis**. The algorithm is stepwise, based on disease severity. Since his BSA is <10% and it doesn't severely impact his quality of life, this is **mild-to-moderate** disease, and the algorithm begins with topical therapy.

Treatment Algorithm

1. **Diagnosis:** Mild-to-moderate Plaque Psoriasis.
2. **Algorithm Step 1 (First-Line):**
   - **Therapy:** Start **Clobetasol 0.05% ointment** (a high-potency topical corticosteroid) to be used BID for 2 weeks *and* **Calcipotriene** (a Vitamin D analog) to be used daily as a steroid-sparing maintenance agent.
3. **Step 2 (Sensitive Areas):** For his scalp, you prescribe a **medicated shampoo (e.g., Ketoconazole 2%)** and a **topical steroid solution**.
4. **Step 3 (Systemic Screen):** Psoriasis is a systemic

inflammatory disease. You must screen him for the most common comorbidity:

- **Action:** You ask, "Do you have any joint pain, stiffness, or swelling in your fingers or back?" to screen for **Psoriatic Arthritis**.

Outcome

Mr. Smith is started on high-potency topical steroids and a Vitamin D analog. He is counseled on the inflammatory nature of his disease and the need to watch for joint symptoms.

DERMATITIS

Dermatitis, or eczema, is a pattern of skin inflammation characterized by erythema, pruritus, and scale. The algorithm varies by the specific etiology.

Atopic Dermatitis (AD)

Pathophysiology

The pathophysiology of Atopic Dermatitis (eczema) is a complex interplay between **skin barrier dysfunction** and **immune dysregulation**. Many patients with AD have a genetic mutation in the **filaggrin (FLG) gene**. Filaggrin is a protein that is crucial for forming the stratum corneum (the skin's "brick wall"). A lack of filaggrin leads to a "leaky" or defective skin barrier (the "mortar" is missing from the wall). This leaky barrier allows: 1) water to escape, leading to xerosis (dry skin), and 2) allergens and irritants to *enter* the skin. These allergens then trigger a T-helper 2 (Th2) dominant immune response (the same response seen in asthma and allergies), releasing cytokines like **IL-4** and **IL-13**. These cytokines cause inflammation (erythema) and, critically, stimulate sensory nerves, causing the intense, defining symptom of AD: **pruritus (itch)**. This leads to the "itch-scratch cycle," where itching causes scratching, which further damages the skin barrier, causing more inflammation and more itching.

Diagnosis and Differential

AD is a chronic, relapsing, highly pruritic inflammatory skin disease. The presentation is age-dependent: infants show facial/extensor involvement, while children/adults show flexural lichenification (antecubital and popliteal fossae). It is associated with a personal or family history of atopy (asthma, allergic rhinitis). The differential includes seborrheic dermatitis (in infants), scabies (intense pruritus, burrows), and allergic contact dermatitis.

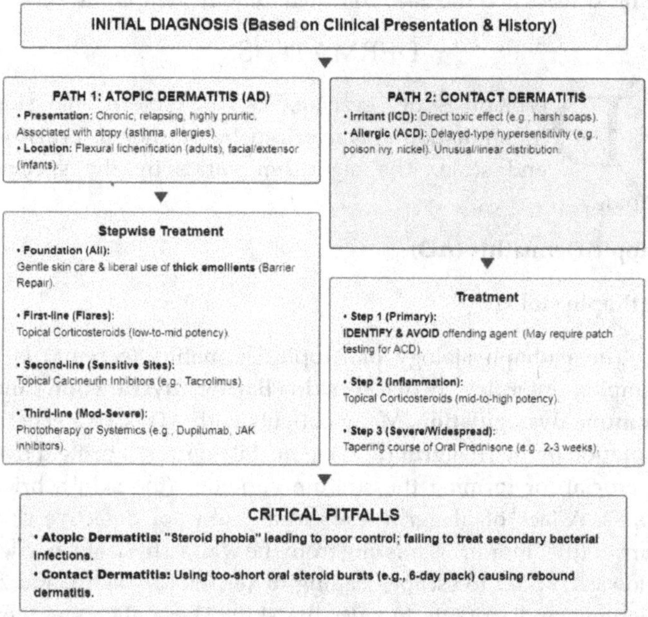

Figure 11.3: Dermatitis - Management Algorithm

Treatment Algorithm

The AD algorithm is a stepwise approach built on a foundation of barrier repair.

- **Foundation (All Patients):** Gentle skin care (e.g., lukewarm baths, mild soap) and liberal use of thick emollients/moisturizers to repair the skin barrier.
- **First-line (Mild-Moderate):** Topical corticosteroids

(low-to-mid potency) for flares.

- **Second-line (Sensitive Sites/Maintenance):** Topical calcineurin inhibitors (e.g., tacrolimus, pimecrolimus) are used, especially for the face and skin folds, to avoid steroid atrophy.
- **Third-line (Moderate-Severe):** For refractory disease, the algorithm moves to phototherapy or systemic agents, including biologics (e.g., dupilumab) or JAK inhibitors.

Table 11.3: Stepwise Algorithm for Atopic Dermatitis (Eczema)

Severity	First-Step (Foundation)	Second-Step (Pharmacological Therapy)	Third-Step (Refractory)
All	**Emollients** (thick creams/ointments), gentle cleansers, trigger avoidance.	---	---
Mild-Mod	All above.	**Topical Corticosteroids** (Low-potency). Topical Calcineurin Inhibitors (e.g., Tacrolimus).	---
Mod-Severe	All above.	**Topical Corticosteroids** (Medium-high potency).	Phototherapy, Systemics (e.g., Dupilumab, JAK-inhibitors).

Monitoring and Follow-Up

Monitoring is clinical, focused on controlling symptoms and preventing flares.

1. **Symptom Score:** Monitoring the patient's (or parent's) report of itch (e.g., on a 1-10 scale), sleep disturbance, and quality of life.
2. **Clinical Exam:** Assessing for signs of active dermatitis (erythema, scale) versus chronic changes (lichenification).
3. **Infection:** Actively monitoring for signs of secondary bacterial infection (*Staph aureus* crusting, "weeping") or viral infection (eczema herpeticum), which are common complications.

Long-Term Management / Secondary Prevention

The entire long-term management algorithm is built on **barrier repair.**

1. **Emollients:** The foundational, non-negotiable management is the daily, liberal use of thick, fragrance-free emollients (creams or ointments, not lotions) to "patch" the leaky skin barrier.
2. **Proactive Therapy:** For patients with frequent flares, the algorithm is to use a "proactive" approach: apply a topical corticosteroid or calcineurin inhibitor (TCI) to "hot spots" 2-3 times per week, *even when the skin is clear,* to prevent the flare from starting.
3. **Trigger Avoidance:** Identifying and avoiding specific triggers, such as harsh soaps, fragrances, wool clothing, or known allergens.

Patient Counseling Points

1. **"Emollients are the 'Medicine,' Steroids are the 'Rescue'":** "The most important part of your treatment is not the steroid cream; it is the *moisturizer*. Your skin has a 'leaky barrier.' The moisturizer acts like the 'mortar' to patch the 'bricks' of your skin. You must apply this *every day, all over,* even when you are not red. The steroid cream is just a 'rescue' to put out the fire

when you have a flare-up."

2. **"Soak and Seal":** "The best way to moisturize is called 'soak and seal.' After a 5-10 minute *lukewarm* (not hot) bath, pat the skin *gently* (don't rub), and then, *while the skin is still damp*, seal in the moisture by applying your thick emollient all over."
3. **"Steroid Phobia":** "I understand you are worried about using steroids. When used *correctly*—as a 'rescue' for a few days to a week on red, itchy skin—they are very safe and very effective. It is *more* harmful to let the eczema get out of control than it is to use the steroid cream properly to stop the itch-scratch cycle."

Common Pitfalls

The most common pitfall is "steroid phobia," where patients or parents under-use topical steroids, leading to poor disease control. Another error is failing to recognize and treat secondary bacterial (staph) or viral (herpes) infections (e.g., eczema herpeticum) that can complicate AD flares.

Contact Dermatitis

Diagnosis and Differential

Contact dermatitis is divided into Irritant (ICD) and Allergic (ACD). ICD is a direct toxic effect (e.g., from harsh soaps, solvents). ACD is a delayed-type hypersensitivity reaction (e.g., to poison ivy, nickel, or preservatives). The main differential is AD, but contact dermatitis often has an unusual, linear, or sharply demarcated distribution corresponding to the exposure.

Treatment Algorithm

- **Step 1: Identification and Avoidance.** The primary algorithm is identifying the causative agent and strictly avoiding it. For ACD, this may require patch testing.
- **Step 2: Inflammation Control.** For acute flares, topical corticosteroids (mid-to-high potency) are used. Severe, widespread cases (e.g., severe poison ivy) may require a 2-3 week tapering course of oral prednisone.

Common Pitfalls

A pitfall in ACD is prescribing a short "med-pack" (6-day) burst of oral steroids, which is often too short and results in rebound dermatitis. Another is failing to identify the allergen, leading to chronic, unresolved dermatitis.

Case Study

A 9-year-old boy (Leo) is brought in by his mother for a "terrible itchy rash." He has a history of asthma and seasonal allergies. On exam, you see dry, scaly, and lichenified (thickened from scratching) plaques in his antecubital fossae (elbow creases) and popliteal fossae (behind the knees).

Discussion

This is the "atopic triad" (asthma, allergies, eczema). The clinical picture—severe pruritus and a "flexural" distribution in a child—is the classic presentation of **Atopic Dermatitis (AD)**. The algorithm is built on a foundation of barrier repair.

Treatment Algorithm

1. **Diagnosis:** Atopic Dermatitis (Eczema).
2. **Algorithm Foundation (Barrier Repair):** This is the most critical part of the algorithm.
   - **Action:** You counsel the parents on "**Soak and Seal**": a 10-minute lukewarm bath, pat dry, and *immediately* apply a **thick, fragrance-free emollient** (e.g., CeraVe or Vaseline ointment) all over to "seal" in the moisture. This must be done daily.
3. **Algorithm Step 1 (Flares):** For the active, red, and itchy plaques.
   - **Therapy:** Prescribe a **medium-potency topical corticosteroid** (e.g., Triamcinolone 0.1% ointment) to be used *only* on the red patches, BID for 1-2 weeks, until the flare resolves.
4. **Counseling:** You address "steroid phobia," explaining that short-term use on active flares is safe and

necessary to break the "itch-scratch cycle."

Outcome

The parents are instructed on the foundational emollient-based algorithm and given a topical steroid for acute flares

SKIN CANCERS

Skin cancer algorithms are dictated by tumor type (melanoma vs. non-melanoma), histologic subtype, location, and patient risk factors.

Non-Melanoma Skin Cancer (BCC, SCC)

Pathophysiology

BCC is the most common cancer in humans. The pathophysiology is a direct result of **ultraviolet (UV) radiation damage** to the DNA of basal keratinocytes, the cells in the lowest layer of the epidermis. The main pathway mutated by UV light is the **Hedgehog (Hh) signaling pathway**. Normally, this pathway is "off" in adult skin. UV-induced mutations (e.g., in the *PTCH1* gene) cause the pathway to become *constitutively "on,"* leading to uncontrolled basal cell proliferation and tumor formation. BCCs are locally invasive and destructive, but have an extremely low metastatic potential, as their growth is dependent on the surrounding stroma (connective tissue).

Monitoring and Follow-Up

Monitoring after treatment is lifelong and twofold:

1. **Site Check:** Monitoring the treatment site (e.g., excision scar, radiation field) for any signs of recurrence (e.g., new papules, ulceration).
2. **Full Body Skin Exam (FBSE):** This is the most important follow-up. A patient with one BCC has a ~40-50% chance of developing a *second, new* BCC within 5 years. This is because their *entire* skin ("field cancerization") has the same UV damage. Patients require a FBSE by a dermatologist every 6-12 months for life.

Long-Term Management / Secondary Prevention

Secondary prevention is the cornerstone of long-term management.

1. **Sun Protection:** This is the most critical intervention. It includes daily use of broad-spectrum (UVA/UVB) sunscreen (SPF 30+), use of sun-protective clothing (hats, UPF shirts), and *avoidance* of peak sun hours (10 am - 4 pm).
2. **Patient Self-Exams:** Teaching the patient to perform a monthly self-skin exam to identify new or changing lesions early.
3. **Topical Chemoprevention:** For patients with extensive "field cancerization" (e.g., numerous pre-cancers), a provider may prescribe topical 5-Fluorouracil or Imiquimod to the entire area to treat subclinical lesions.

Patient Counseling Points

1. **"This is the 'Good' Skin Cancer":** "This is the most common and least dangerous type of skin cancer. It is locally destructive, like a 'termite in the wood,' so we must remove it completely. However, it almost *never* (less than 0.1%) spreads to other parts of your body. We are treating this for a 100% cure."
2. **"This is a 'Warning Shot'":** "Having this one BCC means you have had enough sun damage in your life to make a skin cancer. This puts you at a very high risk of developing *more* of them in the future. The most important thing we do today is start you on a lifelong plan of skin protection."
3. **"Sunscreen is Not Just for the Beach":** "From now on, sun protection must be a daily, non-negotiable habit. This means applying sunscreen to your face and arms every single morning, just like brushing your teeth. 80% of your sun exposure comes from 'incidental' sun, like driving in the car or walking to the mailbox."

Diagnosis and Differential

- **Basal Cell Carcinoma (BCC):** The most common skin cancer. Classically presents as a pearly, translucent papule with telangiectasias. Can also be superficial (scaly pink patch) or nodular.
- **Squamous Cell Carcinoma (SCC):** Presents as a firm, indurated, hyperkeratotic papule or plaque, often with ulceration. Actinic keratosis (AK) is a pre-cancerous lesion that can progress to SCC.
- **Differential:** The differential includes benign lesions like seborrheic keratosis, melanocytic nevus, or inflammatory lesions. Diagnosis is made by skin biopsy (shave or punch).

Treatment Algorithm

The algorithm is based on whether the lesion is low-risk or high-risk (defined by size, location, histology, and patient immune status).

- **Low-Risk BCC/SCC (e.g., small, nodular, on trunk/extremities):**
    - **Standard Excision:** Surgical removal with standard 4-5 mm margins.
    - **Electrodesiccation & Curettage (ED&C):** A common option for low-risk tumors.
    - **Topical Therapy:** For superficial BCC, topical 5-Fluorouracil or Imiquimod can be used.
- **High-Risk BCC/SCC (e.g., large, on face/hands/feet, aggressive histology):**
    - **Mohs Micrographic Surgery:** This is the first-line algorithm for high-risk tumors, as it offers the highest cure rate (by histologically clearing 100% of the margin) while sparing the most tissue.
    - **Radiation Therapy:** An option for non-surgical candidates.

Melanoma

Pathophysiology

Melanoma is a malignancy of **melanocytes**, the pigment-producing cells of the epidermis. The pathophysiology is complex, but it is also strongly linked to **UV radiation**, particularly intense, intermittent "sunburn" exposures. UV light causes DNA damage (e.g., thymidine dimers) that leads to driver mutations in pathways like the **MAPK pathway** (e.g., *BRAF* and *NRAS* mutations). Unlike BCC, which is only locally invasive, melanoma is defined by its high *metastatic potential*. The single most important prognostic factor, **Breslow depth**, is a direct measure of how *deeply* the primary tumor has invaded into the dermis. Once it invades the dermis, it gains access to lymphatics and blood vessels, allowing it to spread to lymph nodes and distant organs.

Diagnosis and Differential

Melanoma is the most dangerous skin cancer. Diagnosis is suspected based on the "ABCDE" criteria (Asymmetry, Border irregularity, Color variegation, Diameter > 6mm, Evolving). The main differential is a benign nevus, seborrheic keratosis, or pigmented BCC. The algorithm requires a full-thickness excisional biopsy for accurate diagnosis and micro-staging.

Treatment Algorithm

The melanoma algorithm is entirely stage-dependent, based on the Breslow thickness (tumor depth) from the initial biopsy.

- **Stage 0 (Melanoma in situ):** Wide local excision with 0.5-1.0 cm margins.
- **Stage I-II (Invasive, Localized):**
    - **Step 1: Wide Local Excision.** Surgical removal with 1-2 cm margins (based on Breslow depth).
    - **Step 2: Sentinel Lymph Node Biopsy (SLNB).** This staging algorithm is offered for most melanomas > 0.8 mm thick to detect microscopic nodal spread.

- **Stage III (Node-Positive):**
  - **Step 1: Complete Lymph Node Dissection** (if clinically positive) or observation (if only positive on SLNB).
  - **Step 2: Adjuvant Therapy.** This algorithm involves systemic immunotherapy (e.g., checkpoint inhibitors like nivolumab) or targeted therapy (if BRAF-mutated) to reduce recurrence risk.
- **Stage IV (Metastatic):** The algorithm is palliative-intent systemic therapy, primarily with immunotherapy (e.g., ipilimumab/nivolumab) or BRAF/MEK inhibitors for BRAF-mutated tumors.

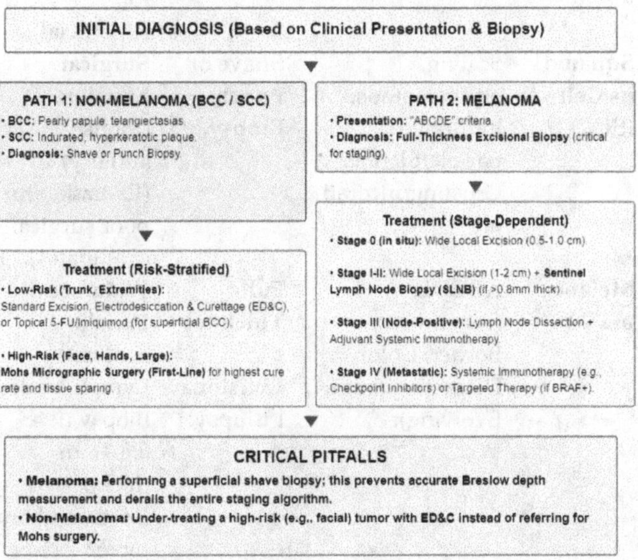

Figure 11.4: Skin Cancers - Management Algorithm

Table 11.4: Management Principles for Common Skin Cancers

Cancer Type	Presentation	Diagnostic Algorithm	Management Algorithm
Basal Cell (BCC)	Pearly papule, telangiectasias, rolled border. Slow-growing.	**Shave or Punch Biopsy.**	**Surgical Excision.** (Mohs surgery for high-risk areas). (Topical 5-FU for superficial).
Squamous Cell (SCC)	Scaling, erythematous, indurated papule/plaque. Crusting/ulceration.	**Shave or Punch Biopsy.**	**Surgical Excision.** (Mohs surgery). (Radiation for poor surgical candidates).
Melanoma	**ABCDEs** (Asymmetry, Border, Color, Diameter >6mm, Evolving).	**Full-Thickness Excisional Biopsy.**	**Wide Local Excision.** Sentinel Lymph Node Biopsy (if > 0.8-1mm thick). (Immunotherapy for metastatic).

Monitoring and Follow-Up

Follow-up for melanoma is the most intensive of all skin cancers and is dictated by the initial stage.

1. **Skin Exams:** Patients require a full-body skin exam by a dermatologist every 3-6 months for the first 2-5 years, then annually for life. They are at high risk for both a

new primary melanoma and a *local recurrence*.

2. **Lymph Node Exams:** A clinical exam of the regional lymph node basins (e.g., neck, axilla, groin) at every visit.
3. **Systemic Surveillance:** For higher-stage (Stage IIB-IV) melanoma, the algorithm includes *routine surveillance imaging* (e.g., CT or PET-CT scans every 6-12 months) to look for distant metastasis, as well as serial bloodwork (e.g., LDH).

Long-Term Management / Secondary Prevention

This is identical to BCC but even more critical: rigorous, lifelong sun protection and monthly self-skin exams. First-degree relatives (parents, siblings, children) should also be counseled to have a baseline full-body skin exam, as there is a genetic component (e.g., *CDKN2A* gene) in ~10% of cases. For patients with Stage II or III disease, **adjuvant systemic therapy** (e.g., immunotherapy with nivolumab) is now a standard part of the long-term management algorithm to reduce the risk of systemic recurrence.

Patient Counseling Points

1. **"This is the 'Serious' Skin Cancer":** "This is a melanoma, which is the most serious type of skin cancer. Unlike other skin cancers, this one has the ability to spread to other parts of the body. Our entire plan is based on the *depth* of the tumor, which we found on your biopsy."
2. **"The Staging Process":** "The first step is a 'wide excision' to remove a wider margin of skin around the biopsy site. At the same time, we will likely perform a 'sentinel lymph node biopsy.' This is a procedure to check the 'first-draining' lymph node to see if any microscopic cells have escaped. This is a *staging* procedure, not a treatment, and it gives us the critical information we need to plan your future care."
3. **"Your Life Has Changed Today":** "A diagnosis of melanoma changes your relationship with the sun, permanently. You must become a 'shade-seeker.' Sun

protection for you is not optional; it is a critical part of your cancer survivorship. You must also commit to regular follow-up with us and learn to do your own monthly skin checks."

Common Pitfalls in Management

A fatal pitfall is performing a superficial shave biopsy on a pigmented lesion suspected to be melanoma; this prevents accurate Breslow depth measurement and derails the entire staging algorithm. In non-melanoma skin cancer, a common error is under-treating a high-risk tumor (e.g., using ED&C on a facial SCC) instead of referring for Mohs surgery. Finally, failing to educate patients on rigorous sun protection and self-skin exams after a skin cancer diagnosis is a missed opportunity for secondary prevention

Case Study

A 45-year-old female (Ms. Miller) with a history of significant sun exposure presents for a skin check. She points to a dark "mole" on her back that her husband noted has been changing. On exam, you note a 7mm pigmented lesion that is **A**symmetric, has an irregular **B**order, and **C**olor variegation (black and brown). It has **E**volved per the patient.

Discussion

This lesion meets multiple "ABCDE" criteria and is highly suspicious for **Malignant Melanoma**. The diagnostic and management algorithm is critical and time-sensitive. A superficial shave biopsy is a pitfall and is contraindicated.

Treatment Algorithm

1. **Diagnosis (Suspected):** Malignant Melanoma.
2. **Algorithm Step 1 (Diagnostic Biopsy):**
    - **Action:** Perform a **full-thickness excisional biopsy** with 1-2 mm margins. This is *required* to get the **Breslow depth**.
3. **Pathology Result:** The biopsy confirms **Invasive Malignant Melanoma, Breslow depth 1.3 mm**, non-

ulcerated.

4. **Algorithm Step 2 (Staging & Treatment):** The algorithm is now dictated by the 1.3 mm depth.
   - **Action 1 (Surgery):** Refer to surgical oncology for a **Wide Local Excision (WLE)** with 1-2 cm margins.
   - **Action 2 (Staging):** Because the depth is > 1.0 mm, the algorithm mandates a **Sentinel Lymph Node Biopsy (SLNB)** to check for microscopic spread.
5. **Follow-up:** The patient will require close surveillance (e.g., full-body skin exams every 3-6 months) for life.

Outcome

Ms. Miller is immediately referred for WLE and SLNB. The results of the SLNB will determine her final stage and if she requires adjuvant immunotherapy (the next step in the Stage III algorithm).

Summary

Common Skin Infections: The algorithm is etiology-driven. Bacterial cellulitis requires oral antibiotics (e.g., cephalexin); purulent abscesses require I&D and MRSA coverage. Fungal tineas are treated topically (e.g., clotrimazole) or orally (e.g., terbinafine) for extensive disease. Viral HSV is managed with episodic or suppressive oral valacyclovir.

Autoimmune Skin Disorders: Psoriasis follows a stepwise algorithm from topicals (steroids, vitamin D analogs) to phototherapy, to systemic biologics. Bullous pemphigoid is managed with high-potency topical or systemic steroids as first-line therapy.

Dermatitis: The algorithm is built on barrier repair. Atopic dermatitis is managed with a foundation of emollients, followed by topical steroids or calcineurin inhibitors. Contact dermatitis requires identification and avoidance of the offending agent, plus topical steroids for flares.

Skin Cancers: Non-melanoma skin cancer (BCC/SCC) algorithms are risk-stratified, with Mohs surgery being the first-line choice for high-risk lesions. The melanoma algorithm is stage-dependent, requiring wide local excision, sentinel node biopsy for staging, and systemic immunotherapy or targeted therapy for advanced disease.

Multiple Choice Questions

1. A patient presents with a tender, 3cm fluctuant nodule on the thigh. Which of the following is the most appropriate first-line algorithm?
   A) Topical mupirocin
   B) Oral cephalexin
   C) Incision and drainage, plus oral trimethoprim-sulfamethoxazole
   D) Oral valacyclovir
2. A patient is diagnosed with onychomycosis of three toenails. What is the most effective first-line treatment algorithm?
   A) Topical clotrimazole cream
   B) Oral terbinafine
   C) Oral cephalexin
   D) High-potency topical steroids
3. A patient with moderate plaque psoriasis is initiated on a high-potency topical corticosteroid and a vitamin D analog (calcipotriene). What comorbidity must be screened for as part of the systemic management algorithm?
   A) Psoriatic arthritis
   B) Celiac disease
   C) Multiple sclerosis
   D) Gout
4. An 80-year-old male presents with intensely pruritic, tense bullae on his trunk and extremities. Oral mucosa is spared. Biopsy with DIF confirms Bullous Pemphigoid. Which is a first-line treatment?
   A) Oral valacyclovir
   B) High-dose oral prednisone
   C) Topical terbinafine
   D) Methotrexate

5. The foundational, non-negotiable step in the treatment algorithm for all severities of atopic dermatitis is:
A) Use of high-potency topical steroids
B) Liberal use of thick emollients
C) Food allergy testing
D) Daily oral antihistamines
6. Which skin cancer is treated with an algorithm that includes Mohs surgery for high-risk lesions on the face? A) Melanoma in situ
B) Basal Cell Carcinoma
C) Kaposi sarcoma
D) Mycosis fungoides
7. A 45-year-old female is diagnosed with a melanoma on her back. The biopsy shows a Breslow depth of 1.2 mm. What is the next step in the staging/treatment algorithm? A) Wide local excision with 1-2 cm margins and a sentinel lymph node biopsy
B) Wide local excision alone
C) Systemic immunotherapy with nivolumab
D) Palliative radiation therapy
8. A patient has a scaling pink patch on their scalp and central face, with "greasy" scale. What is the most likely diagnosis and first-line algorithm?
A) Psoriasis; topical clobetasol
B) Atopic Dermatitis; emollients
C) Seborrheic Dermatitis; ketoconazole shampoo
D) Tinea Capitis; oral griseofulvin
9. A patient is prescribed a "Medrol Dosepak" (6-day steroid taper) for a severe poison ivy reaction. This is a common pitfall because:
A) The dose is too high and will cause atrophy.
B) It will cause a tinea incognito reaction.
C) The duration is too short and can lead to rebound dermatitis.

D) It does not cover potential secondary bacterial infection.

10. A 22-year-old female presents with recurrent, painful vesicular lesions on her genitals 6-8 times per year. What is the best long-term management algorithm?

    A) Episodic topical acyclovir

    B) Daily suppressive oral valacyclovir

    C) Daily topical corticosteroids

    D) Monthly oral fluconazole

Self-Assessment Questions

1. Compare and contrast the first-line treatment algorithm for non-purulent cellulitis versus a purulent skin abscess.
2. A patient has a scaling, annular plaque on their arm. What is the differential, and what diagnostic test would you perform? If it is tinea corporis, what is a major pitfall to avoid?
3. Describe the stepwise treatment algorithm for plaque psoriasis, starting from first-line topical therapy to systemic options.
4. What are the main diagnostic features that differentiate Bullous Pemphigoid from Pemphigus Vulgaris?
5. What is the foundational, non-pharmacological component of the treatment algorithm for all patients with Atopic Dermatitis?
6. A patient presents with a vesicular rash on their hands and forearms 3 days after doing yard work. What is the likely diagnosis, and why is a 6-day steroid pack a common pitfall?
7. What is Mohs micrographic surgery, and what is the algorithm for determining when it is the preferred treatment for a non-melanoma skin cancer?
8. A patient has a new, 5mm dark, irregular papule. Why is a superficial shave biopsy a critical error in the management algorithm?
9. What is the "ABCDE" criteria, and what role does it play in the diagnostic algorithm for skin cancer?
10. Describe the treatment algorithm for a 1.5mm thick melanoma on the back with a negative sentinel lymph node biopsy.

Bibliography

1. Stevens DL, Bisno AL, Chambers HF, Dellinger EP, Goldstein EJ, Gorbach SL, et al. Practice guidelines for the diagnosis and management of skin and soft tissue infections: 2014 update by the Infectious Diseases Society of America. Clin Infect Dis. 2014 Jul 15;59(2):e10–52.
2. Ameen M, Lear JT, Madan V, Mohd Mustapa MF, Richardson M. British Association of Dermatologists' guidelines for the management of tinea capitis 2014. Br J Dermatol. 2014 Nov;171(5):937–58.
3. Workowski KA, Bachmann LH, Chan PA, Johnston CM, Muzny CA, Park I, et al. Sexually Transmitted Infections Treatment Guidelines, 2021. MMWR Recomm Rep. 2021 Jul 23;70(RR-4):1–187.
4. Kim WB, Jerome D, Yeung J. Diagnosis and management of psoriasis. Can Fam Physician. 2017 Apr;63(4):278–85.
5. Menter A, Gelfand JM, Connor C, Armstrong AW, Cordoro KM, Davis DMR, et al. Joint American Academy of Dermatology-National Psoriasis Foundation guidelines of care for the management of psoriasis with biologics. J Am Acad Dermatol. 2020 Aug;83(2):645–6.
6. Venning VA, Taghipour K, Mohd Mustapa MF, Highet AS, Kirtschig G. British Association of Dermatologists' guidelines for the management of bullous pemphigoid 2012. Br J Dermatol. 2012 Sep;167(3):473–84.
7. Wollenberg A, Kinberger M, Roll A, Ehlers A, Schwarz-Friesel C, Bieber T. Eczema/atopic dermatitis. In: Ring J, Przybilla B, Ruzicka T, editors. Handbook of Allergic Diseases. 2nd ed. Munich: Karger; 2009. p. 305–17.
8. Eichenfield LF, Tom WL, Chamlin SL, Feldman SR, Hanifin JM, Simpson EL, et al. Guidelines of care for the management of atopic dermatitis: section 1. Diagnosis and assessment of atopic dermatitis. J Am Acad Dermatol. 2014 Feb;70(2):338–51.
9. Usatine RP, Riojas M. Diagnosis and management of contact dermatitis. Am Fam Physician. 2010 Aug 1;82(3):249–55.
10. National Comprehensive Cancer Network (NCCN). NCCN Clinical Practice Guidelines in Oncology: Basal Cell Skin Cancer. Version 1.2024.
11. National Comprehensive Cancer Network (NCCN). NCCN Clinical Practice Guidelines in Oncology:

Squamous Cell Skin Cancer. Version 1.2024.

12. National Comprehensive Cancer Network (NCCN). NCCN Clinical Practice Guidelines in Oncology: Melanoma: Cutaneous. Version 3.2024.
13. Swetter SM, Tsao H, Bichakjian CK, Curiel-Lewandrowski C, Elder DE, Guild V, et al. Guidelines of care for the management of primary cutaneous melanoma. American Academy of Dermatology. J Am Acad Dermatol. 2019 Jan;80(1):208–50.
14. Bickers DR, Lim HW, Margolis D, Weinstock MA, Goodman C, Faulkner E, et al. The burden of skin diseases: 2004. A joint project of the American Academy of Dermatology Association and the Society for Investigative Dermatology. J Am Acad Dermatol. 2006 Sep;55(3):490–500.
15. Gilson D, L'Eplattenier H, L'Eplattenier J, L'Eplattenier M, L'Eplattenier R, L'Eplattenier S. Tinea incognito. Mycoses. 2019 Nov;62(11):980–91.

CHAPTER 12

TREATMENT ALGORITHMS FOR MEDICAL EMERGENCIES

Author

Mrs. Sunitha Panthagada, Associate Professor, Department of Pharmaceutical Analysis, Koringa College of Pharmacy, Korangi, Tallarevu, Andhra Pradesh, India

Abstract

The management of medical emergencies is dictated by time-sensitive algorithms designed to rapidly stabilize physiology and reverse life-threatening pathology. The Acute Coronary Syndrome (ACS) algorithm bifurcates based on the initial EKG; STEMI requires an immediate reperfusion algorithm, prioritizing primary PCI, while NSTEMI management is guided by risk stratification. The acute stroke algorithm is similarly time-dependent, centered on an immediate non-contrast CT scan to differentiate ischemic from hemorrhagic stroke. Ischemic stroke management is an algorithm of reperfusion, using IV thrombolysis (alteplase) within a 4.5-hour window and mechanical thrombectomy for large vessel occlusion up to 24 hours. The sepsis algorithm is a bundled protocol ("Hour-1 Bundle") mandating lactate measurement, blood cultures, rapid broad-spectrum antibiotic administration, 30 ml/kg crystalloid resuscitation for hypotension, and vasopressors to maintain mean arterial pressure. The anaphylaxis algorithm is linear and prioritized: immediate intramuscular epinephrine is the first-line and life-saving intervention, followed by adjunctive treatments like antihistamines and corticosteroids. The DKA/HHS algorithm is a multi-pronged metabolic resuscitation, balancing three components: aggressive intravenous fluid repletion, continuous insulin infusion (after confirming potassium levels), and vigilant electrolyte (especially potassium) monitoring and replacement.

Keywords: *Sepsis, Stroke, Acute Coronary Syndrome, Anaphylaxis, Diabetic Ketoacidosis, Emergency Medicine*

Learning Objectives

After completion of the chapter, the learners should be able to:

- List the core components of the "Sepsis Hour-1 Bundle."
- Explain the time-sensitive treatment algorithm for acute ischemic stroke, including the indications for thrombolysis and thrombectomy.
- Initiate the correct, immediate treatment algorithm (including dosing) for a patient presenting with anaphylactic shock.
- Compare and contrast the fluid and insulin management algorithms for Diabetic Ketoacidosis (DKA) versus Hyperosmolar Hyperglycemic State (HHS).
- Prioritize the life-saving interventions in the algorithm for a patient with septic shock, managing competing treatment goals.

ACUTE CORONARY SYNDROME

Acute Coronary Syndrome (ACS) refers to a spectrum of conditions where myocardial blood supply is acutely reduced. The management algorithm is one of the most time-critical in medicine, as "time is muscle." This section focuses on the immediate emergency department algorithm (a more detailed cardiology-focused discussion is in Chapter 1).

Pathophysiology

The universal pathophysiology is the **rupture or erosion of an atherosclerotic plaque** within a coronary artery. This rupture exposes the highly thrombogenic lipid core of the plaque to the bloodstream, triggering an immediate coagulation cascade.

Platelets adhere and aggregate, and a fibrin mesh is formed, leading to the development of an occlusive or sub-occlusive **intracoronary thrombus (clot)**.

- In **STEMI**, the thrombus is typically *fully occlusive*, cutting off all blood flow to a large territory of the myocardium. This causes transmural (full-thickness) ischemia and rapid necrosis, visible as ST-segment elevation on an EKG.
- In **NSTEMI/UA**, the thrombus is typically *partially*

occlusive. It limits, but does not completely block, blood flow. This causes subendocardial (partial-thickness) ischemia. In NSTEMI, the ischemia is severe or prolonged enough to cause myocyte necrosis, releasing cardiac troponins. In UA, the ischemia is transient and does *not* cause necrosis (troponins are negative).

Diagnosis and Classification

The initial algorithm begins with any patient presenting with symptoms suggestive of cardiac ischemia (e.g., chest pain, dyspnea, syncope).

- **Step 1: Immediate EKG.** An EKG must be obtained and interpreted within 10 minutes of first medical contact. This is the primary branch point in the algorithm.
- **Step 2: Classification.**
    - **STEMI (ST-Segment Elevation Myocardial Infarction):** The EKG shows ST-segment elevation in two or more contiguous leads or a new left bundle branch block. This indicates a complete, occlusive thrombus.
    - **NSTEMI/UA (Non-ST-Segment Elevation MI / Unstable Angina):** The EKG may show ST-segment depressions, T-wave inversions, or may be non-specific.
- **Step 3: Cardiac Troponins.** Blood is drawn for cardiac troponin levels at presentation and serially. A rise and/or fall in troponin with ischemic symptoms confirms MI (STEMI or NSTEMI).

Differential Diagnosis

The differential diagnosis for acute chest pain includes other life-threatening conditions that must be considered in the initial algorithm:

- **Aortic Dissection:** Severe, tearing, or ripping pain, often radiating to the back.
- **Pulmonary Embolism (PE):** Pleuritic chest pain, dyspnea, and tachycardia.
- **Tension Pneumothorax:** Sudden-onset dyspnea,

tracheal deviation, and hypotension.

- **Esophageal Rupture (Boerhaave Syndrome):** Severe chest pain following forceful vomiting.
- **Pericarditis:** Positional, pleuritic pain, often with diffuse ST elevations.

Treatment Algorithm

The algorithm diverges immediately based on the EKG classification.

STEMI Algorithm (Reperfusion):

- **Goal:** Immediate reperfusion. "Time-to-device" is the main metric.
- **First-line:** Primary Percutaneous Coronary Intervention (PCI) is the preferred algorithm. The goal is a "first medical contact-to-device" time of ≤ 90 minutes (if at a PCI-capable hospital) or ≤ 120 minutes (if requiring transfer).
- **Second-line (Fibrinolysis):** If PCI cannot be performed within these timeframes, the algorithm shifts to intravenous fibrinolytic therapy (e.g., alteplase, tenecteplase). This must be given within 30 minutes of arrival and requires strict screening for contraindications (e.g., prior ICH, recent stroke).
- **Adjunctive Medications:** Immediate aspirin (324 mg chewed), a P2Y12 inhibitor (e.g., ticagrelor, prasugrel), and anticoagulation (e.g., heparin) are given.

NSTEMI/UA Algorithm (Risk Stratification):

- **Goal:** Stabilize, risk-stratify, and determine the need for invasive management.
- **Initial Medications:** Aspirin, a P2Y12 inhibitor (e.g., clopidogrel, ticagrelor), anticoagulation (e.g., enoxaparin, heparin), nitrates (for pain, if not hypotensive), and beta-blockers (if stable).

- **Risk Stratification:** The algorithm uses a risk score (e.g., TIMI or GRACE) to classify patients.
- **Early Invasive Strategy:** Patients with high-risk features (e.g., refractory angina, hemodynamic instability, dynamic EKG changes, high GRACE score) proceed to angiography within 24-48 hours.
- **Conservative Strategy:** Low-risk patients may be managed medically first, followed by non-invasive stress testing to guide further therapy.

Table 12.1: ACS Initial Management Algorithm (STEMI vs. NSTEMI)

ACS Type	EKG Finding	Immediate Treatment Algorithm
STEMI	**ST-Segment Elevation** (in ≥ 2 contiguous leads).	**Immediate Reperfusion:** Primary PCI (if < 90-120 min). (Fibrinolysis if PCI delayed). **MONA-B + DAPT.**
NSTEMI / UA	**ST-Depression** or **T-Wave Inversion.** (No ST elevation).	**MONA-B + DAPT + Anticoagulation.** (Heparin). **Risk Stratify (TIMI/GRACE):** High-Risk → Early Invasive (PCI).

MONA-B: Morphine, Oxygen (if sat < 90%), Nitrates, Aspirin, Beta-blocker. DAPT: Dual Antiplatelet Therapy (Aspirin + P2Y12-I).

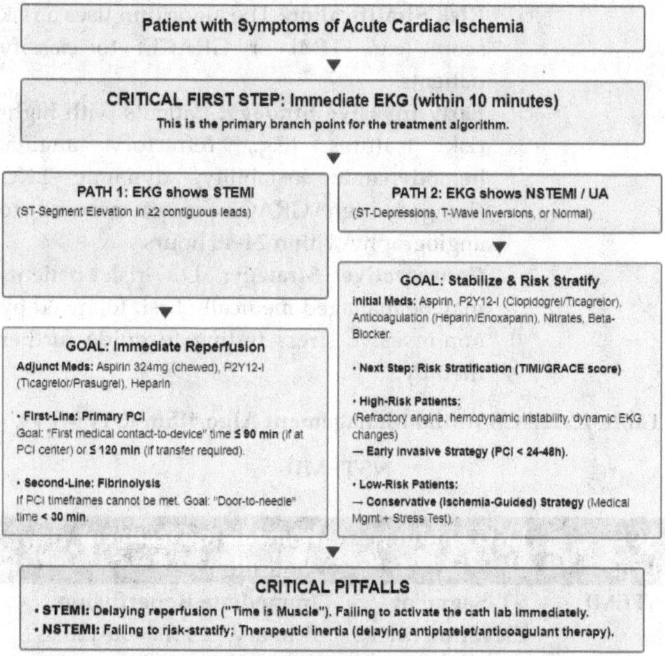

Figure 12.1: Acute Coronary Syndrome - Management Algorithm

Monitoring and Follow-Up

Acute monitoring is intensive and time-sensitive, beginning in the emergency department and continuing in a cardiac/coronary care unit (CCU).

1. **Continuous EKG (Telemetry):** This is the most critical monitoring tool. The primary goals are to watch for **life-threatening arrhythmias** (e.g., Ventricular Fibrillation or Tachycardia, which is the most common cause of death in early STEMI) and to monitor for dynamic ST-T wave changes, which would indicate re-occlusion or ongoing ischemia.
2. **Serial Cardiac Troponins:** Troponin levels are trended (e.g., at 0, 3, and 6 hours). The *peak* of the troponin level correlates with the *size* of the myocardial infarction. A

rapid rise and fall is the classic pattern.

3. **Serial 12-lead EKGs:** In addition to telemetry, full 12-lead EKGs are obtained serially (e.g., on arrival, post-intervention, and for any new chest pain) to assess the evolution of Q-waves, ST segments, and T-wave inversions.
4. **Post-Intervention Monitoring:** After percutaneous coronary intervention (PCI), monitoring is focused on the **catheter access site** (femoral or radial) for bleeding, hematoma, or pseudoaneurysm. Distal pulses and extremity perfusion must also be checked regularly.
5. **Hemodynamic Monitoring:** Vital signs, especially blood pressure and heart rate, are monitored closely to watch for signs of cardiogenic shock (hypotension) or heart failure (tachycardia, hypoxia).

Long-Term Management / Secondary Prevention

This is the cornerstone of post-ACS care. The goal is to prevent re-infarction, heart failure, and death.

1. **Dual Antiplatelet Therapy (DAPT):** This is non-negotiable. Patients receive **Aspirin** (lifelong) plus a **P2Y12 inhibitor** (e.g., clopidogrel, prasugrel, or ticagrelor). The P2Y12 inhibitor is continued for at least 12 months post-stent placement to prevent stent thrombosis.
2. **High-Intensity Statin:** All patients are discharged on a high-intensity statin (e.g., Atorvastatin 80mg, Rosuvastatin 40mg), regardless of their baseline cholesterol. The goal is plaque stabilization.
3. **Beta-Blocker:** Started within 24 hours (if no contraindications) and continued lifelong. Beta-blockers decrease myocardial oxygen demand and reduce the risk of post-MI arrhythmias.
4. **ACE Inhibitor / ARB:** These agents are started, especially in patients with a reduced ejection fraction (EF < 40%), hypertension, or diabetes, to prevent adverse cardiac remodeling and heart failure.
5. **Cardiac Rehabilitation:** A formal, monitored exercise and education program is a critical component of

recovery and secondary prevention.

6. **Risk Factor Modification:** Aggressive management of hypertension, diabetes, and hyperlipidemia, along with absolute smoking cessation.

Patient Counseling Points

1. **"This Was a Heart Attack":** "You had a heart attack. This means one of the arteries that supplies blood to your heart muscle became blocked by a blood clot. We were able to open that artery with a 'stent' (a small metal scaffold), and now the blood is flowing again."
2. **"The 'Holy Trinity' of Medications":** "You will be going home on three essential types of medicine that you must take for at least the next year, and some for life. 1) An **Aspirin** and a '**super-aspirin**' (like Plavix/Clopidogrel). These prevent your new stent from clotting off. Stopping these suddenly can be fatal. 2) A **statin**, which is a high-dose cholesterol pill that 'cools down' the inflammation in all your arteries. 3) A **beta-blocker**, which is a 'heart-protection' pill that lets your heart rest and heal."
3. **Chest Pain "Action Plan":** "If you get chest pain *like this again*: 1) Stop, sit down, and rest. 2) Take one nitroglycerin pill under your tongue. 3) If the pain is *not gone* in 5 minutes, **call emergency services**. Do not take a second pill. Do not drive yourself. Call emergency services."
4. **Cardiac Rehab:** "We will be enrolling you in 'cardiac rehab.' This is an exercise program with nurses and therapists that is the single best way to get your strength back and learn how to protect your heart."

Common Pitfalls in Management

The most critical pitfall in STEMI is delaying reperfusion. Any delay in obtaining the EKG or activating the cath lab is a systems failure. A common diagnostic error is missing a posterior MI (which presents as ST-depressions in V1-V3) or a "STEMI-equivalent." In NSTEMI, a common pitfall is therapeutic inertia, or failing to initiate dual antiplatelet therapy and anticoagulation promptly.

Case Study

A 66-year-old male with diabetes presents with 2 hours of substernal chest pressure. His EKG is obtained in 5 minutes and shows **ST-depressions in leads V4-V6.** His initial Troponin is elevated at 1.8 ng/mL. He has ongoing chest pain despite 3 sublingual nitroglycerin tablets.

Discussion

The EKG (ST-depressions) and positive troponin confirm a **Non-ST-Elevation Myocardial Infarction (NSTEMI).** The algorithm for NSTEMI is to stabilize and then risk-stratify. This patient's **refractory chest pain** places him in the "high-risk" category, which dictates the need for an "early invasive strategy."

Treatment Algorithm

1. **Diagnosis:** High-Risk NSTEMI.
2. **Algorithm (Medical Stabilization):**
    - **Aspirin:** 324 mg chewed.
    - **P2Y12 Inhibitor:** Loading dose of **Ticagrelor 180 mg.**
    - **Anticoagulation:** Start an **IV Heparin infusion.**
    - **Statin:** Administer **Atorvastatin 80 mg.**
    - **Beta-Blocker:** Start oral Metoprolol (once stable).
3. **Algorithm (Risk Stratification):** The patient is "High-Risk" due to refractory angina.
    - **Action:** The algorithm bypasses a conservative "ischemia-guided" strategy. He is scheduled for an **early invasive strategy (cardiac catheterization).**

Outcome

The patient is admitted to the cardiac unit and undergoes angiography within 24 hours, which reveals a 90% blockage in his circumflex artery that is stented.

STROKE

Acute stroke is a neurological emergency caused by disrupted blood flow to the brain. The algorithm is entirely dependent on time from symptom onset and the differentiation between ischemic and hemorrhagic causes. The mantra is "Time is Brain."

Pathophysiology

Stroke is a "brain attack" caused by a sudden disruption of cerebral blood flow.

- **Ischemic Stroke (85%):** The pathophysiology is the acute occlusion of a cerebral artery, leading to a core of irreversible infarction (cell death) surrounded by a ring of salvageable, ischemic tissue called the **penumbra**. The entire treatment algorithm is focused on restoring blood flow to this penumbra before it, too, becomes infarcted. The "time is brain" mantra reflects that millions of neurons die for every minute of occlusion. The occlusion can be **thrombotic** (a clot forming on a local atherosclerotic plaque) or **embolic** (a clot traveling from a distant source, most commonly the heart in atrial fibrillation).
- **Hemorrhagic Stroke (15%):** The pathophysiology is *not* ischemia, but vessel rupture and bleeding.
  - **Intracerebral Hemorrhage (ICH):** A vessel *within* the brain parenchyma ruptures (often due to chronic hypertension). The damage is from the "mass effect" of the expanding hematoma, which compresses and destroys brain tissue.
  - **Subarachnoid Hemorrhage (SAH):** A vessel (most commonly a saccular "berry" aneurysm) ruptures *on the surface* of the brain, spilling blood into the subarachnoid space. This causes a sudden, severe "thunderclap" headache, and the primary neurologic damage is from cerebral vasospasm in the days following the bleed.

Diagnosis and Classification

The algorithm is initiated by a pre-hospital stroke scale (e.g., FAST—Face, Arms, Speech, Time) and confirmed in the emergency department.

- **Step 1: Neurologic Assessment.** A rapid, focused neurologic exam, quantified by the National Institutes of Health Stroke Scale (NIHSS), is performed.
- **Step 2: Immediate Imaging.** The single most important diagnostic step is a non-contrast head CT scan. This must be performed and interpreted within 20 minutes of arrival.
- **Step 3: Classification.**
  - **Ischemic Stroke (85%):** The CT scan is negative for blood. This is caused by a thrombus or embolus.
  - **Hemorrhagic Stroke (15%):** The CT scan shows hyperdensity (white), indicating bleeding. This is sub-classified into Intracerebral Hemorrhage (ICH) or Subarachnoid Hemorrhage (SAH).

Differential Diagnosis

The differential for acute-onset focal neurologic deficits includes "stroke mimics." The most common mimics are:

- **Hypoglycemia:** Must be checked with a finger-stick glucose on all patients.
- **Post-ictal Paralysis (Todd's paresis):** A transient focal weakness following a seizure.
- **Complex Migraine (Hemiplegic Migraine):** Can present with focal weakness or numbness.
- **Bell's Palsy:** A peripheral (LMN) facial droop, as opposed to the central (UMN) droop of a stroke.

Treatment Algorithm

Ischemic Stroke Algorithm (Reperfusion)

  - **Thrombolysis (tPA):** If the patient presents within the 4.5-hour window from "last known normal," is not bleeding on CT, and has no other contraindications, the algorithm is to administer IV alteplase (tPA).

- **Thrombectomy:** For patients with a large vessel occlusion (LVO) identified on CT angiography, mechanical thrombectomy (endovascular clot retrieval) is the standard of care. This algorithm can be initiated up to 6-24 hours from onset in select patients.
- **Blood Pressure:** BP must be controlled *below 185/110 mmHg* before and during tPA. For patients not receiving tPA, "permissive hypertension" (up to 220/120 mmHg) is allowed.

Hemorrhagic Stroke Algorithm (Damage Control)

- **Intracerebral Hemorrhage (ICH):** The algorithm is focused on limiting hematoma expansion. This involves immediate, aggressive blood pressure reduction (e.g., target SBP < 140-160 mmHg) and rapid reversal of any anticoagulation.
- **Subarachnoid Hemorrhage (SAH):** Often from a ruptured aneurysm. The algorithm involves BP control, neurosurgical consultation for aneurysm clipping or coiling, and initiation of nimodipine to prevent cerebral vasospasm.

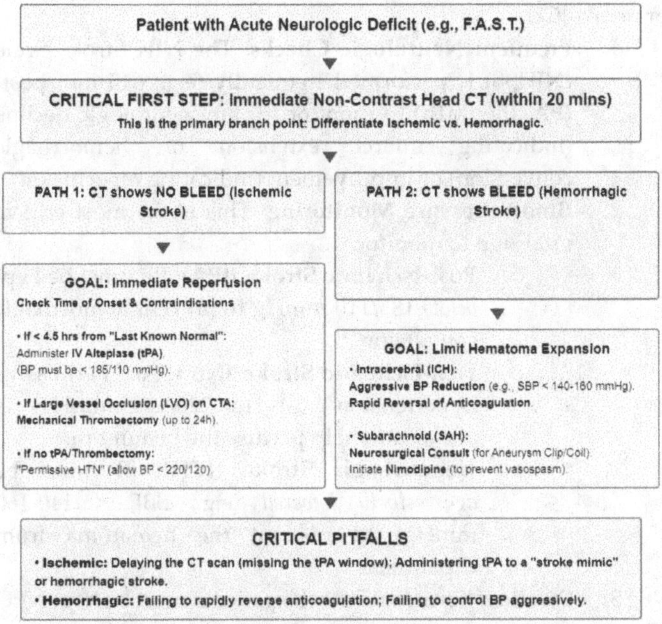

Figure 12.2: Acute Stroke - Management Algorithm

Table 12.2: Acute Stroke Management Algorithm

Stroke Type	Diagnostic Test	Immediate Treatment Algorithm
Ischemic (Acute, ~85%)	**Non-Contrast Head CT** (to *exclude* bleed).	**If < 4.5 hrs:** IV Alteplase (tPA). **If Large Vessel Occlusion:** Mechanical Thrombectomy (up to 24 hrs). Permissive HTN.
Hemorrhagic (ICH / SAH, ~15%)	**Non-Contrast Head CT** (to *confirm* bleed).	**ICH:** Aggressive BP Control (SBP < 140-160). **Reverse** anticoagulation. **SAH:** Neurosurgery consult, Nimodipine.

Monitoring and Follow-Up

Acute monitoring is performed in a specialized stroke unit

or neuro-ICU.

1. **Frequent Neurologic Checks:** The NIH Stroke Scale (NIHSS) is performed frequently (e.g., q15 min post-tPA, then q1h) to monitor for any neurologic decline (indicating infarct extension or hemorrhagic conversion) or improvement (indicating reperfusion).
2. **Blood Pressure Monitoring:** This is the most critical vital sign to monitor.
   - **Post-Ischemic Stroke (tPA):** BP must be kept *below* 185/110 mmHg to prevent hemorrhagic conversion.
   - **Post-Ischemic Stroke (No tPA):** "Permissive hypertension" (up to 220/120 mmHg) is allowed to help perfuse the penumbra.
   - **Hemorrhagic Stroke (ICH):** BP must be *aggressively lowered* (e.g., SBP < 140-160 mmHg) to prevent the hematoma from expanding.
3. **Swallow Screen:** All stroke patients must be kept NPO (nothing by mouth) until a formal bedside swallow screen is performed. Aspiration pneumonia is a common and deadly complication.
4. **DVT Prophylaxis:** Stroke patients are immobile. Sequential compression devices (SCDs) are placed immediately. Anticoagulants (like heparin) are held for the first 24-48 hours, especially post-tPA.

Long-Term Management / Secondary Prevention

The goal is to prevent a second stroke.

1. **Ischemic Stroke (Non-cardioembolic):** Start high-intensity statin and an antiplatelet agent (Aspirin or Clopidogrel).
2. **Ischemic Stroke (Cardioembolic/Afib):** Start long-term anticoagulation (e.g., a DOAC like apixaban) to prevent new clot formation in the heart.
3. **Workup:** All ischemic stroke patients require a "stroke workup" to find the cause: an Echocardiogram (to look for cardiac thrombus or PFO), a Carotid Doppler (to look for carotid stenosis), and telemetry (to look for

occult Afib).

4. **Hemorrhagic Stroke:** The only long-term management is aggressive, lifelong blood pressure control.
5. **Rehabilitation:** All stroke patients require intensive inpatient and outpatient rehabilitation (Physical, Occupational, and Speech Therapy).

Patient Counseling Points

1. **"You Had a 'Brain Attack'":** "This was a stroke. A (blood clot / bleed) in your brain cut off blood flow, which caused your symptoms. We were able to (give a clot-busting medicine / get the clot out / control the bleeding)."
2. **"F.A.S.T.":** "Your family must know the signs of a *new* stroke. Remember F.A.S.T. **F**ace drooping, **A**rm weakness, **S**peech difficulty, **T**ime to call emergency services. *Time is brain.*"
3. **Medication Adherence:** (For ischemic stroke) "The two most important medicines to prevent this from happening again are your **statin** (cholesterol pill) and your **antiplatelet** (aspirin/Plavix) or **anticoagulant** (blood thinner). You must take these for life."
4. **Rehab is Your New Job:** "The brain can re-wire itself, but it takes thousands of repetitions. Your recovery will be a full-time job for the next few months. You must be committed to your physical and speech therapy."

Common Pitfalls in Management

The most tragic pitfall is delaying the non-contrast head CT, which wastes precious time and can exclude a patient from the tPA window. Another critical error is administering tPA to a patient with a "stroke mimic" (e.g., hemorrhagic stroke, aortic dissection) or a contraindication. In hemorrhagic stroke, the most common pitfall is failing to rapidly reverse anticoagulation or lower blood pressure aggressively.

Case Study

A 70-year-old female (Ms. Wei) is brought to the ED by her son. He states she was normal when he spoke to her at 8 PM last night, but he found her at 8 AM this morning with severe right-sided weakness and unable to speak (aphasia). Her "Last Known Normal" (LKN) is 12 hours ago.

Discussion

This is an acute stroke presentation. She is well **outside the 4.5-hour window for IV tPA (alteplase).** The algorithm for this "wake-up stroke" is to immediately get a non-contrast head CT and then advanced imaging (CTA/CTP) to assess for a large vessel occlusion (LVO) and a salvageable penumbra, which would make her a candidate for mechanical thrombectomy.

Treatment Algorithm

1. **Triage:** "Time is Brain." Patient is taken immediately to the CT scanner.
2. **Algorithm Step 1 (CT):** A **Non-Contrast Head CT** is performed. It is **negative for hemorrhage**, confirming an **Ischemic Stroke.**
3. **Algorithm Step 2 (tPA):** She is **NOT a candidate for IV tPA** because her LKN is > 4.5 hours.
4. **Algorithm Step 3 (Advanced Imaging):** A **CT Angiogram (CTA)** is performed, which shows a **Left Middle Cerebral Artery (MCA) occlusion** (a Large Vessel Occlusion).
5. **Algorithm Step 4 (Thrombectomy):** She is within the 24-hour window for thrombectomy. She is taken for emergent **mechanical thrombectomy.**

Outcome

The neuro-interventional team successfully retrieves the clot, restoring blood flow. The patient is admitted to the Stroke Unit for intensive monitoring and rehabilitation.

SEPSIS

Sepsis is a life-threatening organ dysfunction caused by a dysregulated host response to infection. Septic shock is a subset of sepsis with profound circulatory and cellular/metabolic abnormalities.

Pathophysiology

The pathophysiology is not the infection itself, but the body's *overwhelming and self-destructive response* to it. A pathogen (e.g., bacteria) releases PAMPs (pathogen-associated molecular patterns), which are recognized by the immune system. This, combined with tissue damage (releasing DAMPs, or damage-associated molecular patterns), triggers a **cytokine storm**.

This storm of pro-inflammatory cytokines causes:

1. **Widespread Vasodilation:** Capillaries and arterioles dilate, leading to a massive drop in systemic vascular resistance (SVR) and relative hypovolemia.
2. **Capillary Leak:** The endothelium becomes "leaky," allowing fluid and protein to escape from the blood vessels into the tissues, causing massive edema and further depleting intravascular volume.
3. **Endothelial Dysfunction:** A pro-coagulant state is triggered, leading to micro-thrombi (clots) in small vessels, which impairs organ perfusion.

Septic Shock is the endpoint of this process: a state of refractory hypotension (due to vasodilation and leak) and tissue hypoperfusion (due to micro-thrombi and shunting) that requires vasopressors (e.g., norepinephrine) to maintain a survivable blood pressure (MAP > 65). This hypoperfusion leads to multi-organ dysfunction syndrome (MODS).

Diagnosis and Classification

Sepsis is a clinical diagnosis. The algorithm uses screening tools (e.g., SIRS or qSOFA) to identify at-risk patients, and is confirmed by the SOFA score (a measure of organ dysfunction).

- **Sepsis:** Suspected or confirmed infection plus an acute increase in SOFA score ≥ 2 points.
- **Septic Shock:** Sepsis plus the need for vasopressors to

maintain a MAP ≥ 65 mmHg AND a serum lactate > 2 mmol/L, despite adequate fluid resuscitation.

Differential Diagnosis

The differential for a patient presenting with shock (hypotension, tachycardia, end-organ dysfunction) includes other forms of shock:

- **Cardiogenic Shock:** (e.g., massive MI) Will have "cold and wet" features and elevated JVP.
- **Hypovolemic Shock:** (e.g., hemorrhage) Will have "cold and dry" features.
- **Obstructive Shock:** (e.g., massive PE, cardiac tamponade).
- **Anaphylactic Shock:** (see 12.4) Will have rash, wheezing, and rapid onset after exposure.

Treatment Algorithm (Surviving Sepsis Hour-1 Bundle)

The management of sepsis is a time-sensitive, bundled algorithm. All components should be initiated *within one hour* of recognition.

- **Step 1: Measure Lactate Level.** Re-measure if initial lactate is elevated (> 2 mmol/L).
- **Step 2: Obtain Blood Cultures.** Must be drawn *before* administering antibiotics.
- **Step 3: Administer Broad-Spectrum Antibiotics.** This is one of the most critical, time-sensitive steps.
- **Step 4: Begin Rapid Fluid Resuscitation.** For hypotension or lactate > 4 mmol/L, administer 30 ml/kg of intravenous crystalloid.
- **Step 5: Apply Vasopressors.** If the patient remains hypotensive during or after fluid resuscitation, the algorithm is to start vasopressors to maintain a Mean Arterial Pressure (MAP) ≥ 65 mmHg. Norepinephrine is the first-line agent.

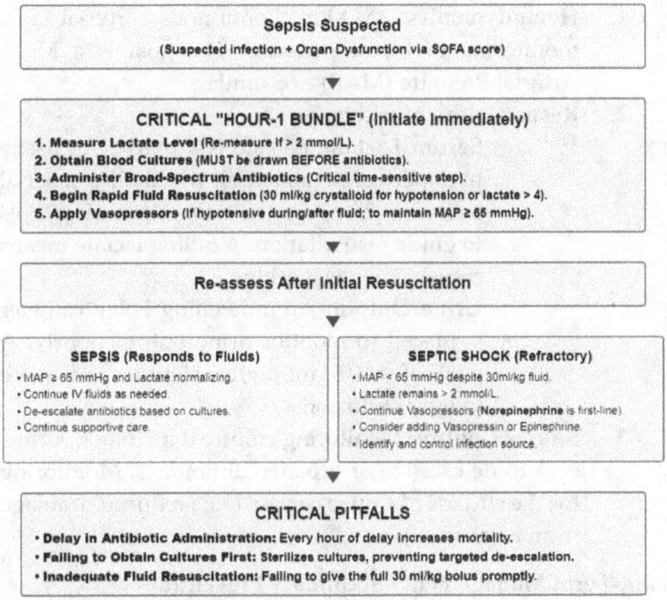

Figure 12.3: Sepsis - Management Algorithm

Table 12.3: Sepsis Hour-1 Bundle (Surviving Sepsis Campaign)

Action	Rationale / Goal
1. Measure Lactate	Identify tissue hypoperfusion. (Remeasure if initial > 2).
2. Blood Cultures	Obtain *before* antibiotics.
3. Broad-Spectrum Antibiotics	Administer ASAP (within 1 hour). Critical mortality benefit.
4. IV Fluid Bolus	**30 mL/kg crystalloid** (e.g., LR or NS) for hypotension or lactate ≥ 4.
5. Vasopressors	Apply if hypotensive during/after fluid (to maintain MAP ≥ 65 mmHg).

Monitoring and Follow-Up

Monitoring is done in an ICU and is guided by the "Surviving Sepsis" guidelines.

1. **Hemodynamics (MAP):** Continuous arterial line monitoring of blood pressure. The goal is a Mean Arterial Pressure (MAP) ≥ 65 mmHg.
2. **Resuscitation Markers:**
   - **Serum Lactate:** Lactate is a marker of tissue hypoperfusion (anaerobic metabolism). Serial lactates (q2-4h) are the *main* monitoring tools to guide resuscitation. A falling lactate means resuscitation is working.
   - **Urine Output:** An indwelling Foley catheter is placed to monitor urine output hourly. A goal of > 0.5 mL/kg/hr signifies adequate kidney perfusion.
3. **Source Control:** Monitoring culture data (blood, urine, etc.) to de-escalate or broaden antibiotics. Monitoring for the success of source control (e.g., reduced drainage from an abscess).

Long-Term Management / Secondary Prevention

This is a new and critical field of "post-sepsis" care.

1. **Post-Sepsis Syndrome (PSS):** The majority of sepsis survivors suffer from PSS. This includes:
   - **Physical:** Profound weakness ("ICU-acquired weakness"), fatigue, and joint pain.
   - **Cognitive:** "Brain fog," memory loss, and difficulty concentrating.
   - **Psychological:** High rates of PTSD, anxiety, and depression.
   - Management involves early physical therapy, cognitive rehabilitation, and mental health screening.
2. **Risk Reduction:** Identifying and vaccinating against preventable infections (influenza, pneumococcus). Managing chronic conditions (like diabetes) that increase infection risk.

Patient Counseling Points

1. **"This Was a Life-Threatening Overreaction":** "You had a severe infection, but the life-threatening part was

your body's *response* to it. Your immune system 'overreacted' and caused a chain reaction that made your blood vessels leak and your blood pressure drop, which started to shut down your organs."

2. **"The 'Hour-1 Bundle'"**: "We had to act very fast. We gave you 1) large volumes of IV *fluid* to fill your 'leaky' pipes, 2) powerful *antibiotics* to fight the infection, and 3) 'pressor' medicine (like norepinephrine) to squeeze your blood vessels and bring your blood pressure back to a safe level."
3. **"The Recovery is Slow (Post-Sepsis Syndrome)"**: "You have been through a war. It is *normal* to feel extremely weak, tired, and 'foggy' in your thinking for weeks or even months. This is called Post-Sepsis Syndrome. It is real, and it will get better, but it takes time. Physical therapy is essential."

Common Pitfalls in Management

The most significant pitfall is a **delay in antibiotic administration**, as every hour of delay increases mortality. Another common error is failing to obtain blood cultures *before* giving antibiotics, which can sterilize the cultures and prevent targeted de-escalation. Inadequate fluid resuscitation (not giving the full 30 ml/kg bolus) is a common error, as is "fluid-creep" or excessive fluid administration in patients who are not fluid-responsive.

Case Study

An 85-year-old male with dementia is brought from a nursing home for "not acting right." He is lethargic and febrile (102.8°F). His vitals: BP **88/50 mmHg**, HR 125, RR 28. His urine is noted to be dark and foul-smelling.

Discussion

This is a classic presentation of **Sepsis** (suspected UTI + altered mental status + fever) leading to **Septic Shock** (hypotension, tachycardia). The algorithm mandates immediate initiation of the **"Hour-1 Bundle."**

Treatment Algorithm (Hour-1 Bundle):

1. **Step 1 (Lactate):** A serum **lactate** is drawn (it comes back at 4.2 mmol/L, indicating hypoperfusion).
2. **Step 2 (Cultures): Two sets of blood cultures** are drawn, and a urinalysis/culture is obtained *before* antibiotics.
3. **Step 3 (Antibiotics):** Broad-spectrum **IV antibiotics** (e.g., Piperacillin-Tazobactam) are administered immediately. **This is the most critical step.**
4. **Step 4 (Fluids):** Because he is hypotensive (BP 88/50), a **30 mL/kg bolus of IV crystalloids** (e.g., 2 liters of Lactated Ringer's) is started immediately.
5. **Step 5 (Pressors):** After the 2L fluid bolus, his BP is still 90/55 (MAP 67). You start a **Norepinephrine infusion** to maintain a MAP ≥ 65 mmHg.

Outcome

The patient is admitted to the ICU, resuscitated with fluids, antibiotics, and vasopressors. His hypotension resolves, and his lactate clears within 6 hours.

ANAPHYLAXIS

Anaphylaxis is an acute, life-threatening, multi-system allergic reaction. The algorithm for management is simple, linear, and must be executed immediately.

Pathophysiology

The pathophysiology is one of catastrophic, explosive mast cell and basophil degranulation. In a sensitized individual, an allergen (e.g., peanut protein) cross-links two **IgE antibodies** on the surface of a mast cell. This single event triggers the immediate release of a flood of pre-formed inflammatory mediators, primarily **histamine**.

Histamine (and other newly synthesized mediators like leukotrienes) acts systemically to cause:

1. **Vasodilation:** Widespread vasodilation and capillary leak, causing a precipitous drop in blood pressure (distributive shock) and flushing.

2. **Bronchoconstriction:** Contraction of smooth muscle in the airways, causing wheezing and shortness of breath.
3. **Angioedema:** Rapid swelling of the submucosal and subcutaneous tissues, particularly the larynx and pharynx, which can lead to fatal airway obstruction.
4. **Urticaria (Hives):** Pruritus and wheals on the skin.

Diagnosis and Classification

Diagnosis is clinical, based on the rapid onset of symptoms in two or more body systems after exposure to a potential allergen.

- **Skin:** Urticaria (hives), angioedema, flushing, pruritus.
- **Respiratory:** Wheezing, stridor, cough, dyspnea, upper airway edema.
- **Cardiovascular:** Hypotension, tachycardia, syncope (shock).
- **GI:** Nausea, vomiting, abdominal cramps, diarrhea.

Differential Diagnosis

- **Severe Asthma Attack:** Presents with wheezing but typically lacks urticaria, angioedema, or hypotension.
- **Vasovagal Syncope:** Presents with pallor, bradycardia, and hypotension, but resolves with supine positioning and lacks allergic features.
- **Panic Attack:** Can have dyspnea and tachycardia, but lacks objective findings like wheezing, hypotension, or urticaria.
- **Flushing Syndromes:** (e.g., Carcinoid, Red Man Syndrome from vancomycin) can mimic the flushing of anaphylaxis.

Treatment Algorithm

- **Step 1: Epinephrine (First-Line and Primary).** This is the single most important step. Administer **Epinephrine 0.3-0.5 mg (of 1:1000 solution) Intramuscularly (IM)** into the anterolateral thigh. This step should not be delayed for any reason. It may be repeated every 5-15 minutes.

- **Step 2: Airway and Oxygen.** Place the patient in a recumbent position (if tolerated), administer high-flow oxygen, and prepare for definitive airway management (intubation) if stridor or respiratory distress is severe.
- **Step 3: Adjunctive (Second-Line) Therapies.** These are given *after* epinephrine to manage secondary symptoms.
    - **H1 Antihistamines:** (e.g., diphenhydramine) for itching and hives.
    - **H2 Antihistamines:** (e.g., famotidine) to complement H1 blockade.
    - **Corticosteroids:** (e.g., methylprednisolone) to potentially prevent a biphasic (late-phase) reaction hours later.
    - **IV Fluids:** A large-bore IV with boluses of normal saline is essential for patients with hypotension.

Monitoring and Follow-Up

Monitoring is acute, in an emergency setting.

1. **A-B-C (Airway, Breathing, Circulation):** The primary monitoring is a constant re-assessment of the airway (for stridor or swelling), breathing (for wheeze or accessory muscle use), and circulation (for blood pressure).
2. **Response to Epinephrine:** Monitoring for resolution of symptoms after epinephrine (e.g., improved BP, reduced wheeze, less swelling).
3. **Biphasic Reaction:** This is the *most critical* monitoring point. A second, "biphasic" wave of anaphylaxis can occur 1-8 hours *after* the initial symptoms have resolved, even without re-exposure. All patients who receive epinephrine for anaphylaxis *must* be observed in a medical setting for at least 4-6 hours.

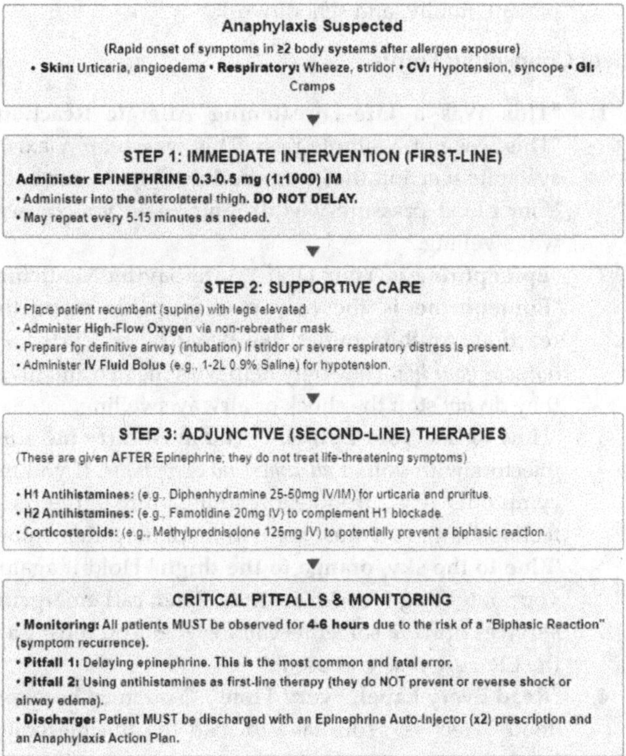

Figure 12.4: Anaphylaxis - Management Algorithm

Long-Term Management / Secondary Prevention

This is focused entirely on prevention and preparedness.

1. **Strict Allergen Avoidance:** This is the primary management.
2. **Referral to Allergist:** For formal allergy testing (skin-prick or RAST) to confirm the trigger.
3. **Epinephrine Auto-Injector (EAI) Prescription:** This is mandatory. The patient must be prescribed *two* EAIs (e.g., EpiPen) and trained on how to use them.
4. **Medical Alert Bracelet:** A bracelet or necklace identifying the severe allergy.
5. **Anaphylaxis Action Plan:** A written plan for the

patient, family, and school/work.

Patient Counseling Points

1. **"This Was a Life-Threatening Allergic Reaction"**: "This was not a simple rash. This was anaphylaxis, a systemic reaction that was shutting down your body. Your blood pressure was dropping and your airway was swelling."
2. **"Epinephrine is Your ONLY Life-Saving Medicine"**: "**Epinephrine** is the *only* medicine that stops this reaction. Antihistamines like Benadryl or Zyrtec *will not save your life*. They only help with the itch and hives; they do *not* stop the shock or airway swelling."
3. **"How to Use Your EpiPen"**: "You must carry *two* auto-injectors with you *at all times, no exceptions*. If you feel symptoms (e.g., trouble breathing, throat tightness, feeling faint), you must use it immediately. Remember: **'Blue to the sky, orange to the thigh.'** Hold it against your outer thigh for 3-5 seconds. **Then call emergency services** or have someone call for you. You must go to the ER *every time* you use it."
4. **"Read Every Label, Every Time"**: "You must become a 'food detective.' You have to read the full ingredient label on *every* packaged food, *every* time, even if you've eaten it before, as ingredients can change."

Common Pitfalls in Management

The most critical and common pitfall is **delaying epinephrine administration** or using antihistamines *as a first-line treatment* for respiratory or cardiovascular symptoms. Antihistamines do nothing to treat life-threatening laryngeal edema or hypotension. Another error is administering epinephrine subcutaneously, which has slower absorption than the IM route. Finally, a pitfall is discharging the patient too early; all patients should be observed for 4-6 hours due to the risk of a biphasic reaction.

Case Study

A 30-year-old male at a restaurant suddenly complains his "throat feels tight" and he is having trouble breathing. He ate a salad that he did not know contained walnuts (he has a known tree nut allergy). He is wheezing, his voice is hoarse (stridor), and he has widespread hives.

Discussion

This is a clear-cut case of **Anaphylaxis** (exposure to a known allergen followed by rapid onset of multi-system symptoms, including airway compromise). The algorithm is linear, and one treatment is paramount.

Treatment Algorithm

1. **Diagnosis:** Anaphylaxis.
2. **Algorithm Step 1 (Primary): EPINEPHRINE.** This is the *only* life-saving step and must not be delayed.
   - **Action:** Immediately administer **Epinephrine 0.5 mg (of 1:1000 solution) IM** into his anterolateral thigh.
3. **Step 2 (Airway/Oxygen):** Place the patient on high-flow oxygen via a non-rebreather mask and call emergency services.
4. **Step 3 (Adjuncts):** *After* epinephrine is given, you can administer second-line therapies for his symptoms.
   - **H1 Blocker:** IV Diphenhydramine (for hives).
   - **H2 Blocker:** IV Famotidine.
   - **Corticosteroid:** IV Methylprednisolone (to prevent a biphasic reaction).
5. **Step 4 (Observe):** He is transported to the ED. The algorithm mandates he be **observed for 4-6 hours** for a potential *biphasic reaction*.

Outcome

The patient's breathing improves dramatically within 2 minutes of the IM epinephrine injection. He is observed in the ED and discharged with a prescription for two new epinephrine auto-injectors.

DKA/HHS

Diabetic Ketoacidosis (DKA) and Hyperosmolar Hyperglycemic State (HHS) are metabolic emergencies of diabetes mellitus. DKA is characterized by hyperglycemia, ketosis, and acidosis. HHS is characterized by profound hyperglycemia and hyperosmolality with minimal or no ketosis.

Pathophysiology

These are two related hyperglycemic emergencies, both driven by insulin deficiency.

- **Diabetic Ketoacidosis (DKA):** This is a state of **absolute insulin deficiency** (seen in Type 1 DM). With no insulin, the body *cannot* use glucose for fuel. It enters a "starvation" state and begins to rapidly break down fat (lipolysis). This fat is converted by the liver into **ketoacids** (beta-hydroxybutyrate). These acids overwhelm the body's buffering system, causing a severe **anion gap metabolic acidosis**. The hyperglycemia itself (from unopposed gluconeogenesis) causes a profound osmotic diuresis, leading to severe dehydration and electrolyte loss.
- **Hyperosmolar Hyperglycemic State (HHS):** This is a state of **relative insulin deficiency** (seen in Type 2 DM). There is *just enough* insulin present to prevent the body from breaking down fat, so **there is no ketosis and no acidosis**. However, without enough insulin to control glucose, the hyperglycemia becomes profound (often > 800 mg/dL). This extreme sugar load in the blood creates a massive osmotic gradient, pulling water out of all body compartments (including the brain) and causing a *severe* osmotic diuresis, leading to profound dehydration and a hyperosmolar state.

Diagnosis and Classification

- **DKA:** Triad of 1) Hyperglycemia (e.g., glucose > 250 mg/dL), 2) High Anion Gap Metabolic Acidosis (pH < 7.3, Bicarb < 18), and 3) Ketones (in urine or serum).

- **HHS:** Characterized by 1) Severe Hyperglycemia (e.g., glucose > 600 mg/dL), 2) High Serum Osmolality (> 320 mOsm/kg), and 3) No or minimal acidosis/ketosis.
- **Overlap:** A mixed DKA/HHS picture is common.

Differential Diagnosis

The differential for a high anion gap metabolic acidosis (in DKA) includes other causes (MUDPILES mnemonic): Methanol, Uremia, DKA, Propylene glycol, Isoniazid, Lactic acidosis, Ethylene glycol, Salicylates. The differential for altered mental status and hyperglycemia (in HHS) includes stroke, sepsis, or other encephalopathies.

Treatment Algorithm

The treatment algorithm for both DKA and HHS is a simultaneous, three-pronged protocol focused on fluids, insulin, and electrolytes.

- **Pillar 1: Intravenous Fluids (Resuscitation).**
  - **Goal:** Restore volume and renal perfusion.
  - **Algorithm:** Start with 0.9% Normal Saline (NS) at a high rate (e.g., 1-2 liters in the first 1-2 hours). Once hemodynamically stable, switch to 0.45% NS (as patients are total-body-water depleted). When serum glucose reaches ~200-250 mg/dL, the algorithm dictates adding dextrose to the fluids (e.g., D5 0.45% NS) to prevent hypoglycemia and allow the insulin drip to continue.
- **Pillar 2: Insulin (Stop Ketosis).**
  - **Goal:** Inhibit ketogenesis and drive glucose into cells.
  - **Algorithm: CRITICAL STEP:** Check serum potassium *before* starting insulin. If K+ is < 3.3 mEq/L, **do not give insulin.** Give potassium first.
  - If K+ is ≥ 3.3, start a continuous IV infusion of regular insulin (e.g., 0.1 U/kg/hr).
- **Pillar 3: Electrolytes (Especially Potassium).**
  - **Goal:** Prevent fatal hypokalemia.

- **Algorithm:** Although patients present with high or normal serum K+, they have a massive *total body* K+ deficit. Insulin will drive K+ into cells, causing serum levels to plummet. The algorithm requires hourly or bi-hourly potassium checks and aggressive replacement, adding K+ to the IV fluids once serum K+ is ≤ 5.2 mEq/L.

The algorithm continues until the anion gap is closed (in DKA) or osmolality and mental status normalize (in HHS).

Table 12.4: Algorithms for Anaphylaxis and DKA/HHS

Emergency	Presentation	Immediate Treatment Algorithm
Anaphylaxis	Rapid onset (mins-hrs) of: **1. Skin** (hives, angioedema) **2. Respiratory** (wheeze, stridor) **3. CV** (hypotension, tachycardia).	**1. EPINEPHRINE (IM)** 1:1000, 0.3-0.5 mg. (Vast. Lateralis). **2. Airway** management. **3. Adjuncts:** H1/H2 Blockers (Diphenhydramine, Famotidine), Steroids.
DKA / HHS	**DKA:** Hyperglycemia, **Ketonemia, Acidosis** (Gap). **HHS: Severe** Hyperglycemia, High Osmolality, No/Min ketones.	**1. FLUIDS:** Aggressive IV Fluids (NS 0.9%). **2. INSULIN:** IV Insulin Drip (close anion gap in DKA). **3. POTASSIUM:** Replete K+ *before* giving insulin (if K+ < 3.3).

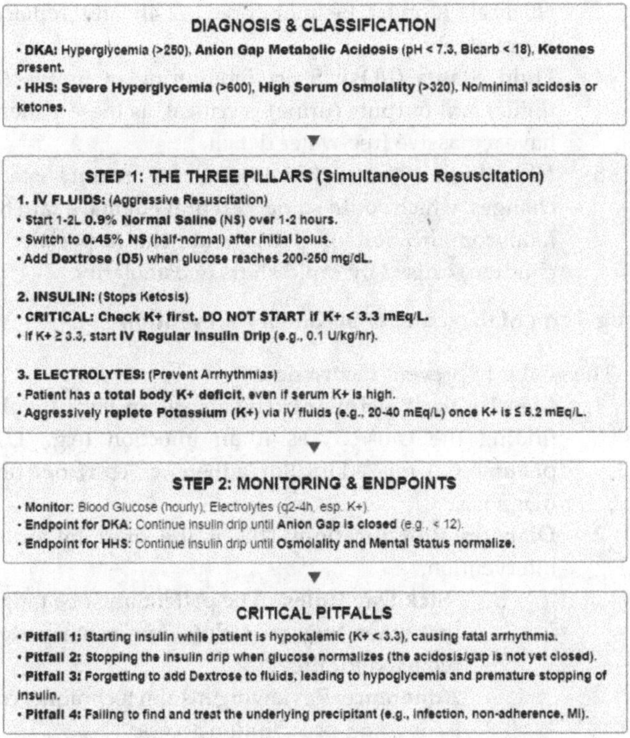

Figure 12.5: DKA / HHS - Management Algorithm

Monitoring and Follow-Up

Monitoring is done in an ICU or step-down unit.

1. **Blood Glucose:** Monitored hourly via fingerstick.
2. **The "Gap" (DKA):** The **anion gap** (Na - (Cl + HCO3)) is the *key* parameter to monitor in DKA. It reflects the level of unmeasured acids (ketones). The goal of therapy is to "close the gap," not just to normalize the glucose.
3. **Potassium:** This is the most dangerous electrolyte to manage. Patients are "total-body potassium depleted," but their serum potassium may be *high* or *normal* on arrival due to the acidosis. As insulin is given (which drives potassium into cells), the serum potassium will

plummet. It must be monitored q2-4h and replaced aggressively.

4. **Fluid Status (I/Os):** Strict monitoring of inputs (IV fluids) and outputs (urine) is critical, as these patients have a massive free-water deficit.
5. **Neurologic Status:** Monitoring for mental status changes, which could signal **cerebral edema**, a rare but fatal complication of DKA treatment (especially in children) caused by rapid shifts in osmolarity.

Long-Term Management / Secondary Prevention

The goal is to prevent recurrence.

1. **Identify the Precipitant:** The algorithm *must* involve finding the cause. Was it an infection (e.g., UTI, pneumonia), missed insulin (adherence, cost), or a new diagnosis?
2. **Diabetes Re-Education:** This is the most important intervention.
    - **"Sick Day Rules":** The patient must be taught that when they are sick (e.Immersive content redacted for brevity.
    - **Adherence:** Reviewing insulin technique, cost issues, and prescription access.
3. **Technology:** Assessing if the patient is a candidate for a Continuous Glucose Monitor (CGM) or an insulin pump to improve control.

Patient Counseling Points

1. **"Your Body Was in a 'Starvation'/'Dehydration' State":** (DKA) "Even though your blood was full of sugar, your body couldn't use it because you didn't have insulin. It thought it was starving, so it burned fat for fuel, which created 'acids' that poisoned your system." (HHS) "Your blood sugar became so high that it acted like a sponge, pulling all the water out of your body's cells, leading to severe dehydration."
2. **"The 'Sick Day Rules'":** "This is the most important lesson. When you are sick (fever, flu, vomiting), your body is stressed and *needs more insulin*, not less. You

must *never* stop taking your insulin, even if you are not eating. You must check your sugar more often, drink fluids, and call us if you're vomiting or your sugar stays high."

3. **Checking Ketones (T1DM):** "If you have Type 1 diabetes and your blood sugar is high (e.g., over 250), you must check your urine or blood for 'ketones.' If you have ketones, you need *more* insulin and you need to call us."
4. **"This Was Preventable":** "This was a very dangerous, but preventable, complication. We will work with you and our diabetes educators to make sure you have a clear plan for your insulin and for what to do when you get sick, so this never happens again."

Common Pitfalls in Management

The most lethal pitfall is **starting insulin before checking potassium** or in a patient with hypokalemia (K+ < 3.3), which can precipitate fatal cardiac arrhythmias. Another critical error is **stopping the insulin infusion** when the blood glucose normalizes; the insulin must be continued until the anion gap is closed (i.e., the acidosis is resolved). A third pitfall is failing to add dextrose to the IV fluids, which forces the premature discontinuation of the insulin drip. Finally, failing to identify and treat the underlying precipitant (e.g., infection, MI, non-adherence) is a common omission.

Case Study: A 19-year-old female with Type 1 Diabetes presents with a 2-day history of vomiting and abdominal pain. She has been "skipping" her insulin doses. She is breathing rapidly and deeply (Kussmaul respirations) and her breath is fruity. Her labs: Glucose 550, pH 7.10, Anion Gap 28, K+ **3.1 mEq/L**.

Discussion: This is a classic presentation of **Diabetic Ketoacidosis (DKA)** (hyperglycemia, acidosis, high anion gap, ketones). The algorithm is to manage the three pillars: Fluids, Insulin, and Electrolytes. Her potassium level is **critically low** (K+ < 3.3), which presents a life-threatening pitfall.

Treatment Algorithm

1. **Diagnosis:** DKA.
2. **Algorithm Pillar 1 (Fluids):**
   - **Action:** Start aggressive **IV fluid resuscitation** with **0.9% Normal Saline** (e.g., 1L in the first hour).
3. **Algorithm Pillar 2 (Potassium):** This is the most critical step.
   - **CRITICAL PITFALL:** Her K+ is 3.1 mEq/L. **DO NOT START INSULIN.** Insulin will drive this low K+ into the cells, causing a fatal arrhythmia.
   - **Action:** Add **40 mEq of Potassium** to the first liter of IV fluids and start replacement.
4. **Algorithm Pillar 3 (Insulin):**
   - **Action:** Hold the insulin drip. Re-check the potassium level in 1 hour. Once the K+ is ≥ **3.3 mEq/L**, you can safely begin the **IV regular insulin infusion** (e.g., at 0.1 U/kg/hr).
5. **Monitoring:** The algorithm dictates hourly glucose checks and checking the anion gap and potassium every 2-4 hours. The goal is to "**close the gap,**" not just to lower the glucose.

Outcome: The patient's potassium is repleted, and the insulin drip is safely started 1 hour later. She is admitted to the ICU for DKA management.

Summary

Acute Coronary Syndrome: The algorithm is EKG-driven. STEMI requires an immediate reperfusion algorithm (PCI or lytics). NSTEMI requires an algorithm of medical stabilization and risk stratification.

Stroke: The algorithm is CT-driven. Ischemic stroke (negative CT) is managed with a time-sensitive reperfusion algorithm (tPA and/or thrombectomy). Hemorrhagic stroke (positive CT) is managed with an algorithm of BP control and anticoagulation reversal.

Sepsis: The algorithm is a "bundle" of care. The Hour-1 Bundle mandates cultures, lactate measurement, rapid broad-spectrum antibiotics, and 30 ml/kg fluid resuscitation followed by vasopressors if needed.

Anaphylaxis: The algorithm is linear and prioritized. IM Epinephrine is the non-negotiable first-line treatment, followed by adjunctive therapies (antihistamines, steroids, IV fluids).

DKA/HHS: The algorithm is a metabolic resuscitation balancing three pillars: aggressive IV fluid replacement, continuous IV insulin (after K+ is confirmed $\geq$ 3.3), and vigilant potassium repletion.

Multiple Choice Questions

1. A 55-year-old male presents with chest pain. An EKG obtained within 10 minutes shows ST-segment elevations. The hospital is not PCI-capable, and the nearest PCI center is 3 hours away. What is the most appropriate algorithm?

   A) Administer aspirin and heparin, and transport to the PCI center.

   B) Administer IV fibrinolytic therapy (e.g., alteplase) within 30 minutes, if no contraindications.

   C) Perform an emergency echocardiogram to guide therapy.

   D) Administer aspirin, clopidogrel, and observe with serial EKGs.

2. A 70-year-old female presents with acute left-sided weakness. "Last known normal" was 2 hours ago. A non-contrast head CT is negative for blood. Her BP is 170/95 mmHg. What is the next step?

   A) Administer IV alteplase (tPA).

   B) Administer IV labetalol to lower SBP to < 140 mmHg.

   C) Perform a CT angiogram to look for LVO.

   D) Administer aspirin 325 mg.

3. A 40-year-old male presents with severe, watery diarrhea, a fever of 102.5°F, and a BP of 85/50 mmHg. Sepsis is suspected. Which of the following is the most appropriate *first* step?

   A) Start a norepinephrine infusion.

   B) Administer a 30 ml/kg bolus of 0.9% Normal Saline.

   C) Administer broad-spectrum antibiotics (e.g., piperacillin-tazobactam).

   D) Obtain blood cultures and measure serum lactate.

4. A patient in the ED develops acute-onset stridor and hypotension 5 minutes after receiving an IV antibiotic. What is the *first* and *most important* action?

   A) Administer IV diphenhydramine.

   B) Administer IV methylprednisolone.

C) Administer Epinephrine 0.3 mg IM in the anterolateral thigh.

D) Secure the airway with intubation.

5. A 25-year-old with Type 1 Diabetes presents with nausea, vomiting, and confusion. Labs: Glucose 450, pH 7.15, Anion Gap 24, Serum K+ 2.9 mEq/L. What is the most appropriate initial algorithm?

   A) Start an IV insulin infusion at 0.1 U/kg/hr.

   B) Administer a 1L bolus of 0.9% NS and administer IV potassium. *Do not start insulin*

   C) Administer a 1L bolus of 0.9% NS and start an IV insulin infusion.

   D) Administer IV sodium bicarbonate to correct the acidosis.

6. In the management of septic shock, what is the first-line vasopressor if a patient remains hypotensive after adequate fluid resuscitation?

   A) Epinephrine

   B) Vasopressin

   C) Dopamine

   D) Norepinephrine

7. A 60-year-old male presents with a "thunderclap headache." A non-contrast head CT is negative. What is the most critical pitfall to avoid?

   A) Discharging the patient with a diagnosis of migraine.

   B) Administering tPA.

   C) Failing to perform a lumbar puncture to rule out SAH.

   D) Giving nimodipine.

8. A patient is successfully treated for anaphylaxis and is now symptom-free. What is the most appropriate disposition algorithm?

   A) Discharge immediately with an EpiPen prescription.

   B) Discharge after 1 hour of observation.

C) Observe for 4-6 hours due to the risk of a biphasic reaction. D) Admit to the hospital for 48 hours of IV steroids.

9. When treating a patient with DKA, the IV insulin infusion should be continued until which of the following endpoints is met?
   A) The blood glucose is < 200 mg/dL.
   B) The anion gap is closed.
   C) The serum ketones are negative.
   D) The patient is able to eat.
10. A patient presents with acute chest pain. EKG shows ST-depressions in V2-V4. Troponin is 5.2 ng/mL. The patient has refractory chest pain despite nitrates. What is the algorithm?
   A) Administer IV fibrinolytics.
   B) Proceed to an early invasive strategy (cardiac catheterization).
   C) Perform an emergency stress test.
   D) Discharge with follow-up, as this is Unstable Angina.

Self-Assessment Questions

1. What is the single most important diagnostic test in the acute stroke algorithm, and how does its result bifurcate the entire treatment pathway?
2. A patient presents with a STEMI. What is the preferred reperfusion algorithm, and what are the main time-to-treatment goals?
3. Describe the five components of the "Hour-1 Bundle" for sepsis management. Which two are the most time-sensitive for improving mortality?
4. A patient presents with acute-onset urticaria, wheezing, and hypotension after a bee sting. What is the first-line treatment, and what is the critical pitfall to avoid?
5. What are the three pillars of the DKA treatment algorithm? What is the most critical electrolyte check to perform before initiating one of these pillars, and why?
6. Compare and contrast the immediate treatment algorithm for a STEMI versus an NSTEMI.
7. What is the "permissive hypertension" algorithm in ischemic stroke, and how does the administration of tPA change this algorithm?
8. A patient with septic shock remains hypotensive (MAP 60 mmHg) after a 30 ml/kg crystalloid bolus. What is the next step in the algorithm?
9. Why are corticosteroids and antihistamines considered "adjunctive" or "second-line" therapies in anaphylaxis, and what is their role?
10. What is the primary goal of the insulin infusion in DKA (i.e., what metabolic parameter is being "treated"), and when is it safe to transition to subcutaneous insulin?

Bibliography

1. Lawton JS, Tamis-Holland JE, Bangalore S, Bates ER, Beckie TM, Bischoff JM, et al. 2021 ACC/AHA/SCAI guideline for coronary artery revascularization: a report of the American College of Cardiology/American Heart Association Joint Committee on Clinical Practice Guidelines. J Am Coll Cardiol. 2022 Jan 18;79(2):e21–129.
2. Collet JP, Thiele H, Barbato E, Barthélémy O, Bauersachs J, Bhatt DL, et al. 2020 ESC Guidelines for the management of acute coronary syndromes in patients presenting without persistent ST-segment elevation. Eur Heart J. 2021 Apr 7;42(14):1289–367.
3. Powers WJ, Rabinstein AA, Ackerson T, Adeoye OM, Bambakidis NC, Becker K, et al. Guidelines for the early management of patients with acute ischemic stroke: 2019 update to the 2018 guidelines for the early management of acute ischemic stroke: a guideline for healthcare professionals from the American Heart Association/American Stroke Association. Stroke. 2019 Dec;50(12):e344–418.
4. Nogueira RG, Jadhav AP, Haussen DC, Bonafe A, Budzik RF, Bhuva P, et al. Thrombectomy 6 to 24 hours after stroke with a mismatch between deficit and infarct. N Engl J Med. 2018 Jan 4;378(1):11–21.
5. Hemphill JC 3rd, Greenberg SM, Anderson CS, Becker K, Bendok BR, Cushman M, et al. Guidelines for the management of spontaneous intracerebral hemorrhage: a guideline for healthcare professionals from the American Heart Association/American Stroke Association. Stroke. 2015 Jul;46(7):2032–60.
6. Connolly ES Jr, Rabinstein AA, Carhuapoma JR, Derdeyn CP, Dion J, Higashida RT, et al. Guidelines for the management of aneurysmal subarachnoid hemorrhage: a guideline for healthcare professionals from the American Heart Association/American stroke association. Stroke. 2012 Jun;43(6):1711–37.
7. Evans L, Rhodes A, Alhazzani W, Antonelli M, Coopersmith CM, De Backer D, et al. Surviving sepsis campaign: international guidelines for management of sepsis and septic shock 2021. Intensive Care Med. 2021 Nov;47(11):1181–247.
8. Singer M, Deutschman CS, Seymour CW, Shankar-Hari M, Annane D, Bauer M, et al. The Third International Consensus Definitions for Sepsis and Septic Shock (Sepsis-3). JAMA. 2016 Feb 23;315(8):801–10.
9. Shaker MS, Wallace DV, Golden DBK, Oppenheimer J, Bernstein JA, Campbell RL, et al. Anaphylaxis—a 2020 practice parameter update, systematic review, and Grading of Recommendations, Assessment, Development and Evaluation (GRADE) analysis. J Allergy Clin Immunol. 2020 Apr;145(4):1082–123.
10. Dybvik H, Dybvik M, Dybvik E, Dybvik K. Anaphylaxis: a 2021 update. J Am Coll Emerg Physicians Open. 2021 Jul 15;2(4):e12503.
11. Kitabchi AE, Umpierrez GE, Miles JM, Fisher JN. Hyperglycemic

crises in adult patients with diabetes. Diabetes Care. 2009 Jul;32(7):1335–43.

12. Umpierrez GE, Korytkowski M. Diabetic emergencies - ketoacidosis, hyperglycaemic hyperosmolar state and hypoglycaemia. Nat Rev Endocrinol. 2016 Apr;12(4):222–32.
13. Fayfman M, Pasquel FJ, Umpierrez GE. Management of hyperglycemic crises: diabetic ketoacidosis and hyperglycemic hyperosmolar state. Med Clin North Am. 2017 May;101(3):587–606.
14. The GUSTO investigators. An international randomized trial comparing four thrombolytic strategies for acute myocardial infarction. N Engl J Med. 1993 Sep 2;329(10):673–82.
15. Seymour CW, Gesten F, Prescott HC, Friedrich ME, Iwashyna TJ, Phillips GS, et al. Time to treatment and mortality during mandated emergency care for sepsis. N Engl J Med. 2017 Jun 8;376(23):2235–44.

APPENDICES

APPENDIX A: COMMON LABORATORY VALUES

These ranges are illustrative and may vary significantly based on the laboratory, patient population, and testing methodology. All values must be interpreted in the context of the individual patient and the specific laboratory's reference range.

Hematology (Complete Blood Count)

- White Blood Cell (WBC) Count: 4.0–11.0 x 10^9/L
- Red Blood Cell (RBC) Count:
    - Male: 4.3–5.7 x 10^{12}/L
    - Female: 3.8–5.1 x 10^{12}/L
- Hemoglobin (Hgb):
    - Male: 13.5–17.5 g/dL
    - Female: 12.0–15.5 g/dL
- Hematocrit (Hct):
    - Male: 40%–52%
    - Female: 36%–48%
- Platelet (Plt) Count: 150–450 x 10^9/L
- Mean Corpuscular Volume (MCV): 80–100 fL

Basic Metabolic Panel (BMP / Chem-7)

- Sodium (Na^+): 135–145 mEq/L
- Potassium (K^+): 3.5–5.0 mEq/L
- Chloride (Cl^-): 98–107 mEq/L
- Bicarbonate (HCO_3^-/CO_2): 22–29 mEq/L
- Blood Urea Nitrogen (BUN): 7–20 mg/dL
- Serum Creatinine (SCr): 0.6–1.2 mg/dL
- Glucose (fasting): 70–100 mg/dL

Comprehensive Metabolic Panel (CMP)

- All BMP components plus:
- Albumin: 3.5–5.0 g/dL
- Total Protein: 6.0–8.3 g/dL
- Alkaline Phosphatase (ALP): 40–120 U/L
- Alanine Aminotransferase (ALT): 7–56 U/L
- Aspartate Aminotransferase (AST): 10–40 U/L

- Total Bilirubin: 0.1–1.2 mg/dL

Coagulation Panel

- Prothrombin Time (PT): 11–13.5 seconds
- International Normalized Ratio (INR) (uncoagulated): < 1.1
- Activated Partial Thromboplastin Time (aPTT): 25–35 seconds

Lipid Panel (Fasting)

- Total Cholesterol: < 200 mg/dL (Desirable)
- Low-Density Lipoprotein (LDL) Cholesterol: < 100 mg/dL (Optimal)
- High-Density Lipoprotein (HDL) Cholesterol: > 40 mg/dL (Male), > 50 mg/dL (Female) (Protective)
- Triglycerides: < 150 mg/dL

Thyroid Function

- Thyroid-Stimulating Hormone (TSH): 0.4–4.0 mIU/L
- Free Thyroxine (Free T4): 0.8–1.8 ng/dL

Cardiac Markers

- Troponin I (High-Sensitivity): Varies by assay. Must be interpreted by the lab-specific 99th percentile upper reference limit

APPENDIX B: DRUG DOSING GUIDELINES

DISCLAIMER: This appendix is for educational and illustrative purposes ONLY. It is not a substitute for clinical judgment or official prescribing information (package insert). Drug dosing is highly individualized. NEVER make a clinical decision based on the information below. Always consult official, current resources and institutional protocols.

Principles of Dosing

Dosing algorithms are based on pharmacokinetics (PK) and pharmacodynamics (PD).

1. **Renal Dose Adjustment:** Many drugs are cleared by the kidneys. Dosing must be adjusted in patients with chronic kidney disease (CKD) or acute kidney injury (AKI). Adjustments are typically based on calculated Creatinine Clearance (CrCl) (e.g., Cockcroft-Gault equation) or estimated Glomerular Filtration Rate (eGFR). Common drugs requiring renal adjustment include gabapentin, many antibiotics (e.g., penicillin, cephalosporins, vancomycin), and LMWH (e.g., enoxaparin).
2. **Hepatic Dose Adjustment:** Dosing for drugs metabolized by the liver is more complex. Adjustments are often guided by the Child-Pugh score in patients with cirrhosis. Many benzodiazepines, opioids, and beta-blockers require dose reduction.
3. **Loading Doses:** Used to rapidly achieve a therapeutic steady-state concentration for drugs with a long half-life (e.g., amiodarone, digoxin, phenytoin).
4. **Titration:** Many drugs, especially for cardiovascular or neurologic conditions, are started at a low dose and titrated up to effect or tolerance to minimize side effects (e.g., carvedilol, TCAs, SSRIs).

Example Dosing for Common Conditions

Drug	Class	Common Indication	Typical Adult Dose	Adjustment Notes
Lisinopril	ACE Inhibitor	Hypertension, HFrEF	**HTN:** Start 10 mg PO daily, titrate to 40 mg. **HFrEF:** Start 2.5-5 mg PO daily, titrate to 20-40 mg.	**Renal:** Reduce dose if CrCl < 30 mL/min. Monitor K^+, SCr.
Metoprolol Succinate	Beta-Blocker	HFrEF, Hypertension	**HFrEF:** Start 12.5-25 mg PO daily, double dose every 2 weeks to target 200 mg daily.	Titrate slowly.
Atorvastatin	HMG-CoA Reductase Inhibitor	ACS (High-Intensity)	80 mg PO daily.	---
Furosemide	Loop Diuretic	ADHF (Congestion)	40-80 mg IV bolus. (Typically 2-2.5x patient's	Dose is based on volume status, not a fixed

Drug	Class	Common Indication	Typical Adult Dose	Adjustment Notes
			home oral dose).	algorithm.
Amoxicillin	Penicillin Antibiotic	Strep Pharyngitis	1 g PO daily or 500 mg PO BID.	**Renal:** Adjust for severe impairment.
Azithromycin	Macrolide Antibiotic	CAP (Outpatient)	500 mg PO on Day 1, then 250 mg PO daily on Days 2-5.	No renal adjustment. High risk for QT prolongation.
Ceftriaxone	3rd Gen. Cephalosporin	Sepsis (Inpatient CAP)	1-2 g IV every 24 hours.	**No renal adjustment.**
Epinephrine	Adrenergic Agonist	Anaphylaxis	0.3-0.5 mg (of 1:1000 solution) IM. Repeat every 5-15 min.	IM route is critical.

Drug	Class	Common Indication	Typical Adult Dose	Adjustment Notes
Alteplase (tPA)	Fibrinolytic	Ischemic Stroke	0.9 mg/kg IV total (max 90 mg). 10% as bolus over 1 min, rest as infusion over 60 min.	Strict time windows and contraindications.
Insulin, Regular	Insulin	DKA/HHS	0.1 U/kg/hr continuous IV infusion.	**DO NOT START** if K^+ < 3.3 mEq/L.

APPENDIX C: DRUG INTERACTIONS

CRITICAL DISCLAIMER: This information is for educational purposes ONLY. It highlights common interaction mechanisms and is not an exhaustive list. Always use a drug-interaction checker (e.g., in the EMR or pharmacy software) before prescribing or dispensing.

Principles of Drug Interactions

1. **Pharmacodynamic Interactions:** Two drugs have additive or antagonistic effects at the same or a similar receptor. The effect is often predictable.
2. **Pharmacokinetic Interactions:** One drug alters the Absorption, Distribution, Metabolism, or Excretion (ADME) of another. The most common mechanism involves the **Cytochrome P450 (CYP450)** enzyme system in the liver.

Pharmacokinetic (CYP450) Interactions

The CYP450 system metabolizes the majority of drugs.

- **Inhibitors** *decrease* enzyme activity, leading to *increased* levels of the substrate drug and risk of toxicity.
- **Inducers** *increase* enzyme activity, leading to *decreased* levels of the substrate drug and risk of therapeutic failure.

High-Yield CYP450 Inducers (Decrease substrate levels)

Indu3cer	Substrates Affected (Examples)
Rifampin	Warfarin, Oral Contraceptives, DOACs, Antifungals
Phenytoin	Warfarin, Oral Contraceptives, Statins
Carbamazepine	Warfarin, Oral Contraceptives, Antidepressants
Phenobarbital	Warfarin, Oral Contraceptives, Benzodiazepines
St. John's Wort	SSRIs, Warfarin, Oral Contraceptives, Digoxin

High-Yield CYP450 Inhibitors (Increase substrate levels)

Inhibitor	Enzyme (Typical)	Substrates Affected (Examples)
Amiodarone	CYP2C9, 2D6, 3A4	Warfarin, Digoxin, Simvastatin
Azole Antifungals (e.g., Fluconazole)	CYP2C9, 3A4	Warfarin, Phenytoin, Statins, DOACs
Macrolides (Clarithro/Erythro)	CYP3A4	Statins (Simva/Atorva), Warfarin, DOACs
Non-DHP CCBs (Verapamil, Diltiazem)	CYP3A4	Statins, Digoxin
Protease Inhibitors (e.t., Ritonavir)	CYP3A4 (Strong)	Numerous
Grapefruit Juice	CYP3A4	Statins, CCBs

Pharmacodynamic (Additive Effect) Interactions

Interaction Type	Drug Class 1	Drug Class 2 (+ Class 3)	Clinical Consequence
Serotonin Syndrome	SSRIs / SNRIs (e.g., Fluoxetine)	MAOIs, Tramadol, Linezolid, Triptans	Confusion, fever, hyperreflexia, autonomic instability. Potentially fatal.
Hyperkalemia	ACE Inhibitor or ARB	Potassium-Sparing Diuretic (Spironolactone) + K^+ Supplement	Severe hyperkalemia leading to cardiac arrhythmia.

Interaction Type	Drug Class 1	Drug Class 2 (+ Class 3)	Clinical Consequence
Bleeding Risk	Anticoagulant (Warfarin, DOAC)	Antiplatelet (Aspirin, Clopidogrel) + NSAID (Ibuprofen)	Synergistic increase in major bleeding risk, GI bleeding.
QT Prolongation	Antiarrhythmics (Amiodarone)	Antipsychotics (Ziprasidone) + Antibiotics (Azithromycin, FQ) + Antiemetics (Ondansetron)	Increased risk of Torsades de Pointes (TdP), a life-threatening ventricular arrhythmia.
CNS Depression	Opioids (Oxycodone)	Benzodiazepines (Lorazepam) + Alcohol	Additive sedation, respiratory depression, coma, and death.
Hypotension	Alpha-blockers (Tamsulosin)	PDE-5 Inhibitors (Sildenafil) + Nitrates	Severe, refractory hypotension and syncope.

ANSWERS TO THE MCQS

Chapter 1: 1. C 2. B 3. C 4. A 5. C 6. B 7. D 8. C 9. A 10. B

Chapter 2: 1. C 2. B 3. D 4. C 5. A 6. C 7. A 8. A 9. A 10. B

Chapter 3: 1. C 2. C 3. A 4. B 5. C 6. B 7. B 8. A 9. C 10. C

Chapter 4: 1. B 2. D 3. C 4. B 5. C 6. C 7. B 8. B 9. C 10. D

Chapter 5: 1. A 2. C 3. A 4. D 5. B 6. B 7. A 8. B 9. B 10. D

Chapter 6: 1. D 2. A 3. A 4. B 5. B 6. A 7. C 8. C 9. A 10. A

Chapter 7: 1. C 2. B 3. C 4. B 5. B 6. C 7. D 8. B 9. B 10. B

Chapter 8: 1. A 2. B 3. B 4. A 5. B 6. B 7. B 8. B 9. B 10. C

Chapter 9: 1. C 2. B 3. C 4. A 5. B 6. B 7. B 8. B 9. C 10. B

Chapter 10: 1. C 2. A 3. B 4. B 5. D 6. B 7. A 8. A 9. B 10. A

Chapter 11: 1. C 2. B 3. A 4. B 5. B 6. B 7. A 8. C 9. C 10. B

Chapter 12: 1. B 2. A 3. D 4. C 5. B 6. D 7. C 8. C 9. B 10. B

ABOUT THE EDITORS

Dr. SANTHOSH ARUN KUMAR KOMMA

Dr. Santhosh Arun Kumar Komma is a faculty member at A.U. College of Pharmaceutical Sciences, Andhra University, Visakhapatnam, Andhra Pradesh, with over 12 years of teaching and research experience in the area of Clinical Pharmacy Practice. He is one of the first Pharm.D graduates from JSS University, Mysore, and earned his Ph.D. in 2020 from Andhra University. He has published 18 papers and has 3 granted patents to his credit.

Mrs. VINNY THERISSA MANGAM

Mrs. Vinny Therissa Mangam is an Assistant Professor working at Aditya College of Pharmacy, Aditya University with over 5 years of experience in teaching, analytical method development and validation. She published 8 research papers and lifetime member of APT and IPGA. Her expertise lies in optimizing techniques, comparing methods, and transferring procedures to enable enhanced standards in pharmaceutical analysis.

Mrs. SRAVANI RATNAM ARJI

Mrs. Sravani Ratnam Arji, a Lecturer at Government Degree College, Rajahmundry, has a passion for pharmaceutical and biomedical analysis. She has over 5 years of experience in developing analytical methods and techniques for pharmaceuticals.

Dr. SANJAY SAMANTH MANTHENA

Dr. Sanjay Samanth Manthena is a faculty member at A.U. College of Pharmaceutical Sciences, Andhra University, Visakhapatnam, with over 9 years of teaching experience in Clinical Pharmacy Practice. He has authored 2 textbooks, published 14 research papers in various National and International Journals, and has two Indian patents to his credit.

Dr. HEMA ARYA

Dr. Hema Arya is an Assistant Professor in the Department of Pharmaceutical Chemistry, School of Pharmacy, Sharda University, Greater Noida, U.P, India-201306. She is a passionate academician and researcher with 18 years of experience and a strong interest in pharmaceutical sciences. Known for her insightful analysis and commitment to knowledge dissemination, she brings clarity and depth to complex topics. With a keen eye for detail and a dedication to academic excellence, she continues to contribute meaningfully to her field through her writing and scholarly work.

Mr. PRAKASH NATHANIEL KUMAR SARELLA

Mr. Prakash Nathaniel Kumar Sarella is working as an Associate Professor and Controller of Examinations at Aditya College of Pharmacy, Aditya University with over 9 years of experience in teaching and research. His expertise includes nanomedicine, liposomes, polymer therapeutics, antibody-drug conjugates, specialized pharmaceutical packaging solutions, microneedle technologies, and other innovative drug delivery solutions. He published over 42 research papers and life member of APTI and IPGA.

INDEX

www.ingramcontent.com/pod-product-compliance
Lightning Source LLC
Chambersburg PA
CBHW011349230926
51848CB00003B/516
9788198765734